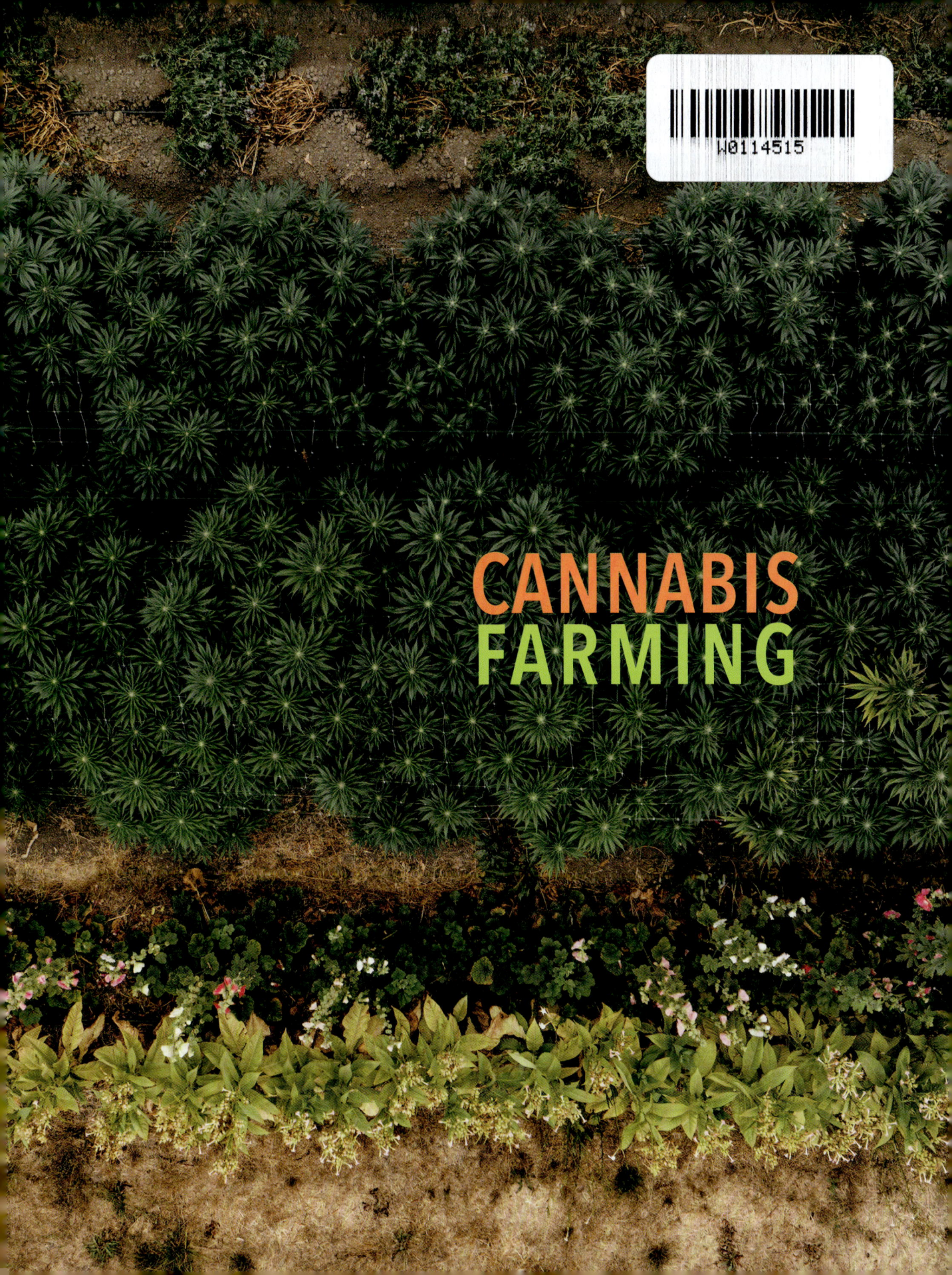

CANNABIS
FARMING

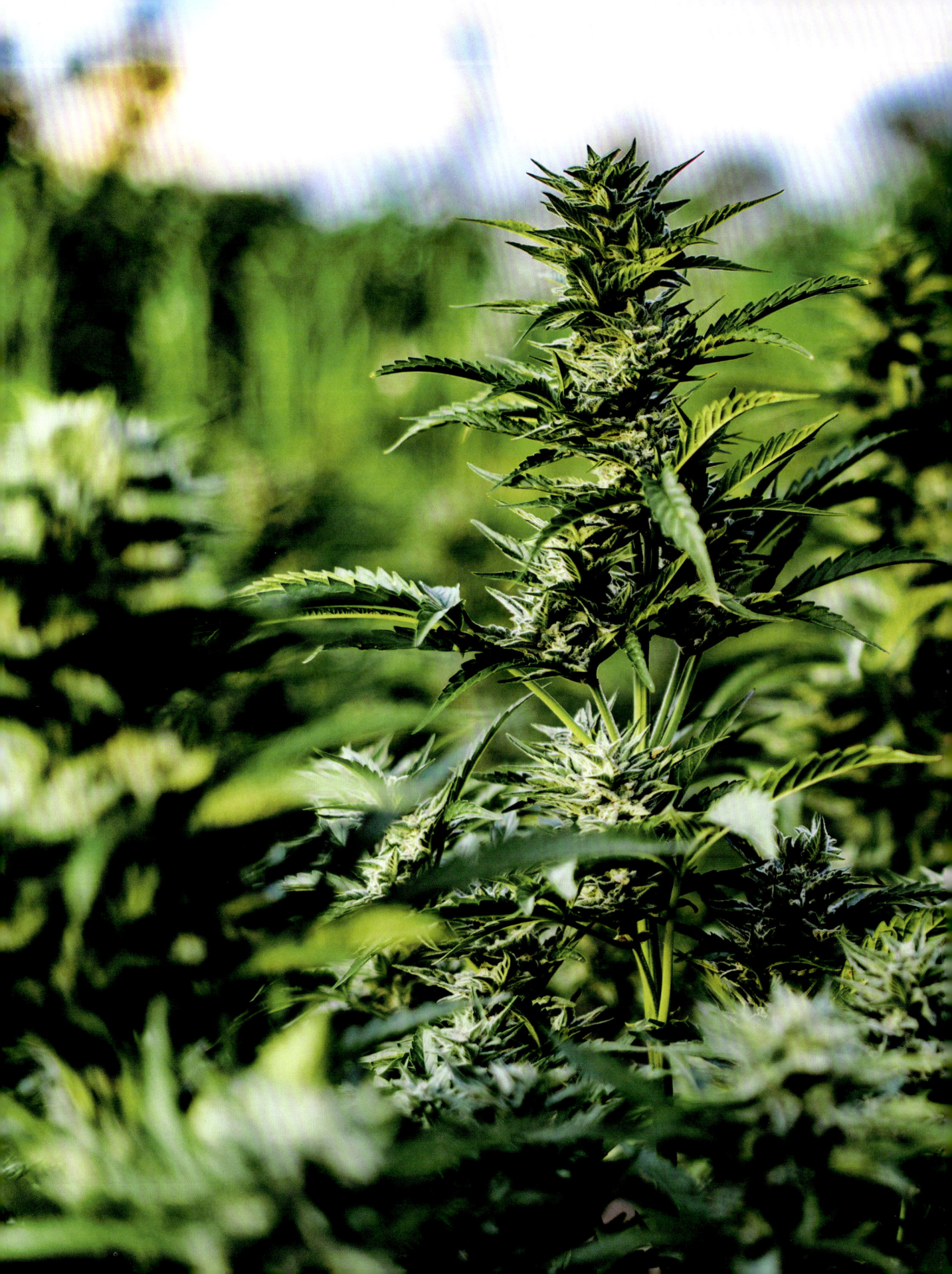

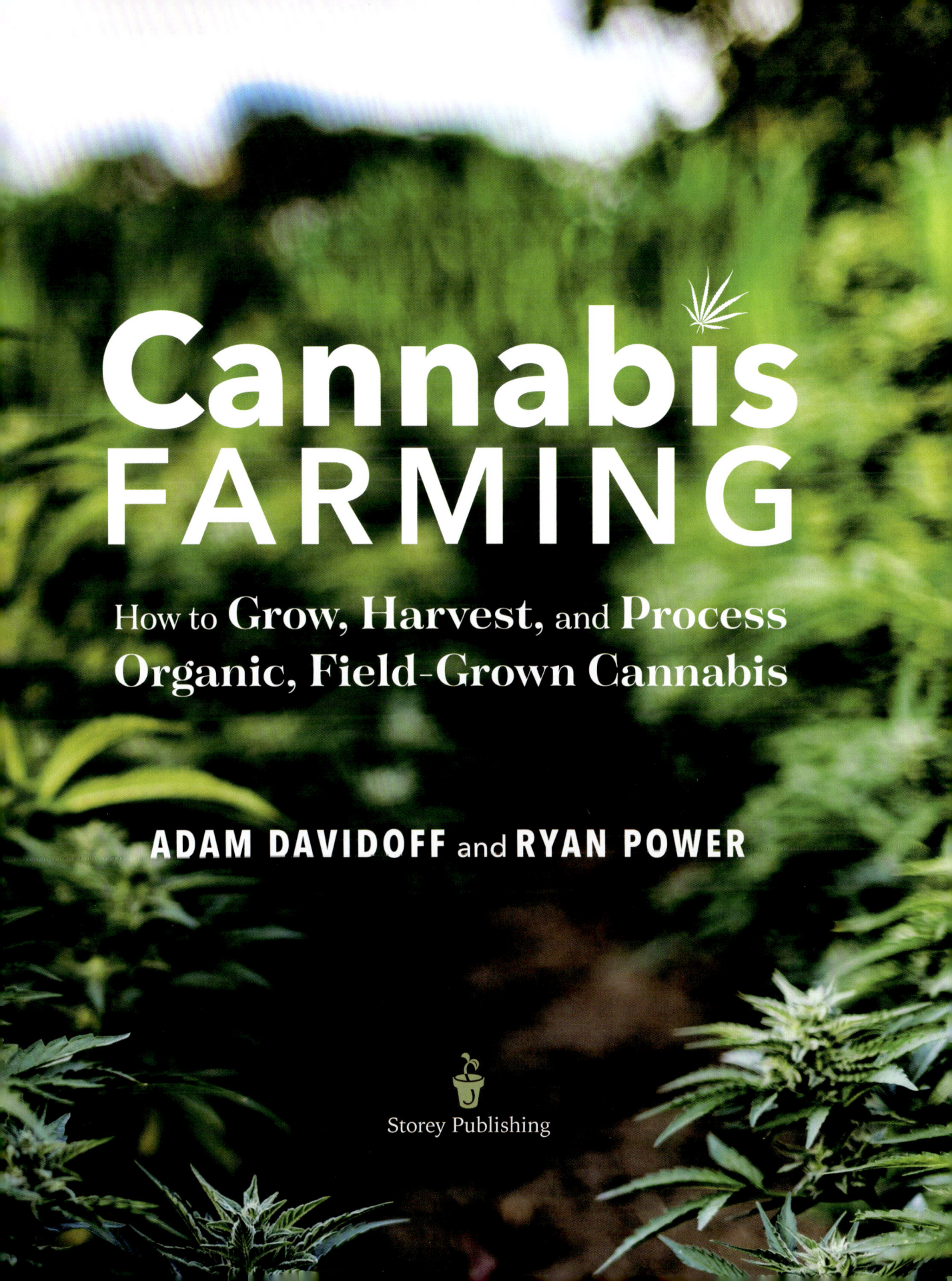

Cannabis FARMING

How to Grow, Harvest, and Process Organic, Field-Grown Cannabis

ADAM DAVIDOFF and **RYAN POWER**

Storey Publishing

The mission of Storey Publishing is to serve our customers by publishing practical information that encourages personal independence in harmony with the environment.

EDITED BY Carleen Madigan and Kristen Hewitt
ART DIRECTION BY Erin Dawson
BOOK DESIGN BY Linda Kocur
TEXT PRODUCTION BY Jennifer Jepson Smith

COVER AND INTERIOR PHOTOGRAPHY BY
© Gary Ottonello
ADDITIONAL PHOTOGRAPHY BY Adam Davidoff, 170, 187, 191; © Andrew Koturanov/Shutterstock.com, 53 t.; © Danita Delimont Creative/Alamy Stock Photo, 128; © Denis Crawford/Alamy Stock Photo, 74 r.; © funnyangel/Shutterstock.com, 50; © Holly Mazour/Shutterstock.com, 143; © JiriLancaric/Shutterstock.com, 186; © Kimberly Boyles/Shutterstock.com, 190; © M1randje/Shutterstock.com, 142; © MJfotografie.cz/Shutterstock.com, 53 b.; © PHILIPPE MONTIGNY/Shutterstock.com, 130; © Pong Pong/Shutterstock.com, 73, 74 l., 76; © PRO Stock Professional/Shutterstock.com, 161; Ryan Power, 18; © Smit/Shutterstock.com, 40; © steve polter/iStock.com, 92; Whitney Cranshaw, Colorado State University, Bugwood.org/CC BY 3.0 US, 75 l.; © ZenkyPhoto/Shutterstock.com, 62
ILLUSTRATIONS BY © Michael Gellatly

TEXT © 2025 by Adam Davidoff, Ryan Power, and William Hancock

The information in this book is true and complete to the best of our knowledge. All recommendations are made without guarantee on the part of the authors or Storey Publishing. The authors and publisher disclaim any liability in connection with the use of this information.

The publisher is not responsible for websites (or their content) that are not owned by the publisher.

Storey books may be purchased in bulk for business, educational, or promotional use. Special editions or book excerpts can also be created to specification. For details, please contact your local bookseller or the Hachette Book Group Special Markets Department at special.markets@hbgusa.com.

Storey Publishing
210 MASS MoCA Way
North Adams, MA 01247
storey.com

Storey Publishing is an imprint of Workman Publishing, a division of Hachette Book Group, Inc., 1290 Avenue of the Americas, New York, NY 10104. The Storey Publishing name and logo are registered trademarks of Hachette Book Group, Inc.

ISBNs: 978-1-63586-826-5 (paperback);
978-1-63586-827-2 (ebook)

Printed in Thailand through Asia Pacific Offset on paper from responsible sources
10 9 8 7 6 5 4 3 2 1

APO

Library of Congress Cataloging-in-Publication Data on file

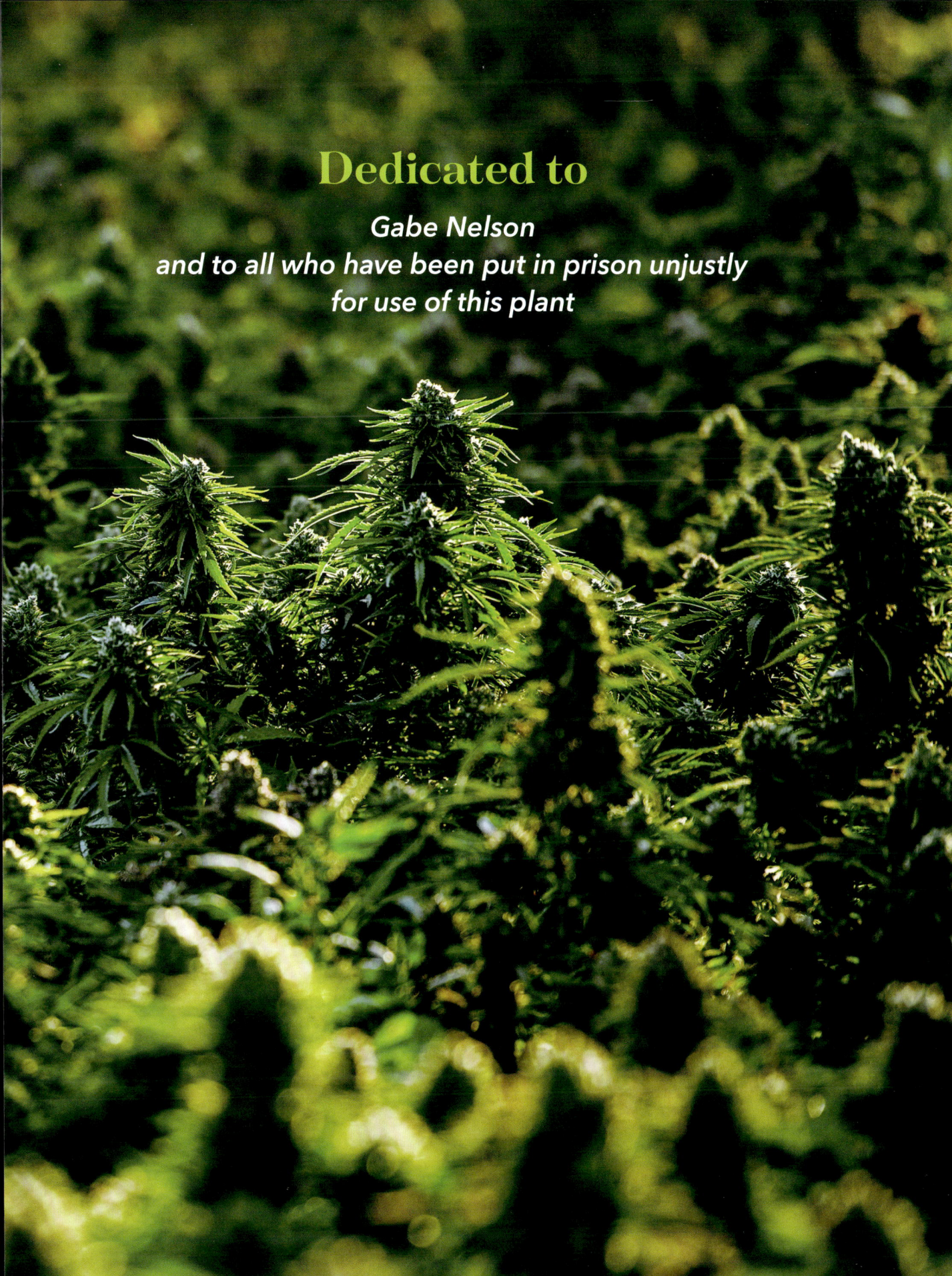

Dedicated to

Gabe Nelson
and to all who have been put in prison unjustly
for use of this plant

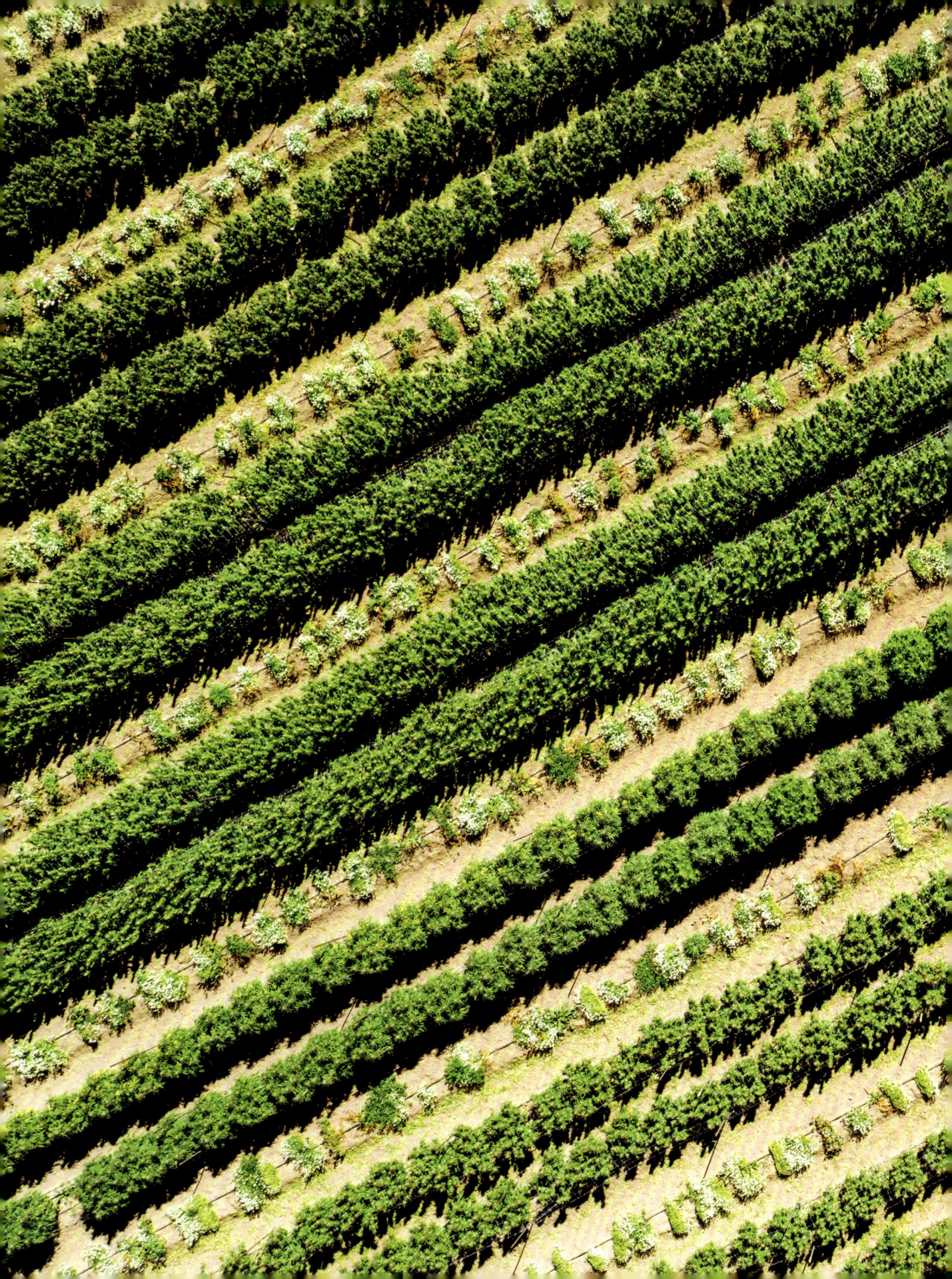

CONTENTS

SECTION 1:
Planning–Late Winter to Early Spring   25

SECTION 2:
Planting–Spring 81

SECTION 3:
Crop Management–Summer 119

SECTION 4: Harvest, Storage, and Processing–Fall and Winter 153

Authors and Atlas Seed
cofounders Adam Davidoff
(left) and Ryan Power (right)

Our Origin Story

We met in middle school, became best friends in high school, and went to college together. At the University of California, Santa Cruz (UCSC) we both enrolled in environmental studies with a focus in sustainable agriculture. The program proved to be part inspirational and part depressing, and by the end we were both clear: We wanted to put our energy into work that would make the world a better place. Then *bam!* One night while making an epic homebrew, we decided to start a farm together.

After graduation Ryan did the apprenticeship program at the Center for Agroecology and Sustainable Food Systems (CASFS) on the UCSC Farm and Garden. Adam interned there while finishing his degree. In 2010, after several great farming stints around the country–Colorado, New Mexico, and Tennessee–we decided it was time to return home to Northern California and begin New Family Farm.

The initial few years of our farm were beautiful and simple, but they were also a hustle and a grind. We started with a lot of idealism: farming with draft horses and raising way too many animals, including chickens, goats, sheep, pigs, donkeys, and horses. And we tried growing a huge diversity of annual crops, a few of which stuck but most of which we quickly cast aside. We experimented with dry-farming potatoes and tomatoes; we tried rotational grazing with our pigs by allowing them to graze and root in our production fields. At our peak we attended three weekly farmers' markets and supplied eight restaurants and nine grocery stores, delivering everything in an old Dodge Dakota with the paint peeling off. To maximize space in our spiffy delivery vehicle, we modified the lumber rack by wiring boards to the side, which allowed us to safely stack boxes all the way to the top of the rack.

At this point we were doing a little bit of a lot of different things, but we were not doing anything particularly well. The vegetable operation occupied most of our time, yet we needed to make the farm financially profitable. We held on to some of our idealism but had to conform to modernity's orientations: Margins are slim in organic vegetable production, and efficiency is paramount. We reoriented our minds toward running a business, began the process of tooling up, bought a new Kubota tractor, and set out on a quest to transform our farm into one that could turn enough profit to support ourselves and our families.

Practically speaking, this meant carefully planned crop enterprise budgets; thoughtful crop selection (read: Do not grow acres of potatoes if you do not have a mechanical potato digger); judicious use of inputs; efficient use of farm equipment; a professional marketing plan; and, perhaps most important, efficient labor practices. We used to have contests to see who could pick the most bunches of kale in a minute. Adam always won.

After a few years at our original farm location, we bought a piece of land with good water and flat fields on the other side of town. As is common in Northern California, the price tag was high. We ran the numbers and could not find a way to pay for the mortgage only growing vegetables. We found a group of people interested in renting the house on the land and putting in a greenhouse to cultivate cannabis. This arrangement easily covered the costs of owning land and insuring it, allowing us to slowly transition our farming operation. Over the course of that first growing season, we realized that we could incorporate cannabis into our crop plan and grow it more efficiently than most other cultivators. By applying our agricultural, streamlined-cost-of-production mindset to cannabis, we thought we would be able to achieve outstanding yield and profits.

We realized that we could incorporate cannabis into our crop plan and grow it more efficiently than most other cultivators.

As it turns out, cannabis had more to teach us than we could have possibly imagined. We were humbled by many setbacks and mistakes made along the way. We learned more about growing plants in one season than we had in more than five years of raising vegetable crops. In fact, the cultivation of cannabis has changed how we farm altogether.

During that first season we propagated and grew cannabis in almost every possible way—indoors under lights, in raised beds in a light-deprivation greenhouse, outdoors in big pots, and outdoors in native soil. We learned of "autoflowering" (a.k.a. day-neutral) cannabis, which does not need a particular light cycle to initiate flowering. We also learned that *Cannabis ruderalis* is a Siberian landrace that has been crossed into modern *C. sativa* and *indica* varieties to produce plants that will complete their life cycle in 60 to 80 days without any light cycle manipulation. A lightbulb went off in our heads. The potential to incorporate autoflowering genetics into row-cropping systems is much higher than with normal photoperiod lines.

Autoflowers can be propagated in seedling trays just like cabbages, and the growing plants require no trellising. They allow for predictable and successive harvests. We brought in autoflowering seeds from Canada and Europe and tried growing them all in the fields. For photoperiod lines, we sourced clones of some of the top genetics

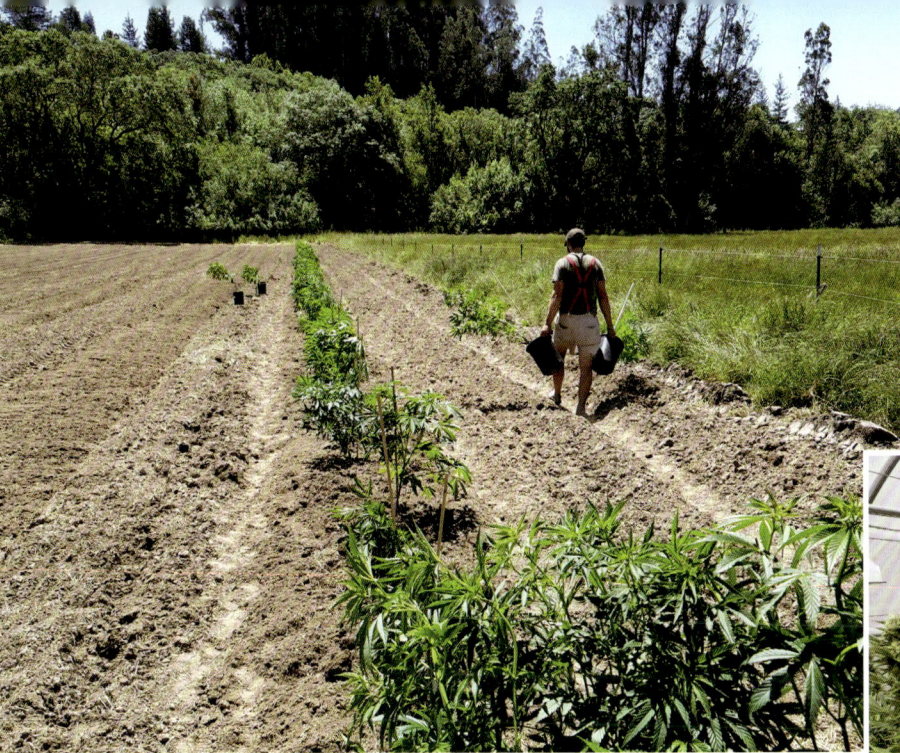

We have experimented with propagating and growing cannabis in almost every possible way—indoors under lights, in raised beds in a light-deprivation greenhouse, outdoors in big pots, and outdoors in native soil.

available in California at that time. Nothing performed as we hoped. Until then, cannabis had not yet been grown outdoors in the open in row-cropping systems, and breeders had not had the opportunity to develop seed in that setting. After one season we learned that the genetics we needed didn't exist.

While we developed our acumen with field-scale cannabis production, we simultaneously started Atlas Seed to breed genetics for agricultural applications. By selecting traits that lend themselves to an efficient production system, we created lines that perform exceptionally under field conditions and environments that vary drastically. In the fields our flower production system goes hand in hand with our genetic development program. It has been a journey to incorporate cannabis into a diverse farm ecosystem. From cultural practices to genetics, we have made significant headway.

Why We Wrote This Book

We wrote this book in part for ourselves, to codify and systematize the knowledge and experience we've developed over the past few years, and in part for the future of the industry and growers everywhere. Our farm business benefited immensely from clearly

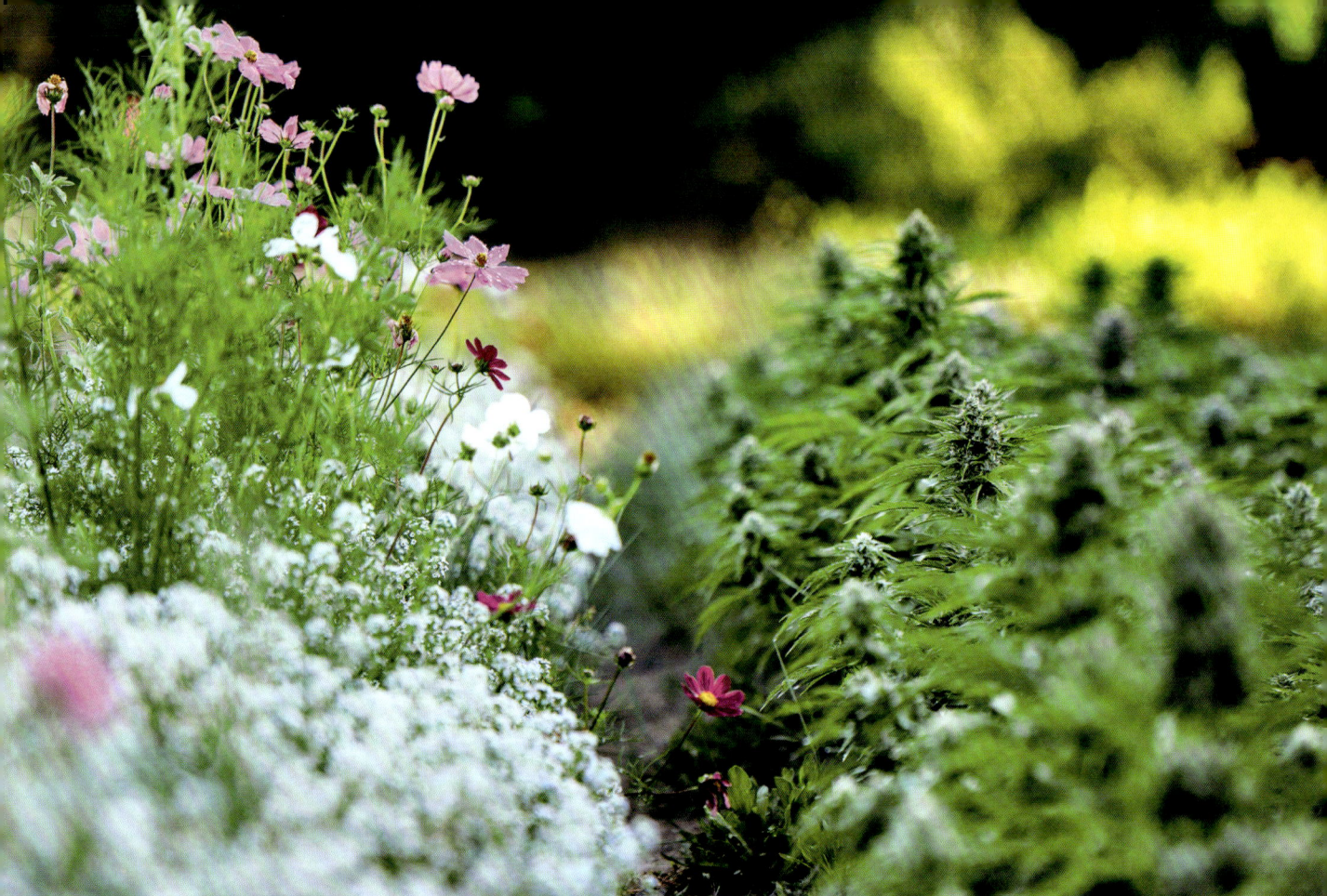

written, practical books about the practice and business of farming, such as Richard Wiswall's *The Organic Farmer's Business Handbook* and Eliot Coleman's *The New Organic Grower*. We wanted a book for those already growing cannabis as well as those considering it. Growing cannabis in modern agricultural systems is relatively new, so view this manual as a dynamic document that inevitably will change over time. That said, the methods and principles we outline are rooted in the agronomy of today's agriculture and are comprehensive enough to qualify as a manual, version 1.0. Employing the system outlined in these pages can lower production costs per pound well below the current industry average.

This book is written for those with at least some experience in farming or in growing cannabis. It is a technical manual that assumes basic to intermediate knowledge of cannabis botany and farming systems. Readers familiar with terpenes or drip irrigation, for example, can hit the ground running with this book.

We cover the outdoor, row-crop cultivation of cannabis grown primarily for its flower, which applies to flowers grown for their THC content (what is called cannabis or weed) and/or for CBD content (known as hemp, CBD flower, or smokable hemp).

Our focus on this distinctive way of growing means that you won't find information on industrial hemp production, indoor cultivation, light-deprivation greenhouses, extraction technologies, or other methods. We do not spend pages introducing cannabis botany, as do some exuberantly colorful cannabis growing "manuals," but highlight only those features directly related to an agricultural application. And we do not outline clonal propagation, because we do not consider cloning to be economical for the future of scaled cannabis production. Finally, though we do not explicitly describe using open-ended hoop houses, most, if not all, of the concepts outlined in this book still apply in covered outdoor systems.

Though relatively brief compared to our entire farming journey, the seasons marking the beginning of legal cannabis cultivation in the twenty-first century have felt very long–packed tightly with intense learning curves, regulatory hoop–jumping, and a rodeo-level momentum. It's hard to believe how much the industry has changed in only a few years and how challenging it has been adapting row-cropping systems for this beautiful and enchanting plant.

Cannabis is a plant. There is a mystique surrounding it that is largely due to its historic illegalization and ensuing development underground. Our hats go off to the caretakers, growers, and breeders of this amazing plant throughout prohibition and their steady dedication to craft, and to the immense benefits cannabis has to offer people. Our aim is to bring cannabis into traditional agricultural systems. With an eye to the future, this book provides a thorough account of what we have learned and how we learned it, complete with detailed descriptions of every step of our cannabis production model. For an overview of how laws and regulations have shaped cannabis horticulture and our perspective on the current industry, see Appendix I, page 195.

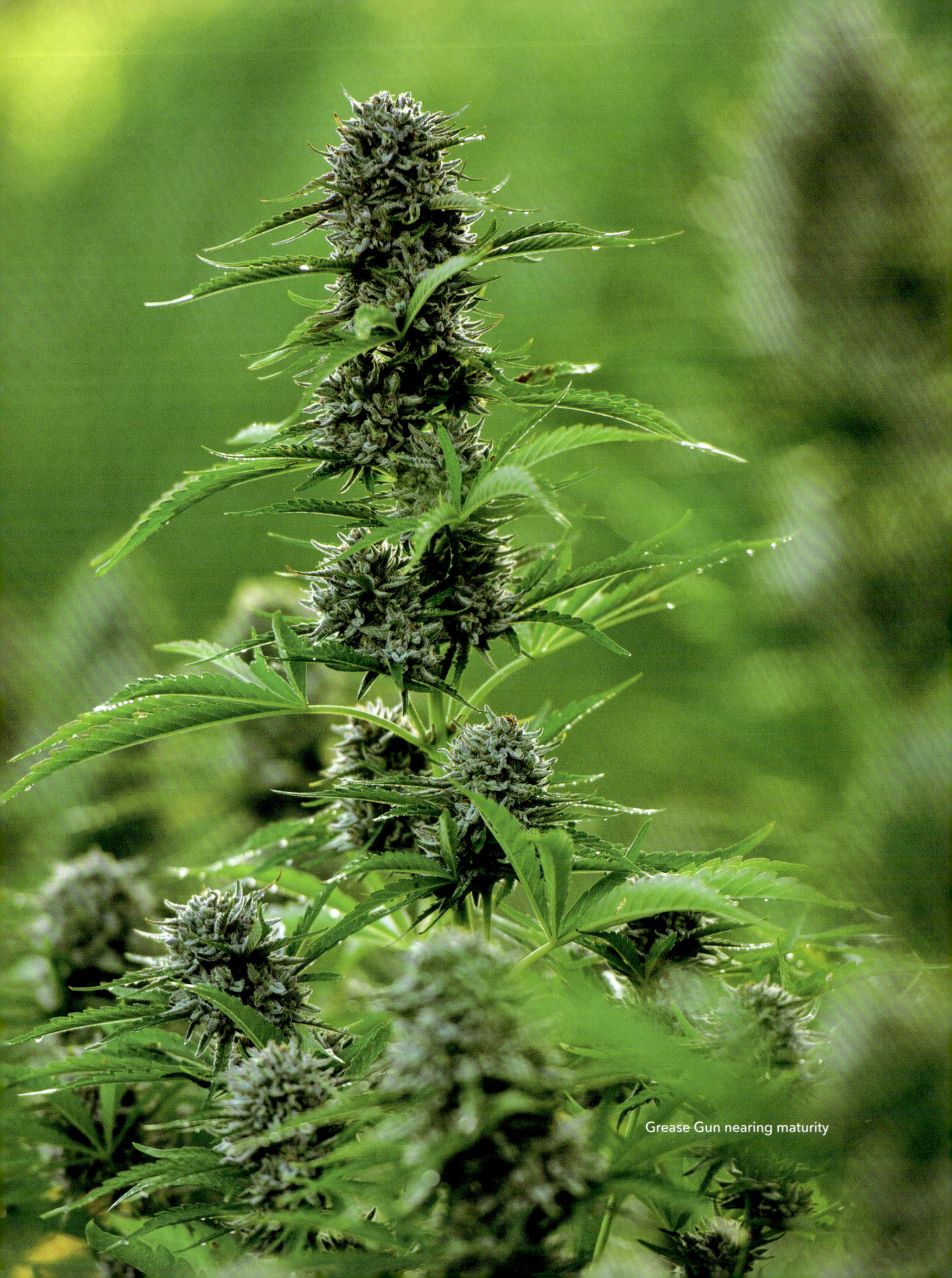

Grease Gun nearing maturity

It Helps to Have Chutzpah

All farmers are gamblers. Many wouldn't view themselves that way, but it's true. Farming (and life, for that matter) requires surrendering control, as many of the variables required to grow a successful crop are simply not controllable. Farmers are at the mercy of the wind, rain, sun, climate, insect life cycles, markets, and innumerable other variables that are outside of their control. Perhaps we just felt like the risk of farming alone was risk enough, so when we first started our farm we purposely avoided growing cannabis. We were farming vegetables with a team of draft horses and took a puritanical approach. We didn't need cannabis and all the additional hoopla that accompanied the crop (though we certainly could have used the money). But we only resisted for so long, until year five, when we decided we would grow four or five plants out back behind the barn.

At this point we also raised feeder hogs for sale and had several sows for breeding, including a spunky and sweet one named Bertha. Bertha was due to farrow at the end of September—prime harvest season on our farm. One Friday as we left to sell at a nearby farmers' market, we noticed signs that Bertha was going into labor. Later that evening, as we backed the truck into the barn, we saw that our organized, stacked boxes of freshly picked tomatoes were disheveled, with half-eaten tomatoes all around them. An immediate check on Bertha revealed five healthy and suckling piglets and a dead one she had rolled on. Back in the barn, the destruction was extensive. She had knocked over several stacks, eaten parts of four cases of

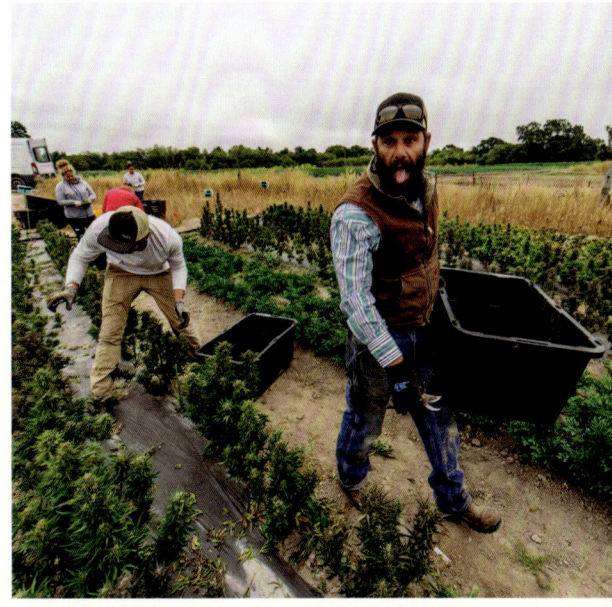

Cannabis farming requires a bit of a defiant spirit.

17

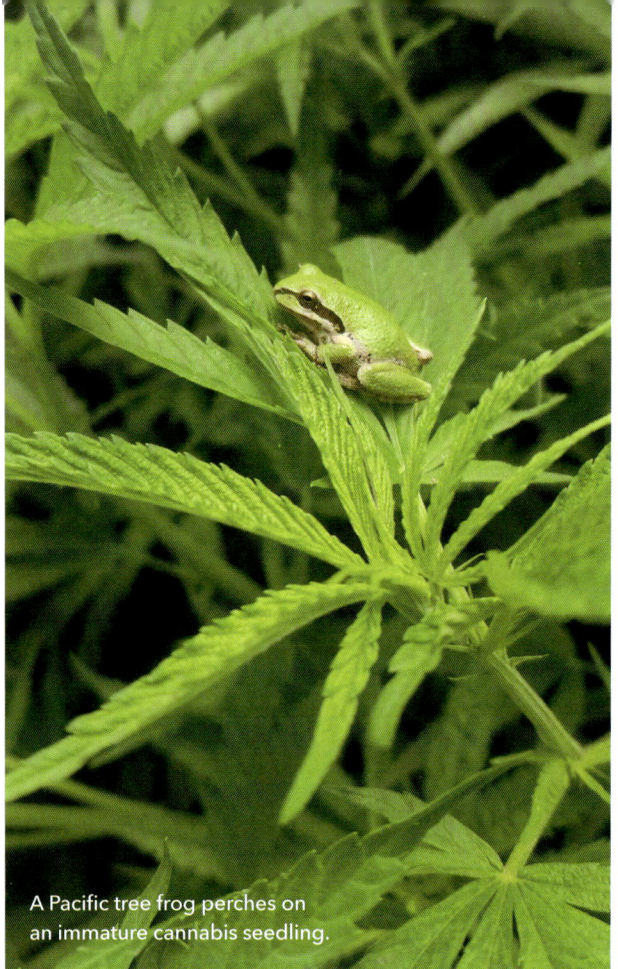

A Pacific tree frog perches on an immature cannabis seedling.

tomatoes, and sprayed tomato debris and juice over everything. These things happen.

The next day we went to check on our cannabis plants, and they were almost all gone. The remaining stems were nuzzled into a nest pile, and the developing flowers were nowhere to be found. So our first flirtation with cannabis ended with Bertha rampaging through the cannabis plants and chowing down on the tomatoes before delivering her litter. Looking back, it seems appropriate, considering where we are at now.

The threat of pregnant sows destroying your crop is almost nonexistent. However, this story gives perspective on how risky farming is and the increased risks associated with cannabis cultivation. The fact is, cultivating cannabis requires heaps of chutzpah, as there are a litany of hurdles and thus potential risks that would-be growers must leap to succeed.

Historical stigma. Although this is rapidly changing with its recent reclassification from a Schedule I to Schedule III drug, cannabis has been federally illegal for so long that cultivating the plant energetically carries with it some of this historical stigma. Furthermore, it's a potent medicinal plant that has the power to radically alter our brain chemistry. It is important to respect the plant's power and energy and not take for granted its healing properties and historical usage.

Theft and security issues. Due to their longtime illegal status, cannabis crops have historically carried a high value, and theft in agricultural settings is real. Some farmers go to great lengths to protect their crops by installing tall barbed-wire fences, putting in video surveillance, or hiring private security. In other cases, licensing bodies have specific or onerous security requirements just for a farmer to be able to cultivate. As long as cannabis remains a high-value crop, threat of theft will continue to be a consideration.

Bureaucratic hurdles. Regardless of the location, obtaining any licensing related to cannabis cultivation has been fraught with uncertainty due to a lack of consistency, rapidly shifting rules and regulations, nepotism, and overregulation. When farmers hop on the permitting roller coaster, they are often held up at some point in the process for weeks, months, or literally years in the worst instances. They are granted permits that are later revoked for no apparent reason. Countless farmers are stymied in expensive and uncertain attempts to obtain permits and end up in permit purgatory. The risk and uncertainty associated with obtaining and keeping permits to cultivate cannabis cannot be understated.

Open pollination. Cannabis rapidly loses value for both extraction and/or processing when it is pollinated and seeded (goes to seed). The risk to profits posed by unintentional pollination is severe and is another variable that is, in some instances, completely out of the farmer's control. Pollination can occur from hermaphrodites or rogue males within a farmer's own crop. This is the farmer's fault, and they have no one to blame but themselves (see the section on males and herm hunting, page 68). However, pollination can also occur from a neighbor's crop, and under the right conditions a "neighbor" can be as far as 10 miles away. Hemp males grown en masse have been known to pollinate outdoor cannabis crops on a statewide scale in Oregon, for instance.

Inconsistent genetics. The marketplace for cannabis genetics is fraught with uncertainty. There are many new companies with genetics that underperform. And while many of the genetics out there are acceptable and some great, many of them have not been stress tested or grown out in enough conditions or over a number of years to know how they will react in adverse conditions. While we offer important strategies in our section on vetting genetics (page 32), in this stage of the industry, cannabis genetics are less stable and less predictable than those of corn or cabbage or kale that has been bred and tested for 30-plus years at extensive scales.

Vulnerability to weather. While modern cannabis plants are fairly resilient and vigorous in the vegetative growth stage, inclement weather can cause massive damage overnight. Because of their irregular surface and composition, mature cannabis flowers may either absorb water like a sponge or provide a place for water to gather and sit. Stagnant water and high humidity create ideal conditions for explosive botrytis mold growth. Waterlogged flowers add significant weight to branches, causing them to bend or break. Flowers may bunch together, which encourages mold, or end up on the ground, spoiled by wet soil. High winds near harvesttime, when the plants are top-heavy with mature flowers, can damage plants and reduce yields. Beyond these acute weather events, cannabis crops can be affected drastically simply by poor finishing conditions, namely high humidity. A few days of high humidity during the final stages of growth will affect yield and quality, with the potential to ruin an entire crop.

Limits on business practices. Cannabis's evolving legal status still limits the capacity of the industry as a whole. Traditional banking services are difficult, and sometimes impossible, to obtain; insurance and basic business services are even harder; and some vendors refuse to do business with another business that is even associated with cannabis. As a cannabis farmer you never know exactly who is willing to do business with you or provide you with basic services that many businesses need just to keep the doors open.

High start-up costs. The cost to grow a crop of cannabis is high relative to other crops that would be considered high value, such as strawberries. The costs to harvest and dry a crop of cannabis, however, are exorbitant.

Cannabis cultivation practices developed with heavy influence from its status as an illegal or semi-legal crop (see Appendix I, page 195). Growers were forced to sacrifice some intelligent system design to successfully sneak a crop to harvest without getting caught. This has meant that the evolution of cannabis cultivation practices and systems lags far behind those of other agricultural crops. For example, the simultaneous development of the processing tomato and the mechanical tomato harvester was aided significantly by the work done at the ag program at UC Davis. We can only imagine what the industry would be like if cannabis had been cultivated legally out in the open for 50 years and public universities were funding studies of hop latent viroid (HLVd), THC production in plant populations, or any other issues at the forefront of the industry. This process of coming out of the shadows has contributed to a burst of innovation. However, there is still a massive evolution currently taking place, and there will be enormous strides in the development of agronomic systems and an agricultural approach to cannabis cultivation in the years to come.

Agronomic Mindset: Cannabis Is a Crop

Now that cannabis is legal in many states, and with its reclassification, we've had a few years of cultivation with standard agricultural practices. Many of our methods are based in the medium- to large-scale cultivation of vegetables such as brassicas and tomatoes, with additions to meet the specific needs of cannabis. There are no current, regularly practiced conventions in cannabis agriculture yet. Standard agricultural figures, such as planting density and yield per acre, are still in development.

Cannabis is a crop just like any other and has needs like many other heavy-feeding annual plants, such as tomatoes. Applying an agricultural mindset to cannabis cultivation means row cropping in native soil—planting plants in the ground. Row cropping means using standardized processes of field prep, propagation, planting, cultivation, and harvest. In total these practices comprise what we call a crop production system.

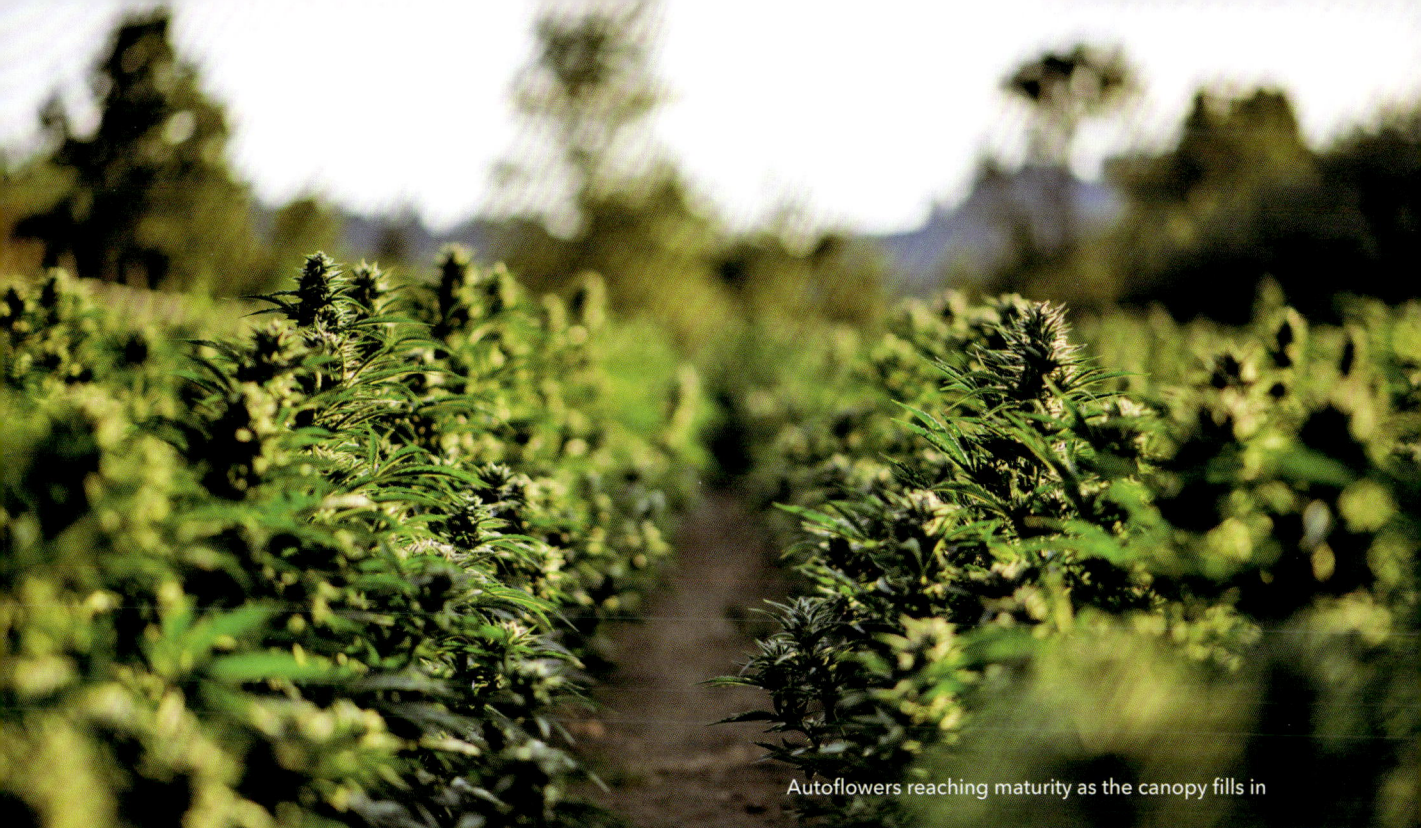

Autoflowers reaching maturity as the canopy fills in

Each piece of the puzzle is as important as the next, and mistakes made or corners cut early in the crop cycle translate to decreased productivity in the end.

A highly efficient farming system must strike a balance between labor efficiency and thoroughness. We want to limit the amount of time required to produce the crop, but we must also meet the needs of the crop to achieve excellent performance. We break this down into the concept of touches, which refers to any time we have to touch the actual plant to get the job done right. Sometimes, when you add up and examine all the touches, you find ways to eliminate one or two and gain efficiency. This concept can be applied to any labor process, such as the storage and acquisition of supplies. Obviously, we want to bring harvest totes into the field using the fewest number of touches possible. Analyzing cultivation and harvest processes through the touch lens is part of the agricultural mindset, and in a multimonth crop cycle its importance cannot be overstated.

The cannabis genome adds distinct variation to the discussion; methods for the cultivation of photoperiod *sativa*-dominant strains differ from *indica*-dominant lines. Clones perform very differently than seeds. Autoflower crop production is entirely distinct from photoperiod full-term, and then there are semi-full-term photoperiods as well. We will make note of these differences throughout the text. Common examples include varied planting densities, planting dates, desired plant size, and finish times.

Finally, in a nascent industry, nobody and everybody is an expert. Tips and tricks abound, but empirically demonstrated agricultural methods are tried and true. Applying these principles to your cannabis operation is sure to create efficiency and standardize success. The goal is to limit the trial and error required to reach excellent, repeatable yield by leaning on time-tested techniques and concepts outlined herein.

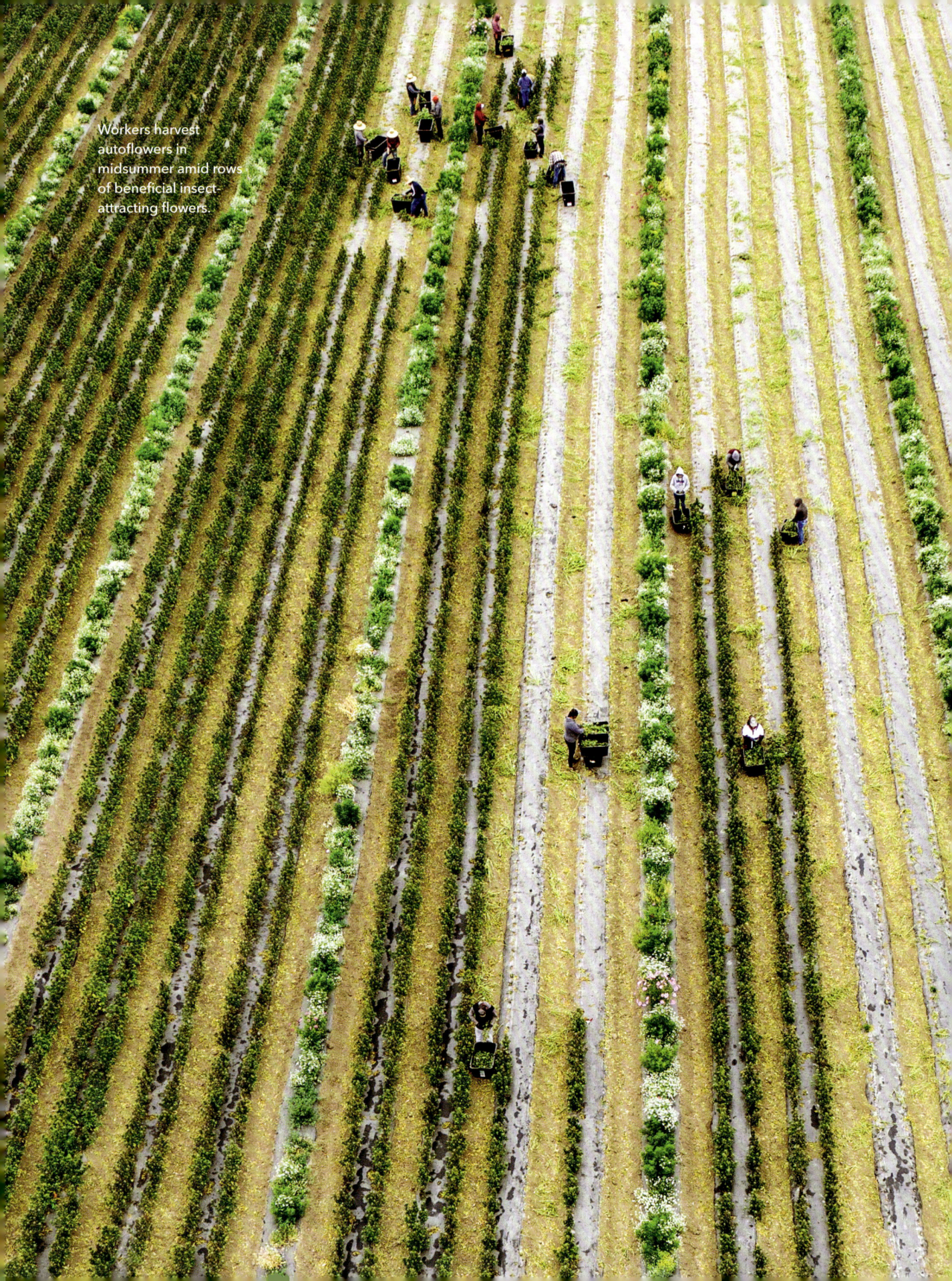

Workers harvest autoflowers in midsummer amid rows of beneficial insect-attracting flowers.

Seasonal Overview of Our Cannabis Farm
WHAT TO DO AND WHEN

WINTER

December
- Review profit and loss for previous year
- Taxes
- Review with staff how the previous season went and talk about employment for the upcoming season
- Make overview of upcoming season: total acreage to plant, variety selection, and building field map
- Address any major changes that need to be made for the upcoming season

January
- Finalize acreage
- Order plants/seeds
- Order supplies/rentals or put on the calendar when to order them

February
- Chill

SPRING

March
- Look longingly at the fields (unless you have hoop houses or an early season)

April
- Review the plan and address any changes
- Begin field work
- Start seeds for first succession

May
- Begin field work
- Start seeds for second succession
- Bedshaping and planting autoflowers
- Close looking

SUMMER

June
- Planting full-terms
- Irrigating
- Weeding
- Close looking

July
- Autoflower harvest
- Irrigating
- Trellising
- Close looking

August
- Irrigating
- Plant maintenance

FALL

September
- Big-leafing
- Harvest begins
- Set up/look carefully at dry space

October
- Harvest
- Drying
- Inventory management
- Plant cover crop

November
- Sales
- Inventory management
- Equipment maintenance

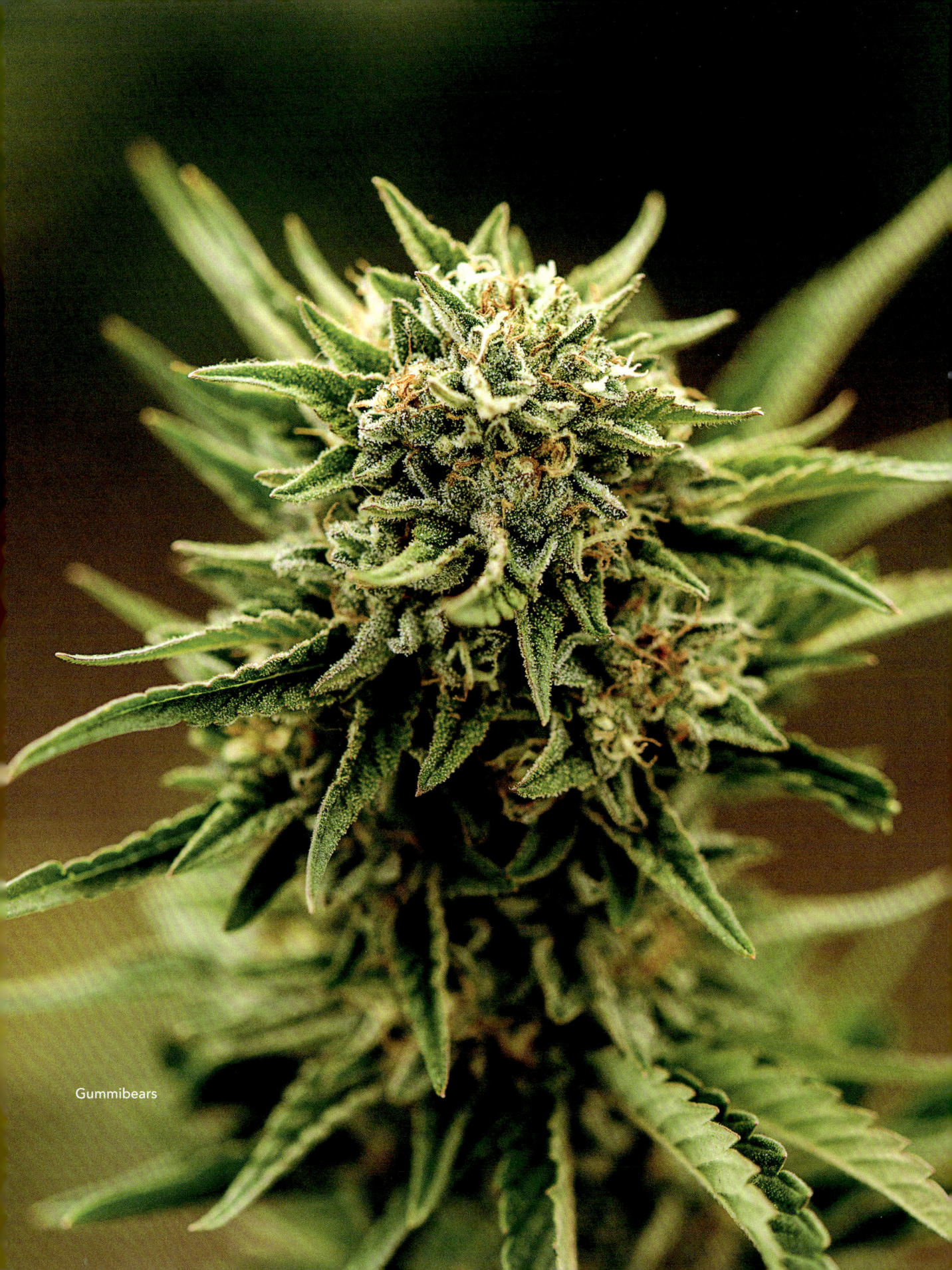

Gummibears

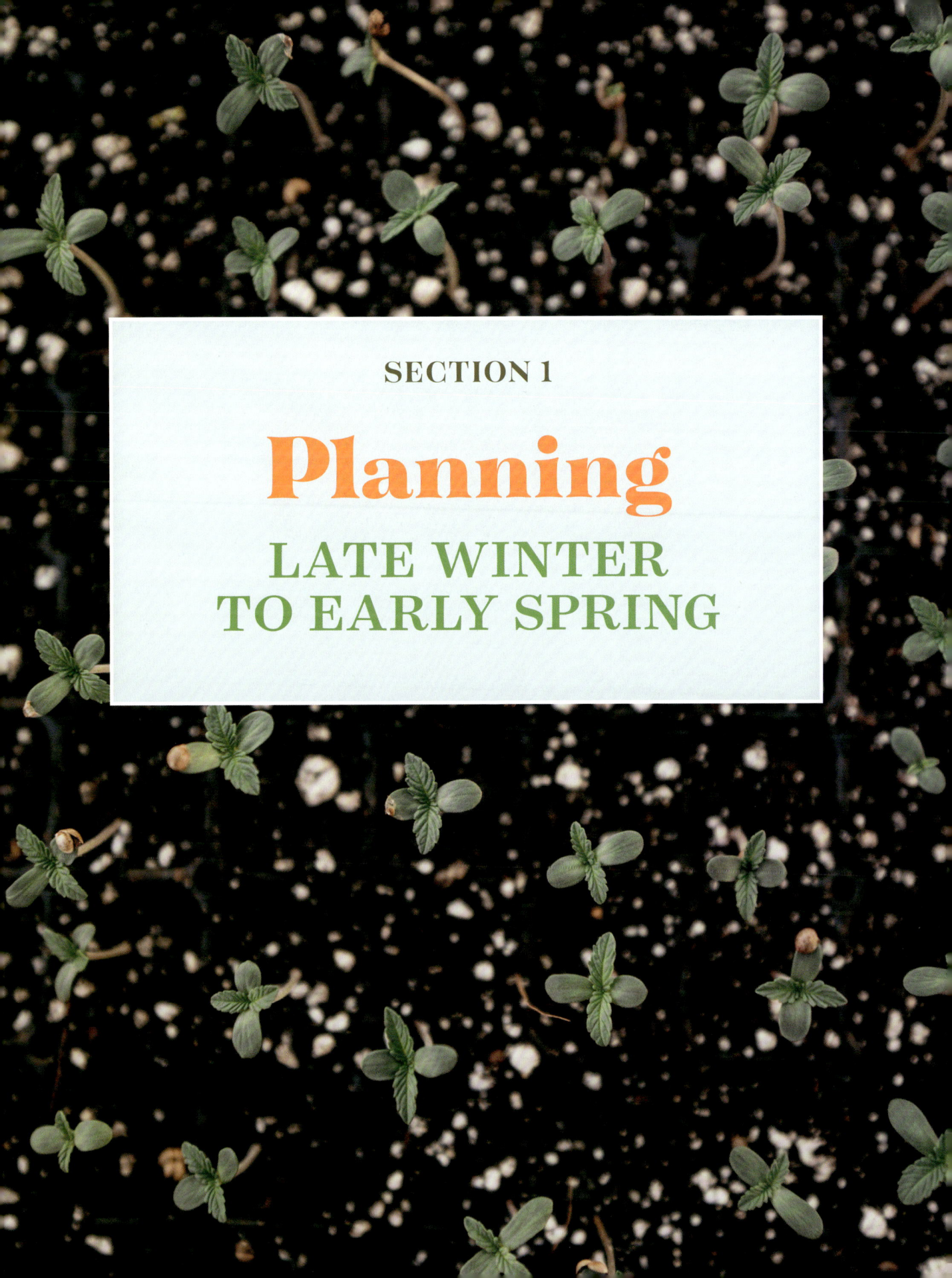

SECTION 1

Planning

LATE WINTER
TO EARLY SPRING

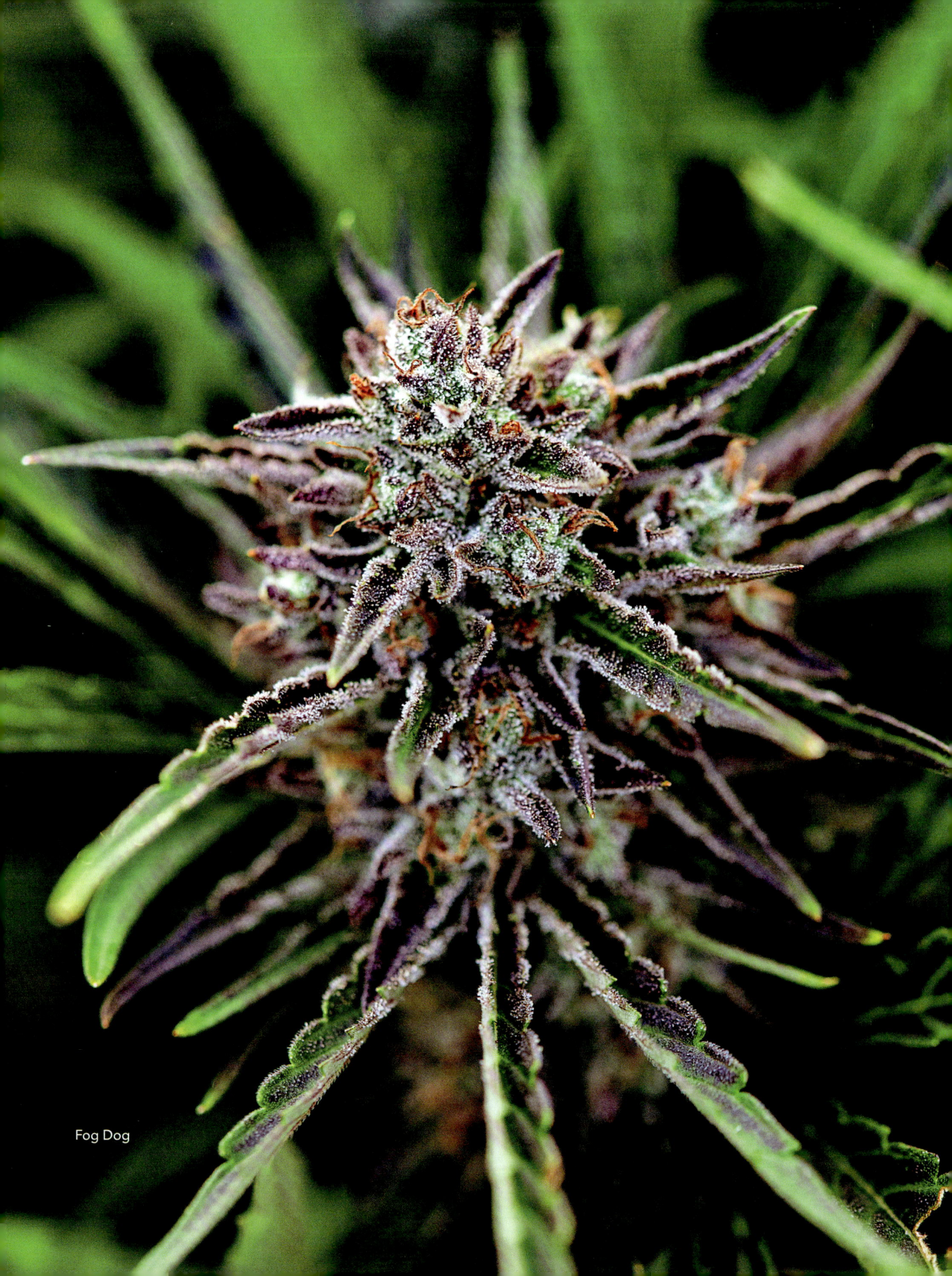

Fog Dog

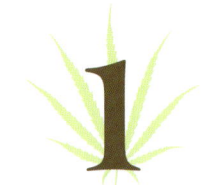

Genetics

The *Cannabis* genus contains a vast diversity of qualities, appearances, chemical constituents, and effects. For the newcomer it can be very confusing. Internet searches will reveal a dizzying array of contradictory information, mostly from the perspective of the consumer. Academic botanical manuals are pedantic and, while interesting, impractical to the field-scale grower. The traditionally used classifications are *Cannabis sativa* and *C. indica*. While these cultivars are indeed quite different, there is much more to consider when planning your operation.

When we started farming cannabis, we were thoroughly confused by the diversity of genetics, their propensities, and how to select them. Seed and clones were expensive, buyers had all kinds of preferences, and nobody knew anything about the agronomics (meaning the field-crop production and soil management needs) of any particular variety. So we tried everything. Very quickly we discovered the idiosyncrasies of cannabis genetics relative to what mattered the most: what grew well for us and what buyers wanted.

We knew seeds would be key to our operation, but seeds were prohibitively expensive, and we realized that the genetics we needed for row cropping—field-scale agriculture—did not yet exist. We launched into the study and practice of breeding and seed production, an endeavor that led to the founding of our seed company, Atlas Seed. Since then we have learned that not only did we need to develop field-scale strains, but we also needed to define and standardize terms relative to the agronomy of cannabis genetics in order to have intelligent conversations in the industry and convey to customers what to expect.

Agronomics and Market Dynamics

AGRONOMICS

- Light cycle/days to maturity
- Mold resistance/susceptibility
- Drought and cold tolerance
- Feminization
- Growth habits:
  Plant height
  Vigor
  Leaf-flower ratio
  Canopy management
  Flower structure
  Yield

MARKET DYNAMICS

- Supply and demand
- Potency
- Time of year
- Terpenes
- Visual appeal
- Hype and trends
- Product categories:
  High end/AAA /top shelf
  Mids/A and B grades
  Value brand/ready to roll/pre-rolls
  Biomass/extraction

We structured this chapter based on what is most useful to us as outdoor and/or at-scale cultivators. To that end we have developed categories to provide an intelligent understanding of cannabis for farmers to appropriately navigate the intersection between agronomic considerations and market dynamics. These considerations are listed in the Agronomics and Market Dynamics table above.

Terpenes

"Terpenes" refers to the unique smell and taste of the flowers. The cannabis plant can produce a very diverse array and varied combinations of terpenes that can smell like gasoline or lemons or cotton candy. These differences characterize the various types of cannabis available (see illustration, facing page). The strength of that odor is colloquially referred to as "how loud the nose is." Each terpene profile also produces different effects when consumed. Buyers and consumers want diversity—a little of this and a little of that. Certain terpenes or smell profiles fall in and out of popularity over the seasons. But it's crucial to understand the main quality all high-quality cannabis products have in common, whether flower, hash, or vape: They all smell good.

When developing a crop plan and choosing genetics, it is important to pay attention to the way plants smell to meet the market's demand for variety. The type of smells your plants will produce is certainly determined by genetics at the base level, but the expression of this trait and the concentration of terpenes produced is also heavily influenced by environment and post-harvest handling. Growers should trial a diversity of genetics on their farm to find what performs best in terpene production. It's beyond the scope of this chapter to go into granular detail on this subject, but see

Atlas Seed's Aroma Families

Our aroma family system provides a framework that connects genetic lineages, terpenes, medicinal effects, and smells, so that farmers can make more informed decisions about what they plant.

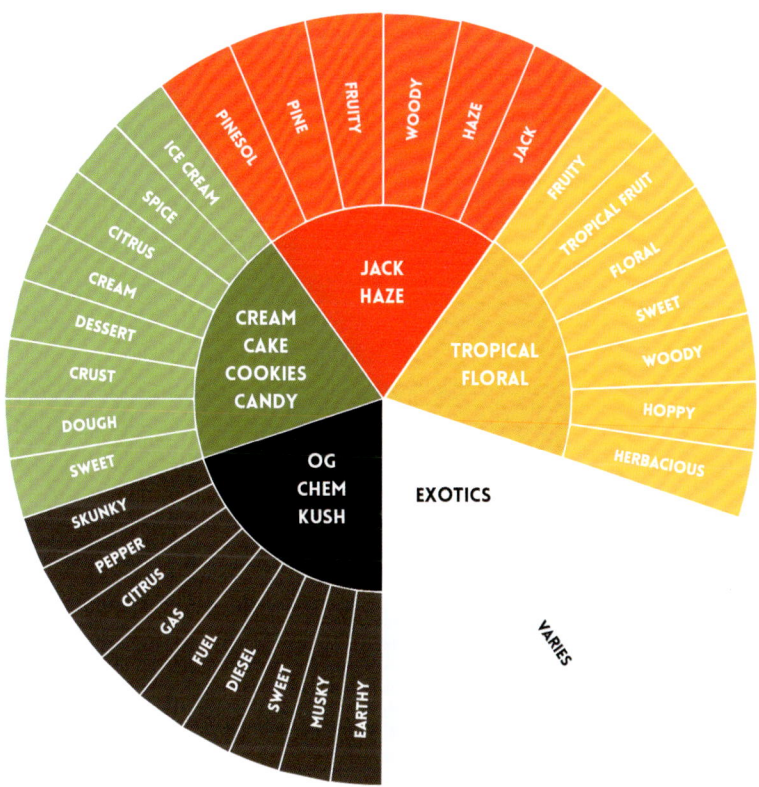

Appendix II: Cannabis Aroma Families (page 201) for a thorough review of genetics and terpene expression if you're looking for help understanding what to plant.

A crucial final point here is that improper or rushed post-harvest will absolutely decimate terpenes. No matter which genetics are chosen, a grower can completely ruin a crop in the drying or curing (dry/cure) phase. For example, terpenes will volatilize at temperatures above 72°F (22°C). The smell of a fresh, growing cola (a single flowering stalk of cannabis) in the field is never what you get in the bag. The best way to preserve terpenes is a "slow and low" dry/cure, which means keeping temperatures low and thus letting the drying process take longer. We cover this more in Chapter 12.

Potency

The second most important factor in market dynamics for a grower is potency, which in this context refers specifically to the percentage of THC and CBD in the flowers (though the concept of "more potent = more high" is the more common understanding). A decade ago, 10 percent THC was an acceptable average. Now buyers balk at anything under 18 percent, and many distributors are expecting to see numbers from 25 to 30 percent THC, an unthinkable demand just a few years ago. As this is the single characteristic in the sales process that is quantified, it exerts huge influence over buyers and consumers. Never mind that, qualitatively, THC percentages are only a piece of the puzzle; while per regulation its potency must be tested, the presence of other cannabinoids is not. Connoisseurs understand that for any strain there is an "entourage effect," which is the cumulative influence of all the different cannabinoids present. There are at least 50 distinct cannabinoids that we know of, and undoubtedly more to be discovered. But in today's marketplace, THC is king.

We have embarked on a potency odyssey both as farmers and breeders over the past years that has revealed many peculiarities of the cannabis plant itself as well as in sampling procedures, lab inconsistencies, and sales negotiations. We found, for example, that THC concentrations vary in a single plant from branch to branch both on plants grown from seed and clones. We also learned that THC production varies within a given population on a bell curve; sampling 50 sibling plants in a row, for example, will yield THC results from 9 to 22 percent.

This presents a unique set of challenges for the breeder, as potency is the single trait that cannot be seen or smelled! We have found, however, that the top-performing plants (those that display exceptional vigor, yield, and appearance) consistently produce the highest potencies. It is therefore not difficult to isolate and breed for potency by selecting for other desirable traits, which is why, in general, THC levels have more than doubled over the past few decades to upwards of 30 percent.

The next step is uniformity of potency in seed lots, a breeding endeavor we are actively working on. Agronomists have explained to us that potassium and calcium are the nutrients that most directly influence potency. Most growers have their own opinions on the matter. In our experience what produces the largest increase in potency (other than selected genetics!) is average temperature. We have grown out clones and

Potency distribution within a seed lot population

All traits are distributed along a bell curve within populations of seed. Breeding reduces the standard deviations from the mean.

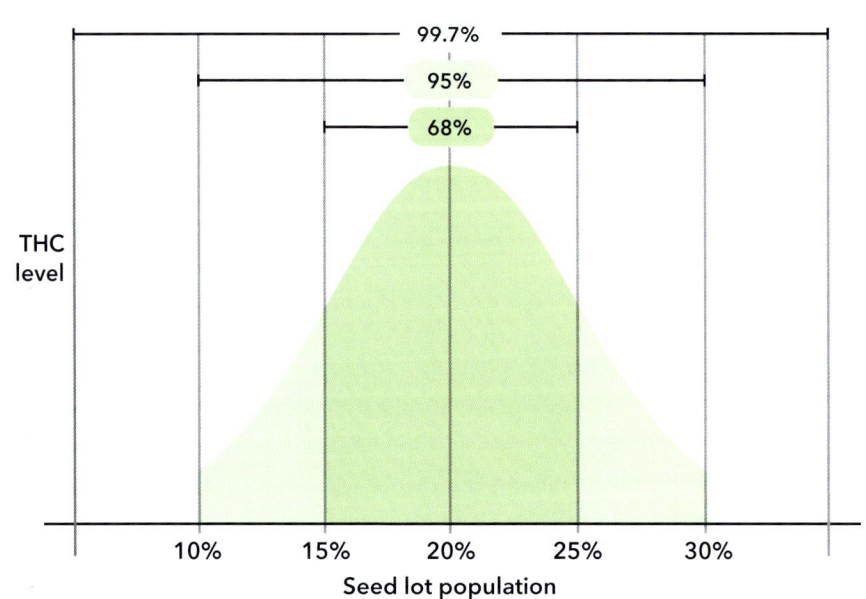

THC level

99.7%

95%

68%

10% 15% 20% 25% 30%

Seed lot population

seed lots that are identical to those grown by our colleagues across the country and have determined time and again that where average temperatures (specifically night temperatures) are higher, potency is also higher. For this reason, and to speed growth in the earlier, colder months, we utilize black plastic mulch (see page 89).

A deeper look into the plant's reasons for producing THC contains some useful insights. Trichomes—the crystalline, sticky, smelly substance on mature flowers—contain the majority of a plant's THC. Cannabis plants produce them as a pest deterrent so insects and animals will not eat their reproductive parts. Therefore, simulating pest pressure can cause plants to produce more trichomes.

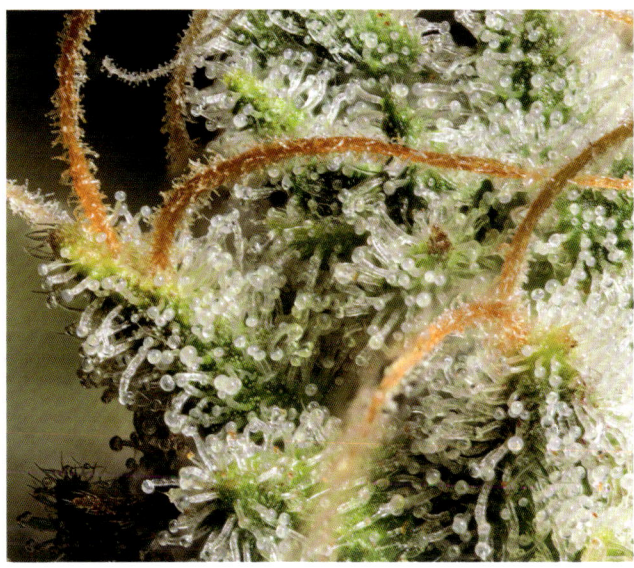

Trichomes on the surface of a flower produce the characteristic "sticky icky" on cannabis flowers.

No matter your chosen genetics, average temperature, or products/nutrients applied, the potency can reach a critical threshold, after which it declines. This is a classic dilution matrix effect: A plant can only produce so much THC. Therefore, the heavier or bigger the flower (more yield), the more diluted the concentration of THC will be. For many varieties this threshold exists beyond the point of ripeness (explained in Chapter 11). But for some plants, and for most autoflowers, the intersection between yield and potency is a sweet spot. Finding it is highly dependent on your environment and experience and may include assessing trichome color and flower density.

A final note on potency that bears mention for the cannabis grower is the mysterious world where laboratory science meets market regulations. Talk to any grower in California and you will hear lamentations about labs. Many people have submitted identical flower samples to different labs and received potency results that vary significantly. Submitting redundant identical samples to a single lab can produce different potency results. Suffice it to say that the laboratory process to determine potency is inaccurate.

How the samples are taken is very important—some buyers will pull samples themselves before purchasing, while others rely on the grower to collect—and individual states will have different testing requirements as well. Ideally the sample represents the entire harvest; but, as noted above, high variation will be present no matter what. The best solution is an average potency reading, which requires combining identical weights taken from flowers from multiple plants—a level of sophistication that is rarely achieved. In the end it's a game. So long as good genetics are chosen, the crop is grown well, and flower quality is high, potency will meet the criteria for market.

How to Select Genetics

Selecting cannabis genetics is done in the planning phase of a given growing season. The process begins with market dynamics—knowing what you can sell. Some farms produce flower biomass specifically for extraction. Some farms grow specialty top-shelf flowers for sale to connoisseurs. Many farms do both and everything in between. As the saying goes: Do not put all your eggs in one basket. We run an autoflower crop for pre-rolls and value brand categories and a full-term crop for higher-quality flower. We love getting two harvests per season. It benefits our pocketbooks and allows us to employ an appropriately sized crew throughout the season.

As we moved into cannabis production, we took many of the lessons we learned from our vegetable operation into consideration when selecting genetics. For example, when you choose seeds, we recommend that you figure out what works and stick with it. For many years we grew tens of thousands of pounds of cabbage for a sauerkraut company, using a tried-and-true variety that never failed and produced uniform cabbages of 3 to 4 pounds. One year we decided to plant 25 percent of our crop with a newly developed kraut variety that was supposed to take a little longer in the field but produce much larger heads between 8 and 10 pounds. This new variety sustained heavy aphid pressure, and we harvested only a small percentage of the crop. It's okay to experiment with new varieties, but we recommend dedicating no more than 25 percent of your production to something new. Use as many breeders, or proven varieties, as you can.

When you're just getting started, a little due diligence goes a long way. Genetic selection should first and foremost be based on your growing climate and region. Start by asking other local growers about what has worked for them. Consider developing relationships with breeders and seed companies and asking them what kind of testing the varieties have seen at scale.

Light Cycle and Flower Maturation

When choosing genetics, an outdoor grower needs to understand the link between flowering light cycle and flower maturation time. You must know when to expect harvest in order to communicate with buyers, plan successions, account for labor and equipment needs, and avoid unfavorable seasonal weather. The *Cannabis* genus is unique in that it has two entirely different light cycle classifications and a cross between them. Most explanations of genetics cover the different genotypic expressions of *Cannabis* and their growth habits and the effects when used. The genotypes *sativa* and *indica*, and hybrids thereof, fall under multiple light cycle categories, however. So we begin with an overview of these categories and then dive into more nuanced agronomic and marketplace considerations. Before jumping in, let's define some terms related to light cycle.

Days to maturity refers to the estimated number of days from when a seed is planted or a clone is taken to the day of harvest. Seed packs come labeled with days to maturity, but that number holds true only under good to great growing conditions at a particular latitude. The actual days to maturity may vary depending on season and latitude (which affect light spectrum and amount), soil temperature and air temperatures, genetic resiliency (how good the genetics are), and major stress events (most commonly over- or under-watering and extreme temperatures).

Initiation refers to the point at which plants begin to form flowers.

Flowering time means the length of time from initiation to mature flowers ready to harvest.

Finish time is the calendar date of maturity. To accurately predict a harvest date, the grower must know the finish time for each cultivar relative to its planting date, which influences the above factors. Another influence on finish time is latitude, which determines the natural light cycle under which the crop is grown. Specifically, photoperiod-determinant genetics will initiate at different dates at different latitudes.

An outdoor grower needs to understand the link between flowering light cycle and flower maturation time.

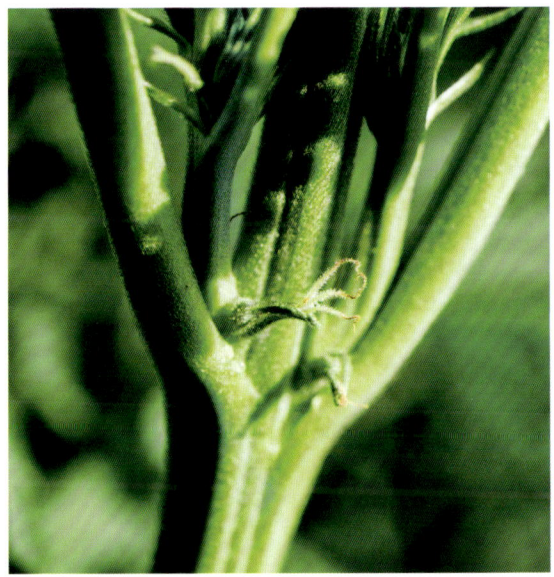 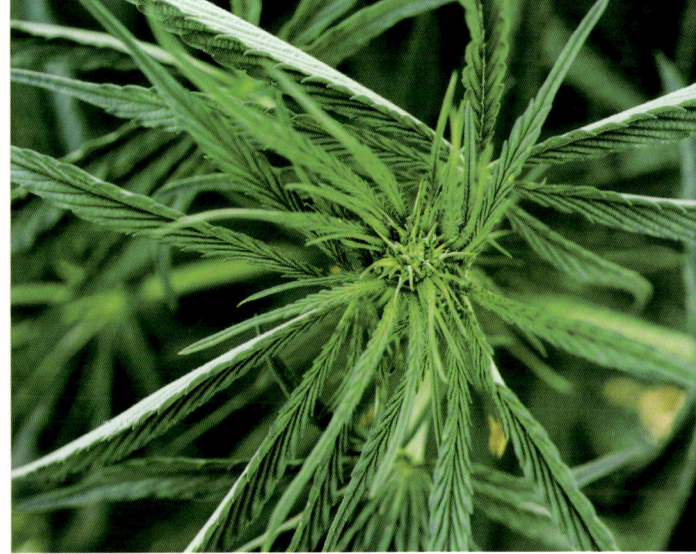

LEFT: A plant shows the first signs of initiation.   RIGHT: A plant roughly 7–10 days after initiation.

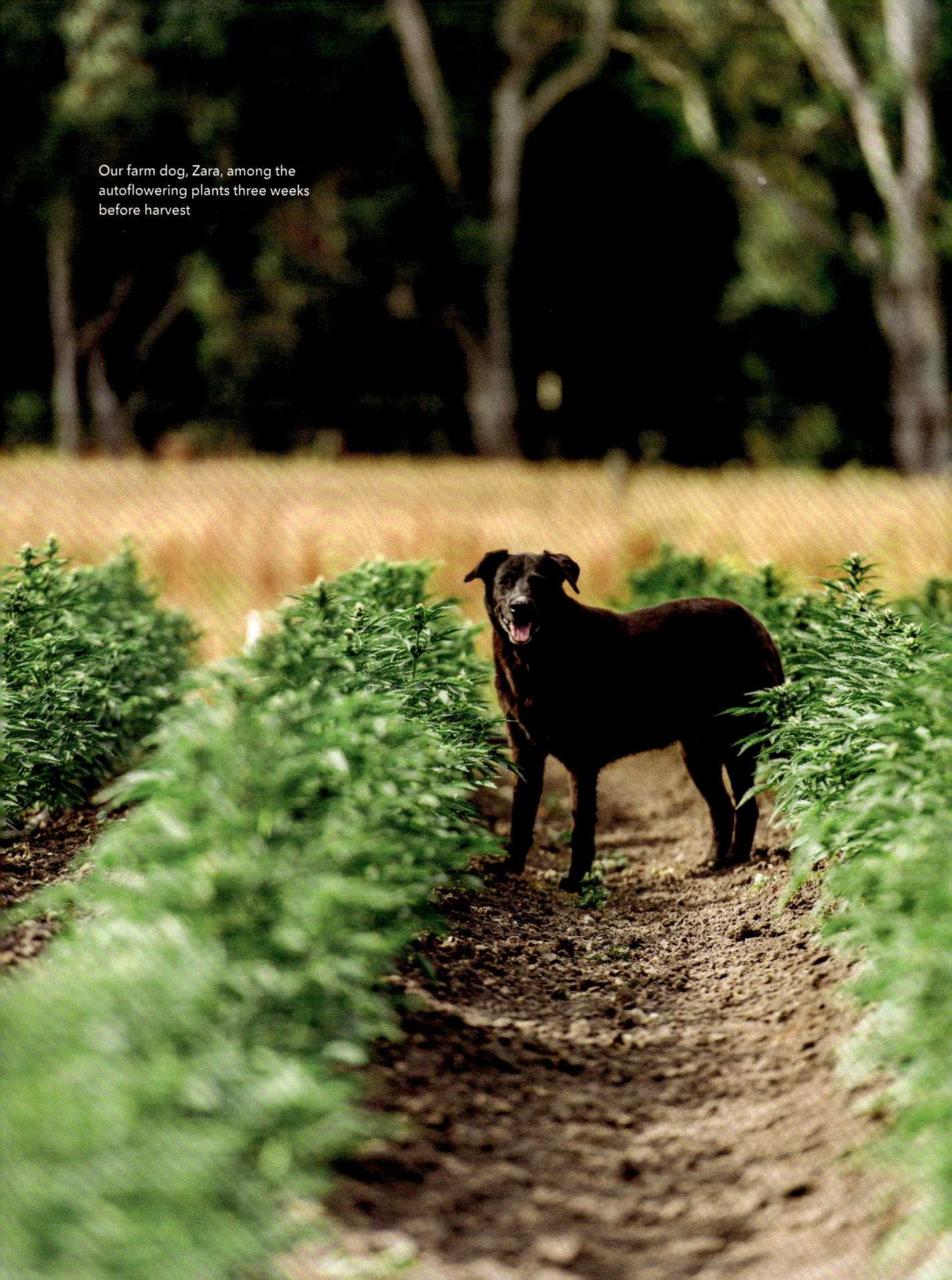

Our farm dog, Zara, among the autoflowering plants three weeks before harvest

Three Light Cycle Types Detailed

Cannabis genetics fall into two general categories: short-day (*Cannabis sativa/indica*) and day-neutral (*Cannabis ruderalis × sativa/indica*). Short-day cannabis is further divided into full-term and semi-full-term varieties. Short-day varieties are known in the industry as full-term/photoperiod determinant, and day-neutral varieties are called autoflowers. Botanically speaking, a plant that requires a long period of darkness is termed a "short-day" (long-night) plant.

Short-day plants form flowers when day length decreases to less than 15 hours. Many fall-flowering plants are short-day plants. Full-term varieties finish in October and sometimes into November. Semi-full-term varieties, which are the first-generation cross between a full-term and an autoflower, finish September to early October. Semi-full-terms initiate earlier in the season and finish their flowering cycle faster than their full-term counterparts. In our side-by-side experience, full-term genetics initiate flowering roughly in the first week of August, and semi-full-term genetics in July. It is important to note that this is not a rubric, as planting date has as much to do with this example as time of year.

Day-neutral cannabis, or autoflower, is *Cannabis ruderalis*, a Siberian subspecies that evolved to flower in the far north where the summer day length is more than 20 hours. It will initiate flowering based on plant maturity and regardless of day length. *Ruderalis* has been crossed and back-crossed and crossed again with *indica* and *sativa* to create the varieties available today. Day-neutral plants typically do not reach more than 4 feet in height, and their days to maturity normally do not exceed 90 days. They are particularly useful because they can be planted in succession with reliable finish times, allowing for efficient use of crew labor and dry/cure space. They also allow growers to complete a big harvest early in the season and then plant a full-term (or another autoflower) crop. In certain climates growers can even get three harvests outdoors in a single calendar year by utilizing day-neutral varieties.

Let's dive into more details pertinent to the grower for each light cycle type.

Full-Term

Full-term genetics express many of the sought-after characteristics in the modern cannabis marketplace: high potencies and strong and diverse terpene profiles. Because of this they will continue to play an important role in the development of genetics and in field-scale production for both the smokable flower market and for extraction.

Full-terms grown from seed or clones require elaborate canopy management—trellising to prevent branches breaking under the weight of maturing flowers, and in most environments pruning (details in Chapter 8). Full-term genetics fall into two subspecies: *sativa* and *indica*, and hybrids between them.

Sativas are generally large plants with generous internodal spacing and light green, long, narrow fan leaves. Flower structure is normally looser than their *indica* counterparts, and flowering time is longer—typically 9 or 10 weeks.

Indicas are shorter, squatter plants with dark green, wide fan leaves and shorter internodal spacing. Flower structure is typically dense, and flowering times are shorter than *sativa*—typically 7 or 8 weeks. Due to the dense flower structure and short internodal spacing, which results in reduced airflow and light penetration, mold is usually more of an issue for *indica* than *sativa*.

As they are bigger plants, sativas usually yield higher than indicas. Yields per acre for full-terms are between 6,000 and 10,000 pounds of biomass.

Cannabis Sativa vs. Cannabis Indica

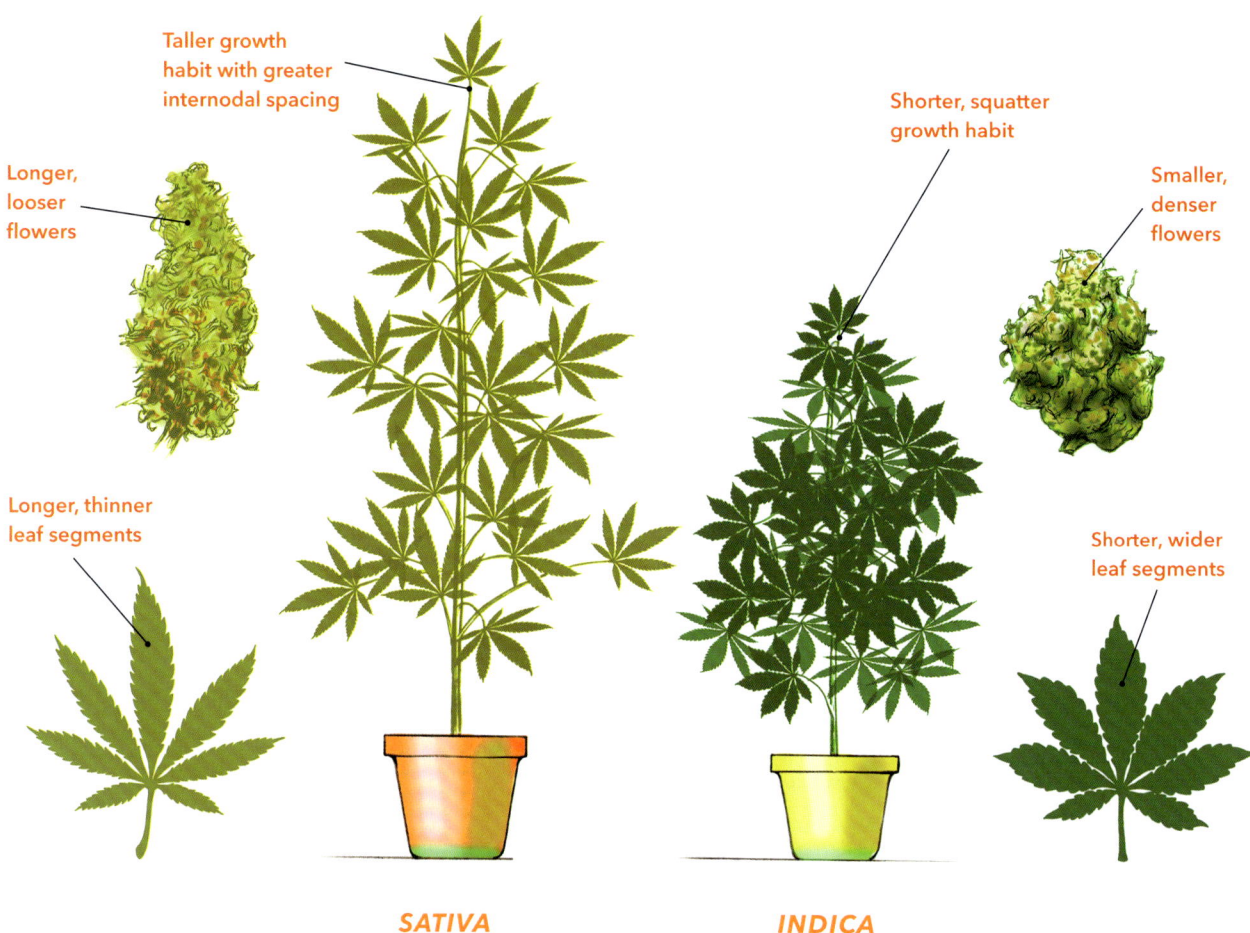

Taller growth habit with greater internodal spacing

Longer, looser flowers

Longer, thinner leaf segments

Shorter, squatter growth habit

Smaller, denser flowers

Shorter, wider leaf segments

SATIVA　　　　**INDICA**

Semi-Full-Term

A semi-full-term is a cross between a photoperiod strain and an autoflower. When we first discovered this category of plant, it was described with a lot of confusing nomenclature geared toward the hobbyist grower and not concerned with precision agricultural models. We therefore came up with the name semi-full-term, which we felt most accurately captured the variation this category offers from a farmer's perspective. Though less commonly known and understood in the legacy and legal markets, semi-full-terms are also referred to as sub-autos, quicks (or quiks), fast-flowering, and fast-finishing photos. Unless a breeder or seed purveyor expressly lists them in their catalog as an auto/photo cross, these terms do not necessarily guarantee that what you're buying is a semi-full-term as defined here; rather, it could be a normal photoperiod plant with a shorter flowering time.

Having a recessive autoflowering gene makes semi-full-term varieties initiate one to three weeks earlier than their full-term parents. When planted into the field in May or early June, semi-full-term varieties will finish sometime in September, with the actual week in September strongly influenced by the flowering time of the full-term parent.

They also possess exceptional vigor relative to both the full-term and autoflowering parents. The predominant advantage of semi-full-term genetics is their earlier harvest date, which enables farmers to avoid cold and wet fall conditions, beat the fall harvest glut, and spread out harvest and post-harvest activities to maximize dry space and minimize crew size. Semi-full-term genetics do not currently produce the superior visual appeal, potency, and terpene content as their full-term parents—though in many instances they are pretty darn close. Yields per acre are similar to those of full-terms.

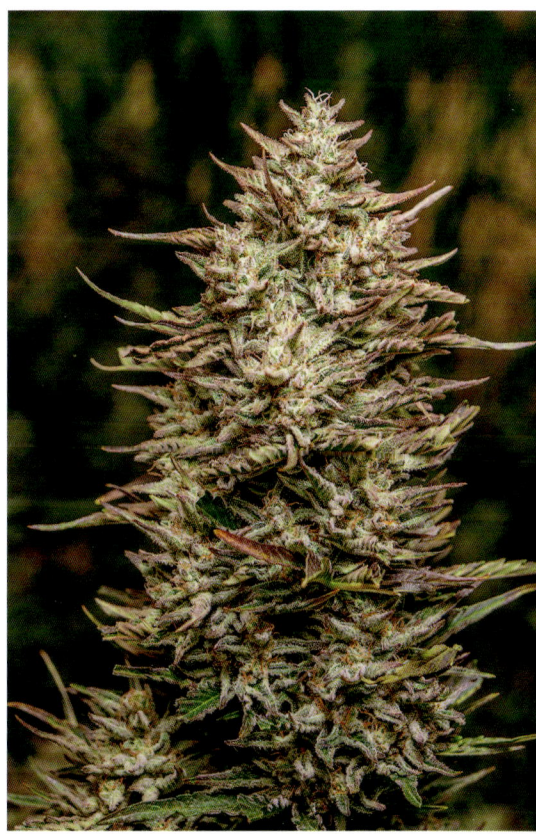

Fog Dog autoflower at maturity

Autoflowers

Autoflowering, or day-neutral, genetics have long had a poor reputation in the industry. They lacked many of the traits desired by the legacy markets of the past, such as dense flowers and a strong terpene profile. However, in the last 10 years we've seen exponential improvement in the quality of autoflowering strains. Some recently released strains, such as our Fog Dog (pictured), look just as good as some full-terms.

Modern autoflower varieties have reliable days to maturity, allowing operations to accurately plan successions and get a harvest in midsummer, or to plan maturation to coincide with ideal climate conditions. Their short stature means no canopy management is needed beyond plant spacing. The harvest is simpler with autoflowers than with large full-term or semi-full-term plants. The flower quality, potency, and terpene content are lower on average than full-terms. They are ideally suited for large acreage and/or to supply the mids, value brand, and biomass product categories. Yields per acre of autoflowers are between 2,000 and 5,000 pounds of biomass.

Autoflowers cannot be cloned and so are available only as seed. These plants will grow vegetatively for 30 to 40 days, then initiate flowering regardless of the light cycle. If you try to clone it, the little cutting just flowers and dies.

The trickiest part about planting autoflowers is their initial establishment phase, especially when transplanting in the multi-acre range. They are built to race to reproduction and thus rapidly develop a taproot that prefers to grow unobstructed throughout its life cycle. If autos experience any root binding in propagation, they will initiate early, and their vegetative and flowering potential will be decimated. Therefore, when you're preparing to propagate and plant autos, you must align the timing of your deployment precisely and address every variable in between, including your tray sizes, field preparation, and available labor. A common mistake we've seen is overeager operations propagating more plugs than they can reasonably hope to transplant with their onsite labor before their seedlings root-bind. Plan carefully and execute this step judiciously for autos to reach their full potential.

Autoflowering Days to Maturity

Relative to planting date, autoflowers take longer to mature when exposed to lower amounts of light and heat. Shorter day lengths and cooler temperatures in the shoulder seasons extend autoflower finishing times.

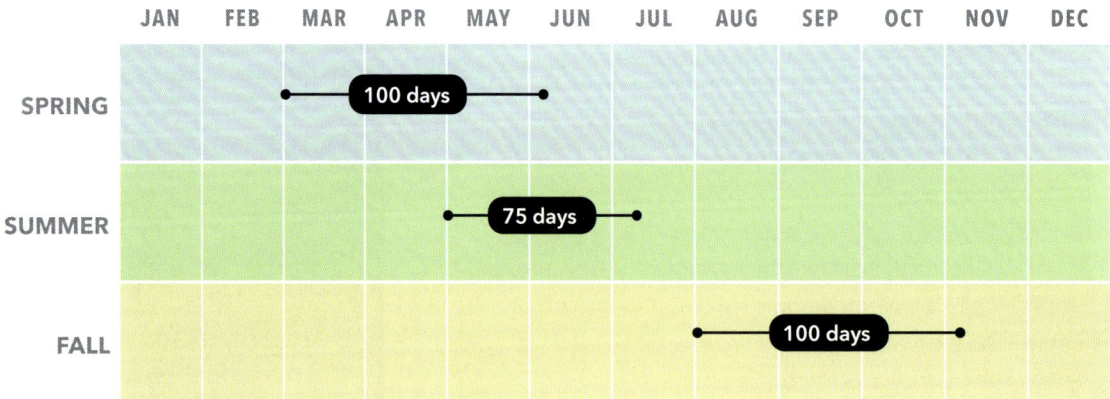

Cannabis Typologies

The *Cannabis* genus has many different expressions that are important to understand from a grower's perspective.

	Autoflowering	Semi-Full-Term	Full-Term
LIGHT CYCLE TYPE	Otherwise known as day neutral, or *ruderalis*, initiates flowering independently of light cycle changes. Can be cultivated under 18/6 or 24-hour light cycles.	First generation (F1) auto/photoperiod cross, light cycle–dependent flowering. Flowers earlier than a pure photoperiod in outdoor setting.	Most common type and otherwise known as "photoperiod," light cycle–dependent flower initiation, longest flowering time.

	Cannabis ruderalis	*Cannabis indica*	*Cannabis sativa*
GENOTYPE	Siberian/northern latitudes; small, squat plants; light cycle–independent; synonymous with autoflowering.	Middle Eastern (Afghanistan/Pakistan); shorter flowering time and smaller plant; shorter, wider leaves; relaxing high.	Eastern Asia, longer flowering time, larger plant, slender finger leaves, energizing high.

	Type I	Type II	Type III
CHEMOTYPE	THC-dominant cannabis.	THC blended cannabis, 2:1/1:1 varieties.	CBD dominant/<3% THC and other various chemovars, CBN/CBG, etc.

Seasonal and Environmental Genetics Considerations

Some genetics are more tolerant of inclement weather than others. It is important to understand the characteristics of your growing season. Ask yourself when the conditions are most ideal for growing, when they are marginal, and when they are potentially catastrophic. Specifically, consider air and soil temperature, rainfall, humidity, wind, and latitude/daylight hours. Bearing in mind that growing in open-ended hoop houses can mitigate many of these considerations, it is still essential to understand how genetics respond to seasonal parameters.

First and last frost dates are the most obvious seasonal markers. Cannabis cultivars vary in their ability to deal with cold. Some may show obvious signs of distress above freezing, whereas others may tolerate multiple heavy frosts and yet others will be fine

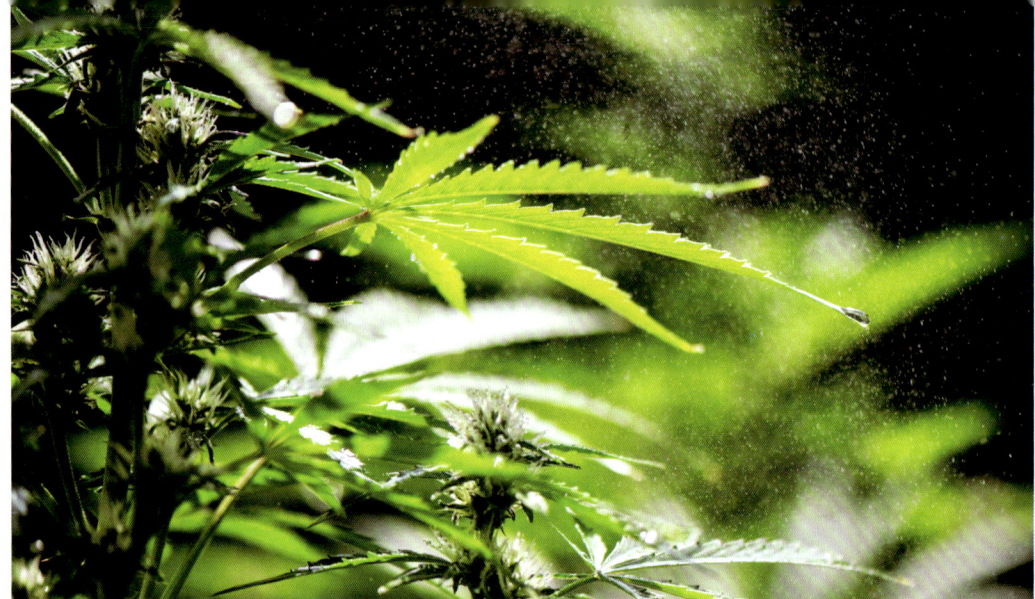

in snow! Several years ago, we were pushing the envelope (as we regularly did), and we had an early-August-planted autoflowering crop that was just coming to maturity in early November when we had hard frosts at roughly 26°F (–3°C) for multiple nights in a row. After the first night, the crop "defrosted" around 10 a.m., and we noticed a slight darkening of the flowers. But the crop still looked in decent shape, and we began harvesting that day.

After the second night of frost, we noticed distinct discoloration and loss of flower density and turgidity. We were concerned, but our team was already harvesting as fast as possible. After the third night of frost, the buds were mostly brown and squishy, like lettuce that had frozen and defrosted. Needless to say, all the remaining flowers on the last day were headed for extraction.

In terms of specifics, many indicas and autoflowering cultivars will tolerate one or more hard frosts, either early in the season while growing vegetatively or late in the season during flower ripening. Sativas, with their equatorial origins, are not as cold hardy and are much more likely to die or suffer significant stress during bouts of cold.

Rain is like frost in that overnight it can change the color, smell, potency, and overall value of your crop. To state it succinctly: Select cultivars with flowering times that match the most favorable growing conditions. Whenever we decide to grow long- or exceptionally long-flowering genetics, we make sure that they are a small percentage (less than 10 percent) of our overall crop to account for expected seasonal variations.

Humidity is another factor in genetic selections. The main cannabis pest, in our opinion, is bud rot (*Botrytis* spp.), which is caused by high humidity and warmth. In regions where high humidity is expected for the duration of the crop, we recommend choosing fast-flowering cultivars with good mold resistance and agronomic traits that support airflow, such as low leaf mass, smaller flowers, and good internodal spacing. In high-humidity regions we've found autoflowers work exceptionally well, because their flowering cycle *and* their overall life cycle are short, which means that there is less time for fungus and pathogens to develop during vegetative growth and thus transfer as flower development progresses. Some regions, such as coastal California, deal with humidity toward the end of the crop cycle in fall. These are the regions where fast-flowering full-term or semi-full-term genetics are suitable.

Wind is an important consideration when making cultivar selections. The increased transpiration caused by consistent dry winds sucks plants dry, causing stress similar to heat stress, not to mention causing structural damage to plants. If you must plant in exceptionally windy areas, select your cultivars carefully. Although all plants suffer under the constant stress of wind and likely experience reduced yields, some cultivars have been selected specifically for resiliency in windy environments. Short, squat, and *indica*-dominant plants plus any autoflowering cultivars deal with wind the best. Taller, lankier, weaker-branched, longer-flowering plants (read: sativas) are more difficult to grow in windy conditions. They require extensive trellising; otherwise you may encounter a high percentage of broken branches or lodged plants (plants that have fallen over).

Latitude is a final key factor when selecting suitable cultivars. This is especially true for growers in far northern or southern latitudes who may face challenging weather conditions come fall. Fast-flowering full-term and semi-full-term plants depend on a certain number of dark hours per day to initiate flower formation. These strains have short flowering cycles and/or will initiate flowering with more light than the traditional 12/12 light-to-dark ratio you hear referenced in cannabis circles. In our latitude and with our climate, for example, our semi-full-term strains transition into flower two to three weeks earlier than our photoperiod strains, thus finishing early.

In more northern regions with more sunlight during the peak of summer, however, strains may grow vegetatively for longer. Most of our semi-full-term strains initiate at or around 14 hours of sunlight per day, which equates to the last 10 days in July. If you compare the amount of daylight on July 22 at our latitude (14 hours 20 minutes) with that of Anchorage, Alaska (17 hours 56 minutes), you can see why it's important to consider latitude when selecting cultivars.

Using Clones

At the time of writing, cannabis clones represent a major portion of the genetics market. Clones are replicas of each other. Clones are made from sexually mature plants, so it is easier to make harvest predictions. They perform nearly identically, and the flower is consistent in terms of appearance and potency. Usually when a nursery offers a clone, a breeder has grown out many seeds and selected the plant that outperformed the others, then taken clones from it. So you know someone has already grown this very plant and the results were worth keeping. Depending on the market you are growing for, flower uniformity at this level may not be necessary, but flower and extract products from clones often are easier to sell because of the benefits outlined on page 42.

Benefits of Clones

Since clones are all direct replicas of each other, they excel in the following ways:

Maturity. Clones all reach maturity at the same time, which makes for an easy harvest flow.

Terpene profile. When grown in the same soil, clones have the same terpene profile. Combined into large bags for sale, plants grown from clones have a stronger and more uniform smell.

Cannabinoid content. When grown in the same soil, clones have very similar cannabinoid content. While cannabinoid content varies at different locations on the same plant, clones should be the same in terms of overall cannabinoid content and the ratios of one type to another.

Canopy height. Because they are genetically the same plant, crops planted from the clone will have a uniform canopy height. This makes spraying, pruning, or other canopy management activities easier.

Genetic preservation. Clones preserve the exact genetic traits that are in high demand by the market. When you find a particular plant that has the exact combination of terpenes, cannabinoids, structure, and vigor that you are looking for, you can maintain that genetic combination through cloning. Although genetic drift can slowly deteriorate the integrity of genetics after many generations of cloning, in general cloning provides a way to keep producing the exact product that your market wants.

Drawbacks of Clones

Despite the advantages, clones do present some drawbacks to be considered.

Cost. Compared to buying seed, maintaining and propagating clones is more expensive.

Risk of pests. Because the mother plants are kept in commercial greenhouses, there is the risk of transmission of pests. We have been shipped clones with aphids on them more than once. A well-known boogeyman pest is the microscopic russet mite. The other "pest" that causes growers to shudder is the hop latent viroid (HLVd), a single-stranded, circular infectious RNA that is completely dependent on its host plant's metabolism for replication (see facing page).

Lack of vigor. Clones are shallow rooters and lack the vigor of seeds. Clones tend to be needier and more delicate than plants grown from seed, which show explosive growth in the field as compared to clones.

Less resilient. Clones are more prone to pest infestation and stunted growth. If a clone is stressed or its light cycle is even slightly affected, such as by the smoky wildfire conditions California often experiences, it can initiate flowering early while a plant grown from seed may not.

Hop Latent Viroid in Cannabis

As the name suggests, hop latent viroid (HLVd) occurs in hops worldwide, but it can also infect hop's relative, cannabis. In the worst cases HLVd will kill the crop, or weaken it to an extent that it is not saleable. However, oftentimes HLVd infection is not obvious, or the effects may not become distinct until later in the crop cycle.

During the vegetative stage, HLVd-infected plants grow shorter with smaller leaves and tighter node spacing. Flowering plants infected with HLVd have smaller, looser buds with many fewer trichomes. One client estimated that cannabis plants infected with HLVd had half the cannabinoid content of healthy plants, and overall yield was reduced 30 percent. We have had plants infected with this viroid more than once. Some strains exhibited stunting, and others didn't at all. During different stages of the growing season, we saw little or no expression of symptoms. Others in the industry have had disastrous experiences with HLVd. As with any sickness or pest, damage done (or not done) is directly related to environmental conditions. We go into detail about healthy ecosystems in Chapter 3.

Tissue Culture

The practice of tissue culture has become increasingly popular in the industry due to pest and disease problems with cloning and the expense of maintaining mother stock perpetually in greenhouse facilities. Tissue culture, also called micropropagation, is the growth of tissues or cells in an artificial medium separate from the parent plant. This technique is typically facilitated via a liquid, semisolid, or solid growth medium, such as broth or agar. Under the right conditions, an entire plant can be regenerated from a single cell. Tissue culture is not novel—it is used with potato tubers and garlic cloves to produce disease-free "seed."

Tissue culture has two distinct value propositions for growers: It purports to be capable of removing hop latent viroid (HLVd) from infected stock, and it renews old and tired mother stock of preferred clones, which tend to lose vigor, performance, and consistency when cloned repeatedly. In some cases nurseries send clones to tissue culture labs to be cleaned and renewed, then use the resulting plants to begin their clone program over again. In other cases growers order tissue culture clones directly so that each plant comes directly from tissue culture. This is quickly becoming an industry standard. It is a highly technological approach that, in our view, is superfluous for outdoor cultivation in most cases. We have ordered tissue culture clones that ended up having HLVd anyway. For indoor and greenhouse growers, however, where the agroecosystem is simpler and thus less resilient, biosecurity is more important, and tissue culturing may still have a place supplying these growers.

Where tissue culture has good applicability is in breeding. It allows breeders to essentially bank parent lines or breeding stock and call up disease-free plants for seed production when ready. "À la carte" working with a third-party lab to actualize this method is still cost prohibitive. Additionally, the safety of breeders' intellectual property is a concern because the industry has a recent history of outright genetics theft, so breeders' putting their prized genetics in third-party facilities is not advisable.

Using Feminized Seed

Seed is the most common and cost-effective way to propagate annual crops. It is the standard in agriculture. Cannabis is an obligate outcrosser—meaning it is highly heterozygous—and thus uniformity can be an issue. Breeders and companies like ours are making strides in breeding for uniformity through practices such as inbreeding parent lines and marker-assisted breeding (using DNA markers to isolate and breed for specific traits). Considerable progress has been made in the past few years.

Producing cannabis seed has another major issue—males. Each plant is dioecious, meaning it is either male or female. The males produce pollen that fertilizes the flowers on female plants, resulting in a seeded crop—and seed production reduces flower quality. Luckily seed companies can produce *feminized* seed, whereby a female plant is "reversed" and produces male flowers. The pollen made in these flowers has only the X chromosome, and in theory progeny from female plants will be 100 percent female. In reality it is 99.99 percent female. This means 1 of every 1,500 to 2,000 plants will be male. We discuss male identification and removal in Chapter 9.

Advantages of Seed

Plants from seed have much higher vigor and better resilience than clones. A seed produces a plant with a thick and strong anchoring taproot. Furthermore, pests cannot be transferred on seed like they can on clones. Some seeds are treated for viral and fungal pathogens. A plant grown from seed is also much easier to propagate and requires little or no repotting into larger containers to achieve a hardened-off transplant ready for the field.

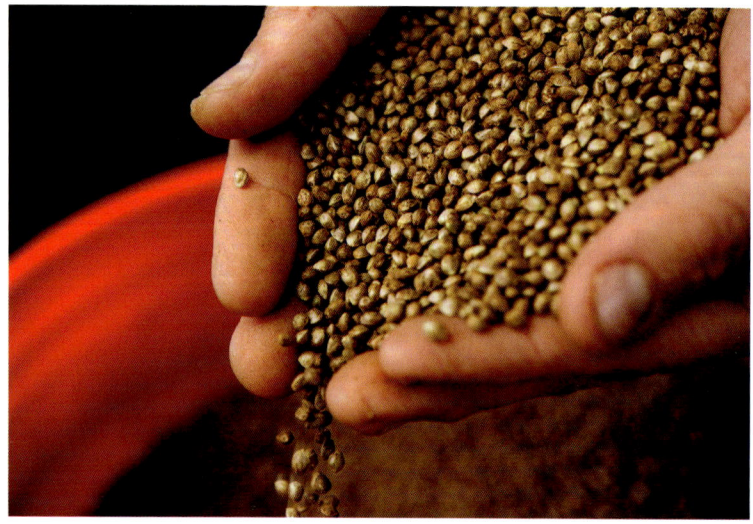

Newly cleaned feminized seed going into storage

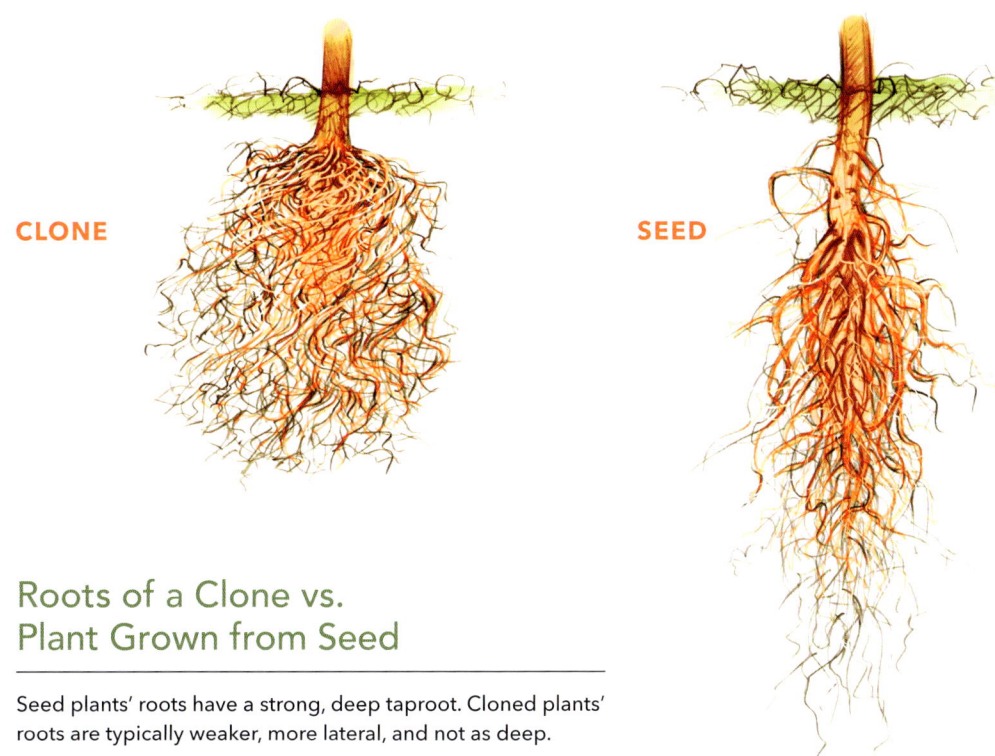

CLONE   **SEED**

Roots of a Clone vs. Plant Grown from Seed

Seed plants' roots have a strong, deep taproot. Cloned plants' roots are typically weaker, more lateral, and not as deep.

Sexual Maturity of Plants Grown from Seed

It's important to understand that plants grown from seed have an internal biological timeline to maturity, whereas clones are already sexually mature, and so harvest timeline predictions can be reliably made. A cannabis plant has reached sexual maturity roughly when leaves change from opposite to alternate. We have grown from seed at every time of year to learn what differences to expect in all seasons. Even when the light cycle outside is within the range that would trigger flowering—less than 14 hours of daylight—a plant grown from seed will not initiate flowering until it reaches maturity.

One year we planted a field of Blue Dream seed on June 15 and harvested the crop well after Thanksgiving. We were lucky that fall was not wet, or much of the crop would have been lost to mold. At the other end of the season, this means that if planted in early spring, plants grown from seed will not go into flower when there are fewer than 14 hours of daylight. At our latitude the length of daylight is more than 14 hours in late May. Therefore, if you plant a full-term seed in April, you do not need to provide additional lighting to keep it from flowering.

What We Do

After considering all the variables above, your decision on which genetics to select and when to plant them is where the rubber meets the road. Your decision will be based on a complicated juxtaposition of factors. Since we've always found it helpful to hear what others are doing, we offer our planting rubric here: We plant our main crop of autoflowers in spring as early as soil moisture and field conditions allow, generally between April 20 and May 1. Planting during this early time slot means we regularly, but not exclusively, use plastic mulch to help the crop succeed.

The main reason we plant this early is for compliance. Exceptionally expensive and restrictive permits in California only allow 1 acre of canopy at a time per parcel—there can be no overlap between the crops. We push the autoflower crop as early as possible so it will have time to finish, even though the planting time isn't ideal. When it finishes at the very end of June or beginning of July (most of our autoflowering varieties are +/– 70 days), we simultaneously harvest the autoflower crop and replant with semi-full-term and full-term varieties. If this regulatory restraint were lifted, we would plant our first autoflower crop later, when the weather is warmer, allowing it to overlap with the semi-full- and full-term planting.

Autoflowers in production in a Central California greenhouse

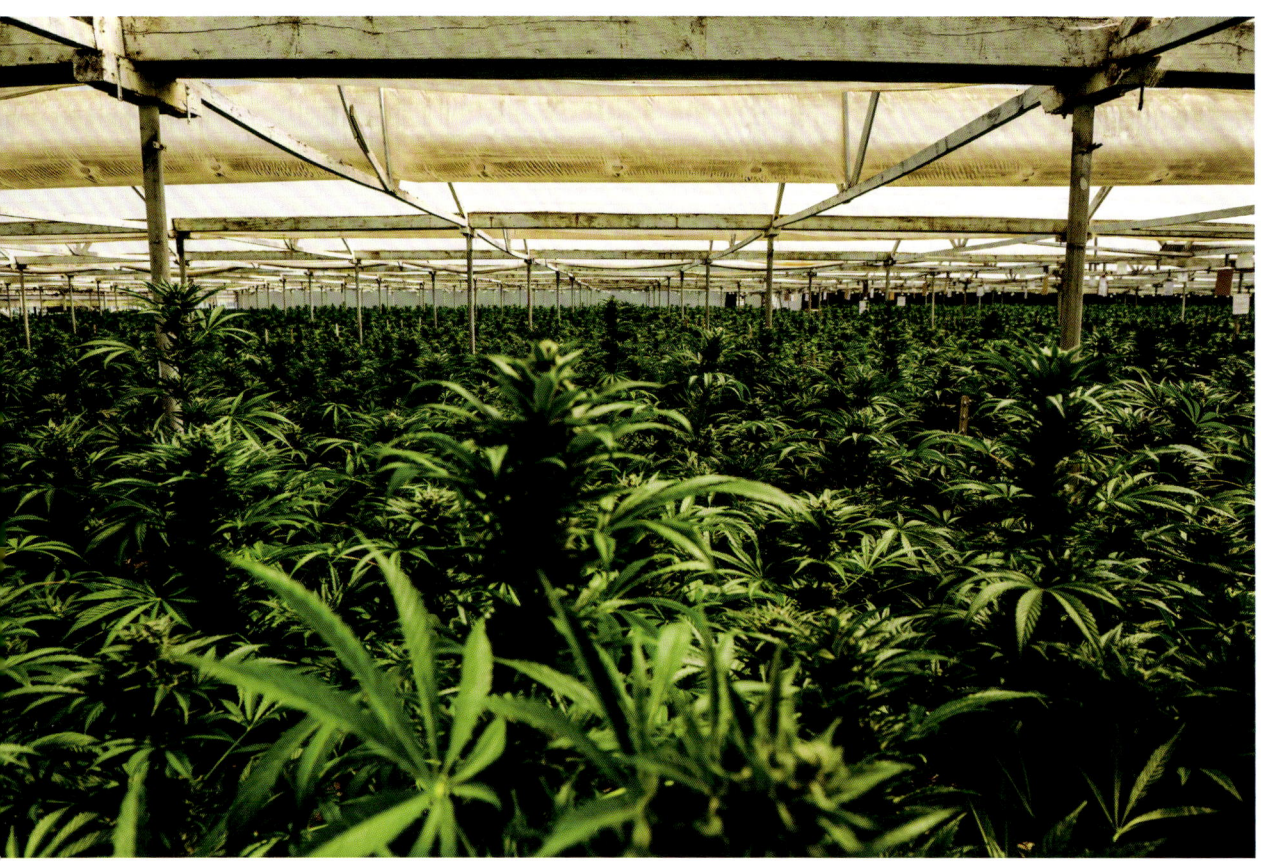

In contrast to our method, consider these interesting anecdotes. A few years ago, a nearby fellow farmer planted the exact same genetics at the same time as we did. The weather and light cycle conditions were nearly identical. However, he was growing in 80-gallon grow bags, and we were growing in native soil. When we went to see his farm in late September, his crop was 10 to 14 days ahead of ours, almost ready to harvest, while ours was surely going to extend into mid-October. We were incredulous that simply constricting root growth by growing in pots could affect the maturity of the crop so drastically.

Similarly, our colleagues and friends at Ladybug Farm in Watsonville grow Atlas Seed autoflowers in one-gallon pots in greenhouses and consistently achieve maturity around 60 days, compared to our experience in the field of 70 to 80 days to maturity.

Finally, market volatility bears mention here. Varieties fall in and out of popularity over time. It does not matter if a chosen variety outperforms everything else if you cannot sell it due to market saturation or consumer preferences. New varieties are released yearly with associated hype. Some companies develop, promote, and protect their own varieties to capture more market share without competition. Supply and demand apply to bulk cannabis flowers broadly, but specifically to varieties as well. We always plant at least eight distinct varieties to account for this.

What This Means for You

The legal US domestic and global cannabis industries are in their infancy, with ample opportunity for cultivators of varying experience levels and capacities to participate. Finding your place and proper genetics in this ever-evolving market with still so many undefined elements requires careful planning on a farm level plus strategic insight at the market level. The selection of the best genetics for your crop plan represents the convergence of your operational capacity to plant, maintain, harvest, and dry; climate; regulatory atmosphere; and overall market trends. It's up to you to sort through these considerations and make the best plan for your farm.

From a sociocultural perspective, cannabis is a plant like any other, and its prohibition to date has merely been political. But for seasoned farmers who are new to cannabis, we hope this chapter has highlighted its differences from your average vegetable and the many accompanying pitfalls that could occur were the all-too-common cowboy grower to go in, guns blazing, without knowing this plant's agronomic distinctions. Now that you've selected your seeds, it's time to look at the best principles and practices for feeding them.

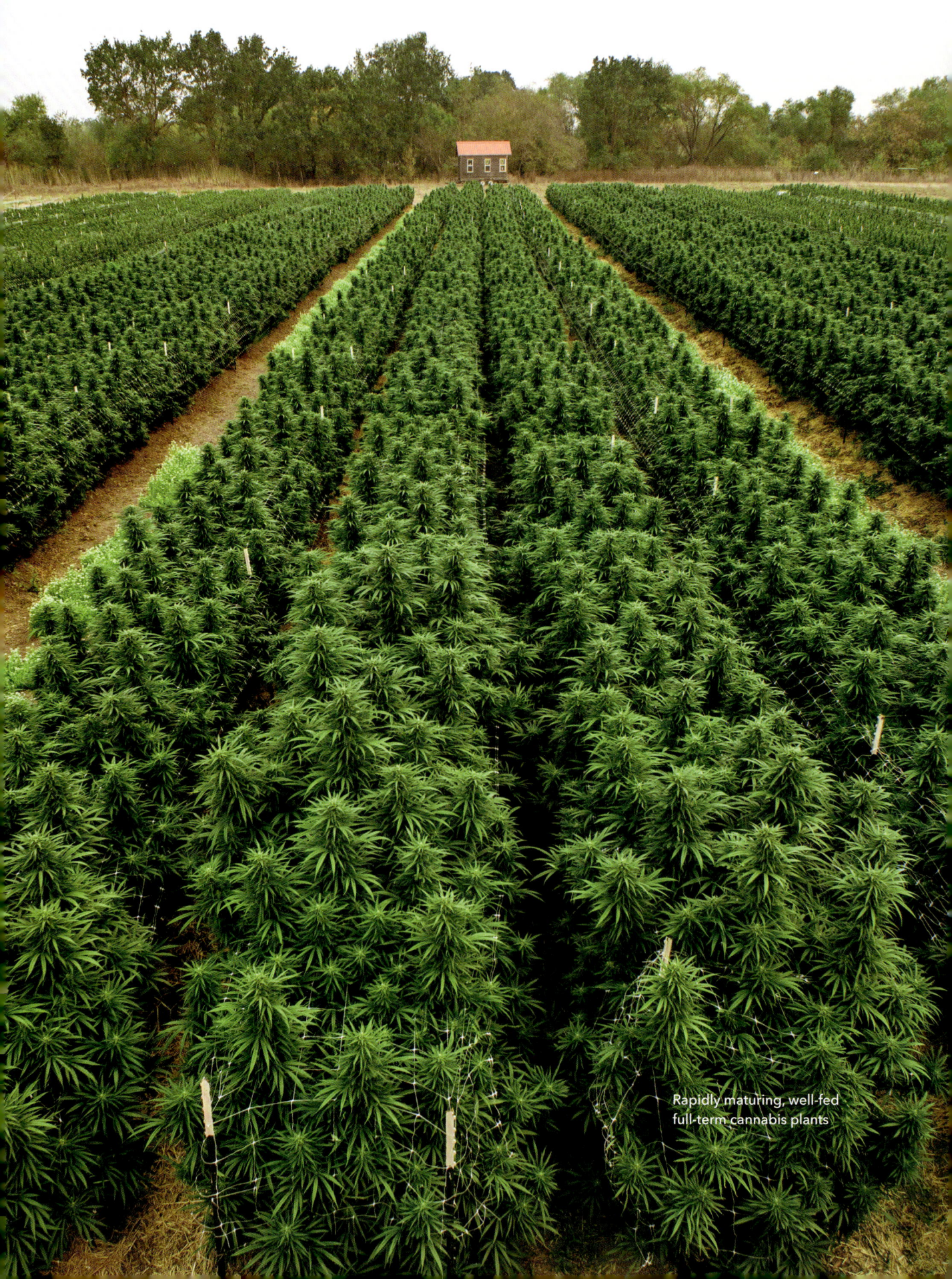

Rapidly maturing, well-fed
full-term cannabis plants

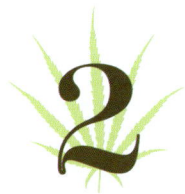

Plant Nutrition and Fertility Management

The specific knowledge base for cannabis's fertility needs is still emerging. The conventional approach has been one of unnecessary, expensive over-fertilization that is potentially harmful to the soil and surrounding environment. Walk into any grow shop and you'll find a large assortment of colorfully branded and expensive fertilizer options. Colloquially referred to as "nutes," these are liquid products, so buyers are primarily paying for water. Traditionally the price of cannabis was high enough to justify their use at scale, but cannabis does not need an overapplication of fertilizers to perform exceptionally.

The plants do exhibit particularly vigorous growth roughly at or just before the middle of their vegetative cycle and just after flower initiation, so it's prudent to ensure an adequate supply of nutrients during those stages of the crop cycle. To accomplish this you must apply the nutrients beforehand or through continual fertigation (fertilizing via irrigation). More important, proper soil management combined with adequate fertilization will produce a high-yielding, high-quality crop. Developing a program for the judicious use of fertilizers and soil amendments in tandem with proper soil management is a process of applied principles rather than a specific recipe. Let's start with the soil.

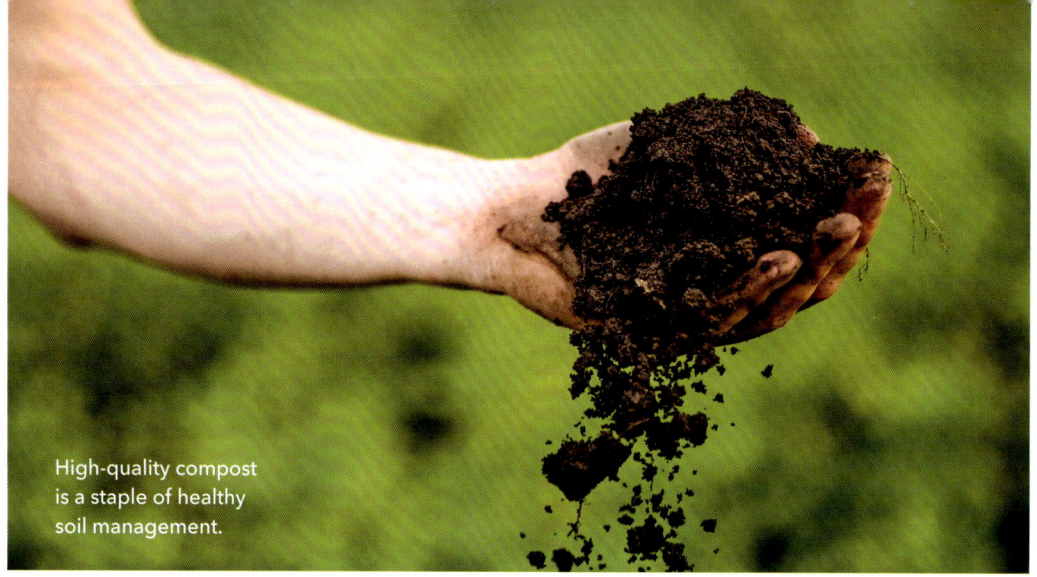

High-quality compost
is a staple of healthy
soil management.

The Living Soil Approach

There are two approaches to planting cannabis directly into native soil. One, which we call "the dead soil approach," views soil as merely a medium for delivering nutrients to plant roots. This approach often uses synthetic salt-based fertilizers and focuses on feeding the plants rather than nourishing the soil. The ideology is like that of many indoor cannabis growers who grow in stone wool or coco peat potting medium. We mention this approach mainly to note that it is a dying modality, because as the market expands, most production is taking place in open-air cultivation.

We prefer to use what we call "the living soils approach," based on the principle that soil is alive and supports a complex web of relationships. We take care of the soil because the soil is what takes care of the crop. And as discussed further in Chapter 3, healthy soils are the foundation of pest and disease mitigation. Simply put, native soils can be managed to provide everything that plants need to thrive. All actions are considered through the lens of what's best for the soil.

In the living soils approach, we:

- Use cover crops.

- Apply amendments, including compost.

- Perform tillage thoughtfully, considering soil moisture and soil type, time of year, tillage equipment, and the needs of the crop.

Many books and university classes cover soil management. (See the bibliography on page 215 for recommendations.) We will describe our program on a practical level without going into meticulous detail. Suffice it to say that the soil is a massively diverse and abundant system of interconnected microorganisms. To focus strictly on what mineral nutrients are present is missing at least half the story. Other factors, such as the amount of compaction and moisture levels at tillage, can decrease or increase biological activity and mineral nutrient availability.

Soil Food Web

Understanding the soil food web helps growers make informed decisions for long-term farm and soil viability.

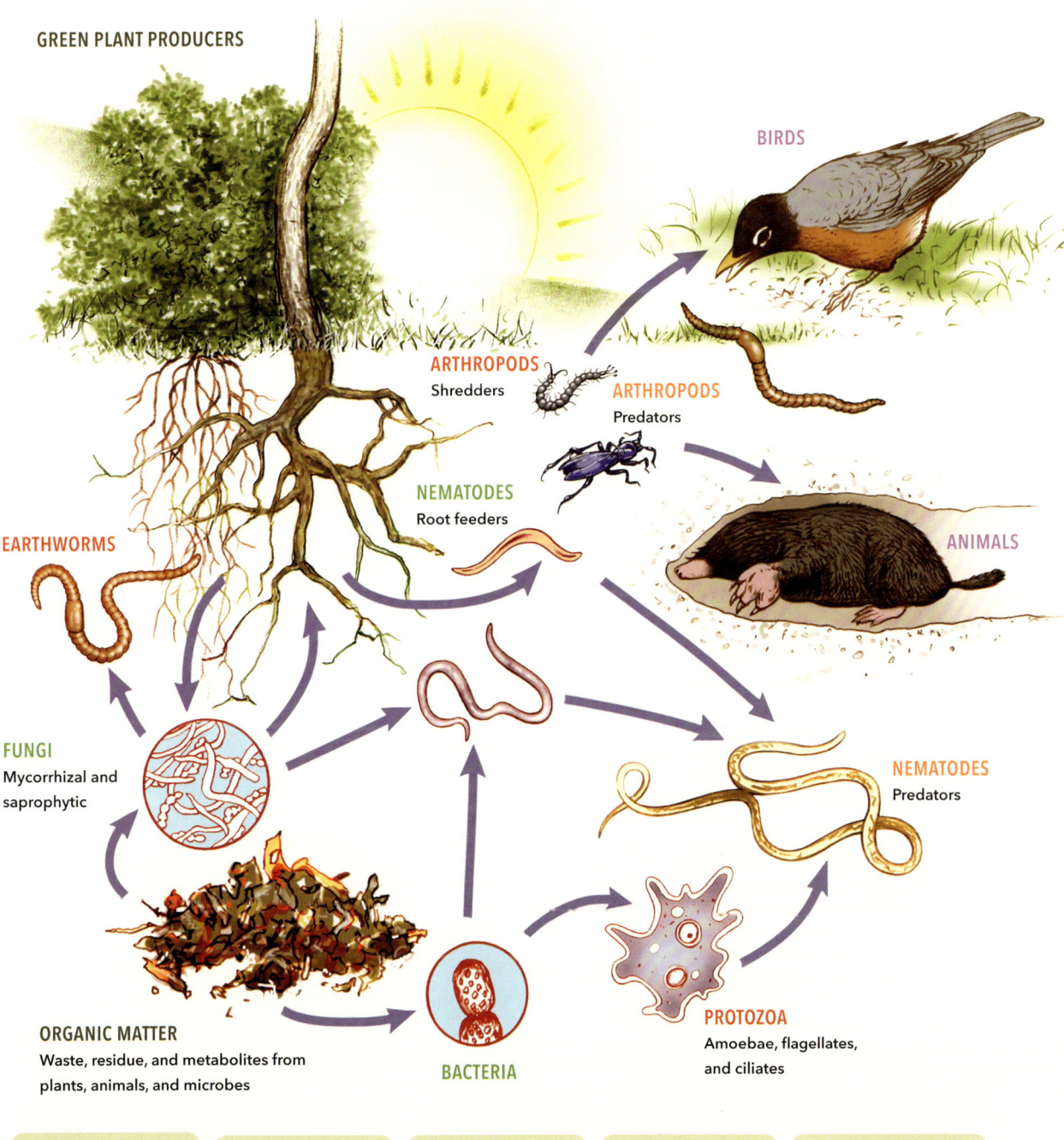

GREEN PLANT PRODUCERS

BIRDS

ARTHROPODS
Shredders

ARTHROPODS
Predators

NEMATODES
Root feeders

ANIMALS

EARTHWORMS

FUNGI
Mycorrhizal and saprophytic

NEMATODES
Predators

PROTOZOA
Amoebae, flagellates, and ciliates

ORGANIC MATTER
Waste, residue, and metabolites from plants, animals, and microbes

BACTERIA

FIRST TROPHIC LEVEL:
Photosynthesizers

SECOND TROPHIC LEVEL:
Decomposers
Mutualists
Parasites
Pathogens
Root feeders

THIRD TROPHIC LEVEL:
Grazers
Predators
Shredders

FOURTH TROPHIC LEVEL:
Higher-level predators

FIFTH AND HIGHER TROPHIC LEVELS:
Higher-level predators

Using Cover Crops

Cover crops are of paramount importance in maintaining and improving soil health. They are a foundational component to regenerative farming systems. The basic concept is that nature never leaves a field bare. A cover crop sends roots deep into the soil to gather nutrients and minerals that have leached beyond the root zone of standard crops. Cover crop roots also perform deep tillage; when the cover crop dies, their roots decompose in place, leaving capillaries connecting soil horizons and, furthermore, turning atmospheric carbon dioxide into organic carbon. When we mow and till (or no-till crimp) the cover crop, the organic matter of the aboveground growth, the roots, and the nutrients brought up from the deep are incorporated into the surface soil to nourish the next cash crop.

Cover crops can be planted any time of year. Many farmers plant winter cover crops for some or all of the following reasons.

- Stabilize the soil and prevent erosion.

- Suppress weeds.

- Provide fertility.

- Foster a healthy soil microbiome.

- Increase soil organic matter.

- Help break pest cycles in conjunction with crop rotation.

- Harvest and upcycle trace minerals or nutrients.

- Provide insectaries for invertebrates and habitat and food for birds.

Choose your cover crop species carefully based on several factors: average winter temperature/number of frosts, soil type, slope, drainage, and expected precipitation by season. Common winter cover crop species include rye grass, oat grass, vetch, peas, bell beans, fava beans, clover, turnips, radishes, rapeseed, and triticale. For winter cover crops, many farmers choose a legume or legume blend that can fix (capture) atmospheric nitrogen. When the residue is incorporated into the soil or crimp-killed in no-till systems, that nitrogen becomes available to your crops. In tillage systems, the nitrogen typically becomes available to plants two to three weeks after tillage.

Though used less frequently than winter cover crops, heat-loving summer cover crops grow fast and provide the same benefits. Common summer cover crops include Sudan grass, cowpeas, buckwheat, millet, and hemp. That's right! Hemp or cannabis is an extremely vigorous nutrient accumulator as well as bioremediator that captures or breaks down organic contaminants (which is why it was planted around the abandoned Chernobyl nuclear power station).

When you incorporate cover crops into the soil is an important decision. Sometimes you can hit the ideal time to work in a cover crop—when soil moisture, weather, and time of year all line up. Other times a stretch of wet or cold weather may delay incorporation until after the ideal window, meaning the cover crops may have set viable

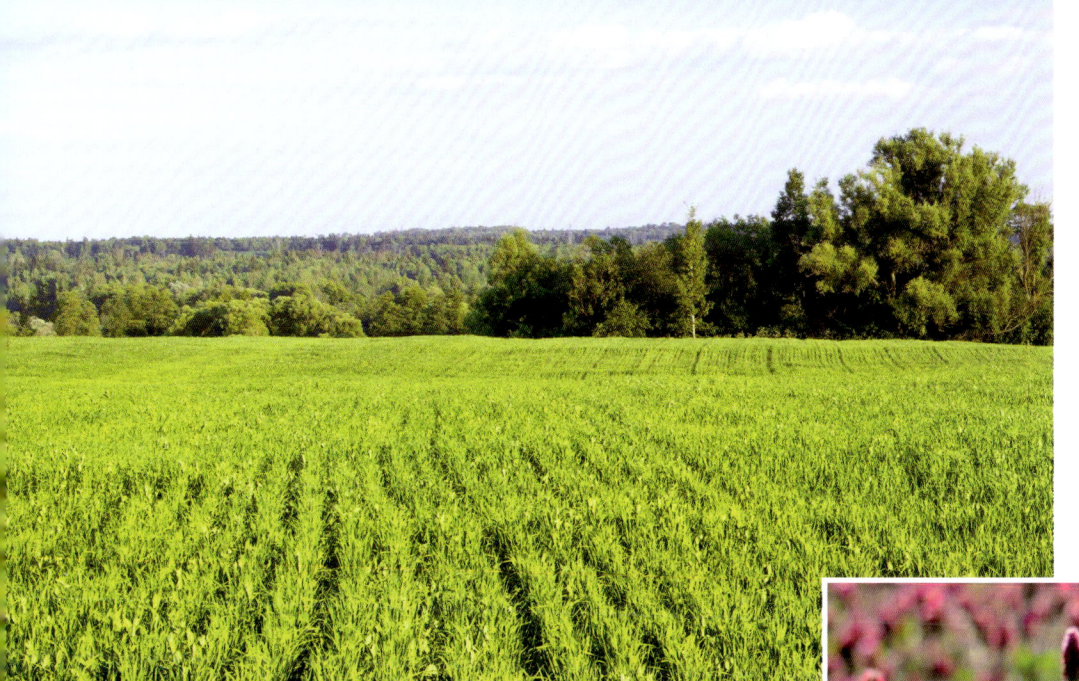

In addition to providing many benefits to the soil, healthy stands of cover crop (oats, left; red clover, below) are just plain beautiful to look at.

seed, had outbreaks of pests (we have often seen three distinct species of aphids on an "overdue" winter cover crop), or started to turn brown and carbonaceous, increasing the time needed for decomposition.

Choosing Amendments

A key component of the living soils approach is using soil tests to determine which specific amendments are required. If you are not proficient in interpreting soil samples, we recommend working with an agronomist or consultant who has extensive experience; or pick up a book on the subject. We prefer to administer these tests in late summer or early fall, which generally allows enough time to incorporate compost or manure and gypsum, lime, or other powdered amendments into the soil well in advance of spring field work.

Amendments fall into three categories: physical/chemical amendments, organic matter, and fertilizers. Chemical amendments alter the soil's chemical composition to be more favorable for crop performance. Organic matter is supplied by decomposed cover crops and the application of composts and/or manures. Fertilizers are solid or liquid products containing specific plant nutrients.

Choosing sources of fertilizer can be overwhelming. Rather than focus on a specific blend or source, start by exploring resources that may be available nearby, particularly when looking for compost or manure. For example, we buy one-ton totes of organic 4-4-2 pelleted chicken manure from a local egg farm. If you're in cattle country, get in touch with a local rancher; if you're in a coastal zone, see if there are by-products from fishing or seaweed operations.

Depending on your governing authority's testing requirements, consider testing your compost for heavy metals and pesticides *before* application on the field. Cannabis and hemp plants are some of the best bioremediators (read: bioaccumulators) and are more than proficient at pulling up long-ago-applied pesticides or heavy metals with a long half-life. For example, we have seen a termite pesticide banned in the 1980s show up in parts per billion in the extracted oil from cannabis grown in a particular field!

Physical and Soil Chemistry Amendments

This class of amendment is designed to alter the physical characteristics of soil and its chemical composition. Compost certainly fits in this category and can be very effective. But sometimes a little more of certain elements is needed.

Common amendments of this type are lime and/or ground oyster shell, and gypsum, all of which are powdered. Both lime and gypsum are mostly calcium. Lime is used to raise soil pH and keep it in the optimum range for plant growth. Soil test reports will indicate what type of lime to apply and at what rate. Gypsum is used to break up clay soils, increasing their workability and softening their structure. We are fortunate to have a compost production facility in our area that will create custom blends, so when we apply compost, we are also putting down lime. Specialized equipment is necessary to apply these powders.

Lime is ideally applied in fall because it can take three to six months for the lime to activate and change the soil pH. Applying lime or gypsum immediately before planting a crop does not produce the desired results. Lime can be especially problematic because of lime burn or "liming injury," where plants are damaged. This occurs when lime is applied just before the crop is planted.

Getting soil pH right is especially important for a high-value crop such as cannabis. Cannabis prefers slightly acidic conditions, with the ideal range being 5.8 to 6.2. It will grow acceptably from pH 5.0 to 7.0, but outside these parameters it will suffer noticeably. Changing soil pH takes time. In our experience, it takes multiple applications (and more material than you would think) to get the pH level where you want it. Be patient and proceed with caution; you can always add more lime, but you cannot take it out. Every soil is different, and it can take years to develop its potential. Consulting with other farmers in the area is always the best place to start.

In some cases, especially in heavy clay soils, even more amendments may be needed to change the physical structure of soil for optimum plant growth. Perlite, lava rocks, and peat moss (not environmentally friendly at scale, however) can also be used for this purpose.

Organic Matter Amendments

A soil's organic matter is a direct measurement of its biological activity, diversity, and health. It also greatly influences the physical structure of soil—for example, by enhancing drainage *and* moisture retention, aeration, and tilth. Cover crops are a crucial component of the production and maintenance of organic matter. Compost, manure, peat moss, coco coir, or materials such as wood chips or leaf mulch can be applied to raise the organic matter of your soil and change its physical characteristics. These materials also contain plant nutrients, but the release of these nutrients into plant-available form is unpredictable, so we do not rely on them as fertilizer.

With organic matter amendments, the timing of application is just as important as the application itself. It takes weeks, and sometimes months, for organic matter to incorporate into and change the soil. Applying it in fall is optimal, as then it has the entire winter to homogenize and settle into your soil. That said, in some years the first autumn rain arrives when we have unharvested crops still in the ground, and the rain is heavy enough to prevent us from getting onto the field with the heavy equipment required to spread compost (we've gotten way too much equipment stuck in our fields over the years). In such circumstances, we've only had the spring for organic matter application.

This brings us to the conundrum of hot compost. In our region, it is essentially impossible to find compost that is not hot—steaming and 100°F (38°C) or higher. Avoid applying hot compost whenever possible! If all locally available compost is delivered hot, purchase it in fall (or well before its intended use), tarp it, and let it settle and cool during winter. The microbiology of fresh, actively decomposing compost is very different from the stable microbiology of healthy soil ready for crops. Sometimes this translates into soilborne disease for the crop. Other times, fresh or hot compost can

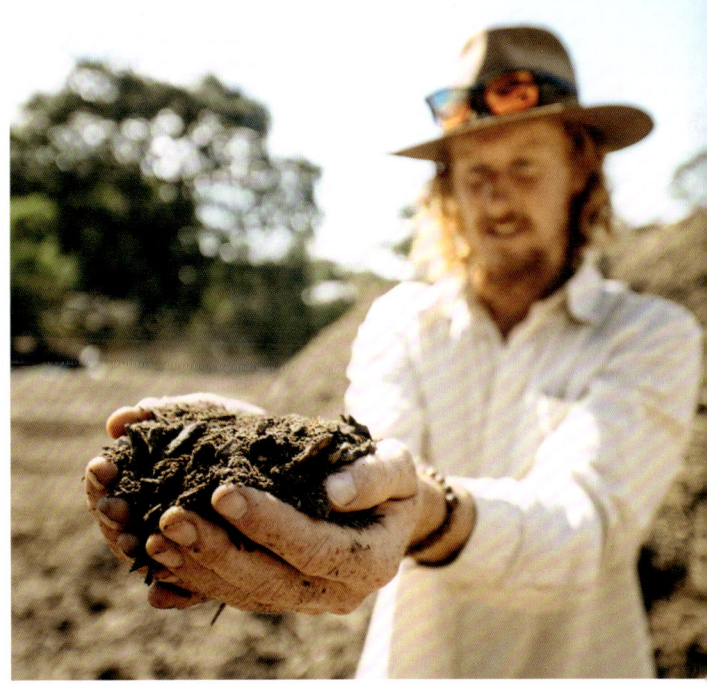

Ryan holding freshly made compost

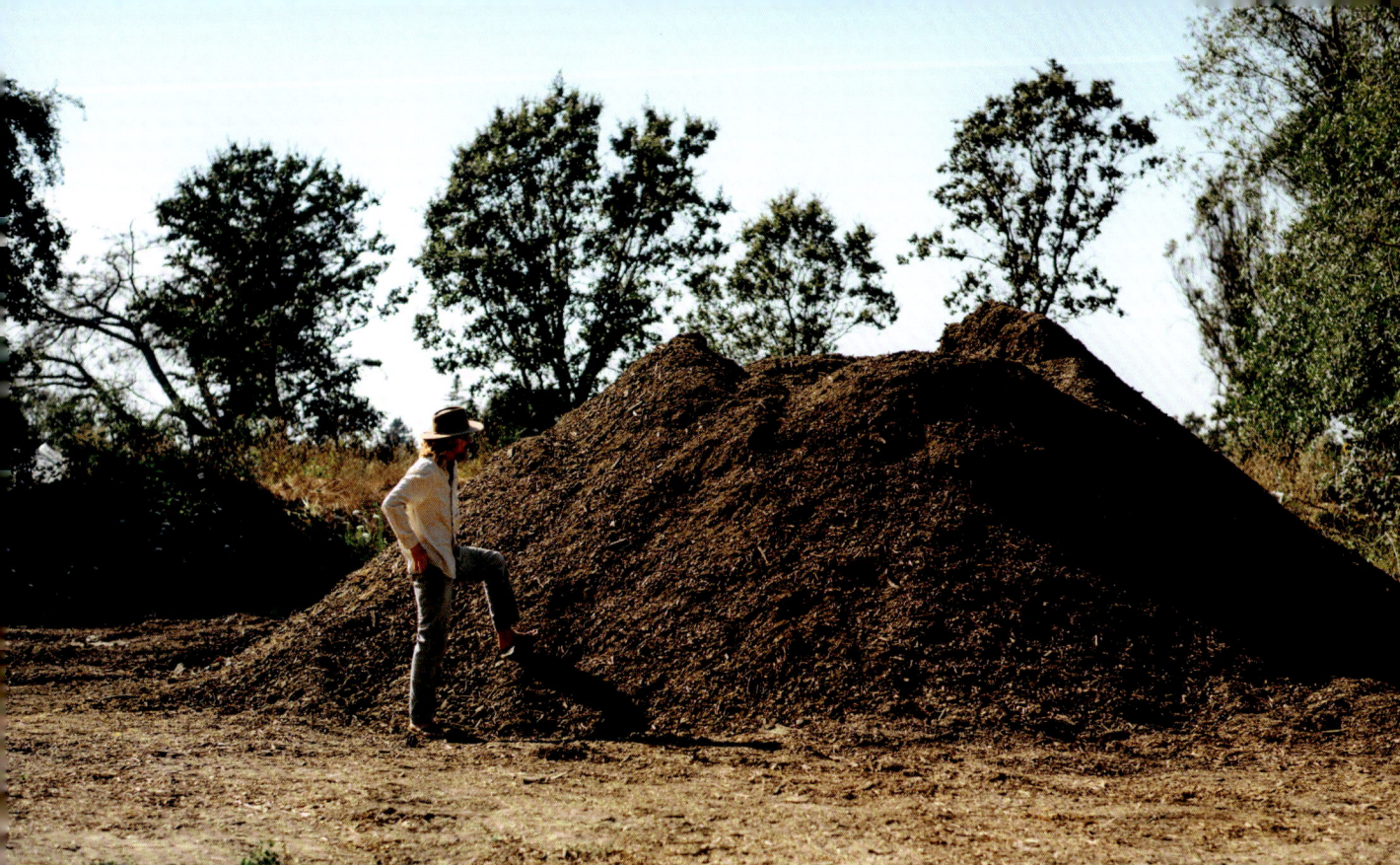

Ryan stands by a pile of farm-made compost consisting of wood chips and horse manure. Compost is integral to healthy agricultural soils.

tie up plant-available nitrogen and deprive your crop of that nutrient the opposite of the intended effect. Never haphazardly apply compost without prior experience with it. Better to wait to apply than to put down a new or hot compost just before planting.

Fertilizers

Fertilizers are inputs specifically intended to feed the crop. They typically do not stick around longer than a single crop cycle or season. The most-applied macronutrients are nitrogen (N), phosphorus (P), and potassium (K), commonly referred to as N-P-K. The N-P-K content of fertilizer is listed on its packaging and refers to how many pounds of each nutrient are present in 100 pounds of fertilizer. Additionally, farmers apply various micronutrients, such as boron or copper. The main concept to keep in mind is that soil is just like a chain: It's only as strong as its weakest link. The law of the minimum, which states that growth is dictated not by total resources available but by the scarcest resource, is very real. So if you have a beautiful loamy soil with great organic matter and drainage that is severely lacking in boron, your crop will not reach its full potential.

There are abundant options for fertilizers. We recommend the KISS (Keep It Simple, Stupid) method when making selections. Solid fertilizers are most easily applied at a field scale before the crop is planted. Keep in mind that small plants require much less fertilizer than do large, mature plants. This is why slow-release fertilizers were developed; they have special coatings that slow down solubility. Slow-release fertilizers are not all created equal, though: We have seen huge price variability based on the effectiveness and/or the brand of the "slow release" formulation. In many row-crop operations, farmers apply fertilizer during cultivations by using injection knives. This mid-crop fertilizer application allows farmers to avoid the higher cost of slow-release fertilizers, add fertility just when the crop is beginning to take off, and make fertility adjustments based on crop performance.

Fortunately, most native soil– and sun-grown cannabis crops are grown using drip irrigation, which makes mid-crop or periodic nutrient applications easy. Watering with liquid fertilizers is called fertigation (fertilize-irrigation). Liquid fertilizers have a place on many (but not all) cannabis farms, but they should be used with care. We consider them an addition or addendum to the healthy soils approach. Liquid fertilizers are expensive, and both the conventional and salt-based options have potentially significant long-term consequences, including destroying the soil microbiome, rapidly changing the soil pH, and leaving salt residues, which inhibit plant growth. Liquid fertilizers specifically work well when plants are in explosive growth phases or for delivering nutrients, such as phosphorus, that plants have a harder time taking up directly from the soil.

Many companies sell certified organic liquid fertilizers. While we are strong proponents of organic, sustainable, and regenerative practices, we understand that in too many instances "organic" just means substituting a conventional product for one with an organic seal of approval, regardless of the externalities of the product or whether it is in fact less destructive to the environment. One example is fish-based products such as fish emulsion. These are produced from overfished seas and are a hallmark of the destructive fisheries industry. Additionally, they are often shipped from across the world, leaving behind a significant carbon footprint. The dubious origin and production process related to these types of certified organic products, plus the fact that they are difficult to get into irrigation solution, gives us pause.

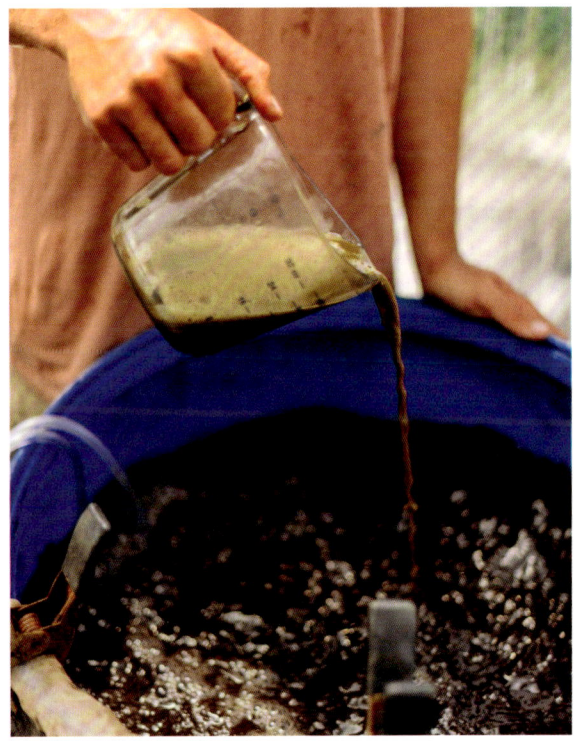

Compost tea is not specifically a fertilizer, but when applied through fertigation, it aids in nutrient availability, crop health, and disease mitigation. We use it religiously.

We have clogged many drip lines (and had to remove them in the field and replace them mid-crop cycle—talk about something that makes you want to rip your hair out!) trying to put down farm-mixed organic inputs. However, it is possible, and many farms do it successfully. We still actively experiment with an array of liquid products, concluding only that fresh-made compost tea is an all-around winner because it unlocks the biology and nutrients already in the soil.

Putting It All Together

Fertility management is not just the science of inputs; it also entails paying close attention. Once the crop is established in the ground, we rely on a set of macro-level visual and intuitive cues to monitor crop health. Are there pests? Is the crop growing vigorously? Is it the correct color? Are the leaves turgid? Does the plant have good posture?

Beyond these macro-level cues, it's helpful to know on a micro level if the crop is uptaking the fertilizers you apply. Taking a cue from the grape industry, many cannabis farmers are turning to tissue analysis to help monitor and/or correct plant health and nutrient uptake.

Many cannabis farmers are turning to tissue analysis to help monitor and/or correct plant health and nutrient uptake.

And how do we pull fertility management together at our farm? With our healthy soils approach, we prefer to front-load fertility as much as possible. We take our soil reports, combine them with our experience from the previous season, and decide what and how much to apply. If we applied sufficient nutrients via fertilizers but did not see the desired performance results, we review the fertility program from the beginning to discern what we can improve. For a full-term crop, we front-load solid fertilizer, usually chicken pellets and sulfate of potash, at a rate of roughly 200-200-200 N-P-K. For autoflowers, the rate is 180-180-180 N-P-K. This is *in addition* to any compost or manure we've applied. We use this rate due to our biointensive approach and high plant density per acre required to maximize yields within California's regulated canopy limits. This front-loading approach has allowed us, in autoflowering crops, to minimize or in some instances completely eliminate the use of liquid fertilizer.

Overall, our fertility program takes a year-round, holistic approach. In fall we apply compost and then seed cover crop using rye or a vetch/bell beans/rye mixture. In spring we apply sulfate of potash, monoammonium phosphate, and 4-4-2 chicken pellets sufficient to meet our desired application rates listed above. Due to our heavy clay soil, most years we apply gypsum. Finally, we use liquid fertilizers during the crop cycle as needed.

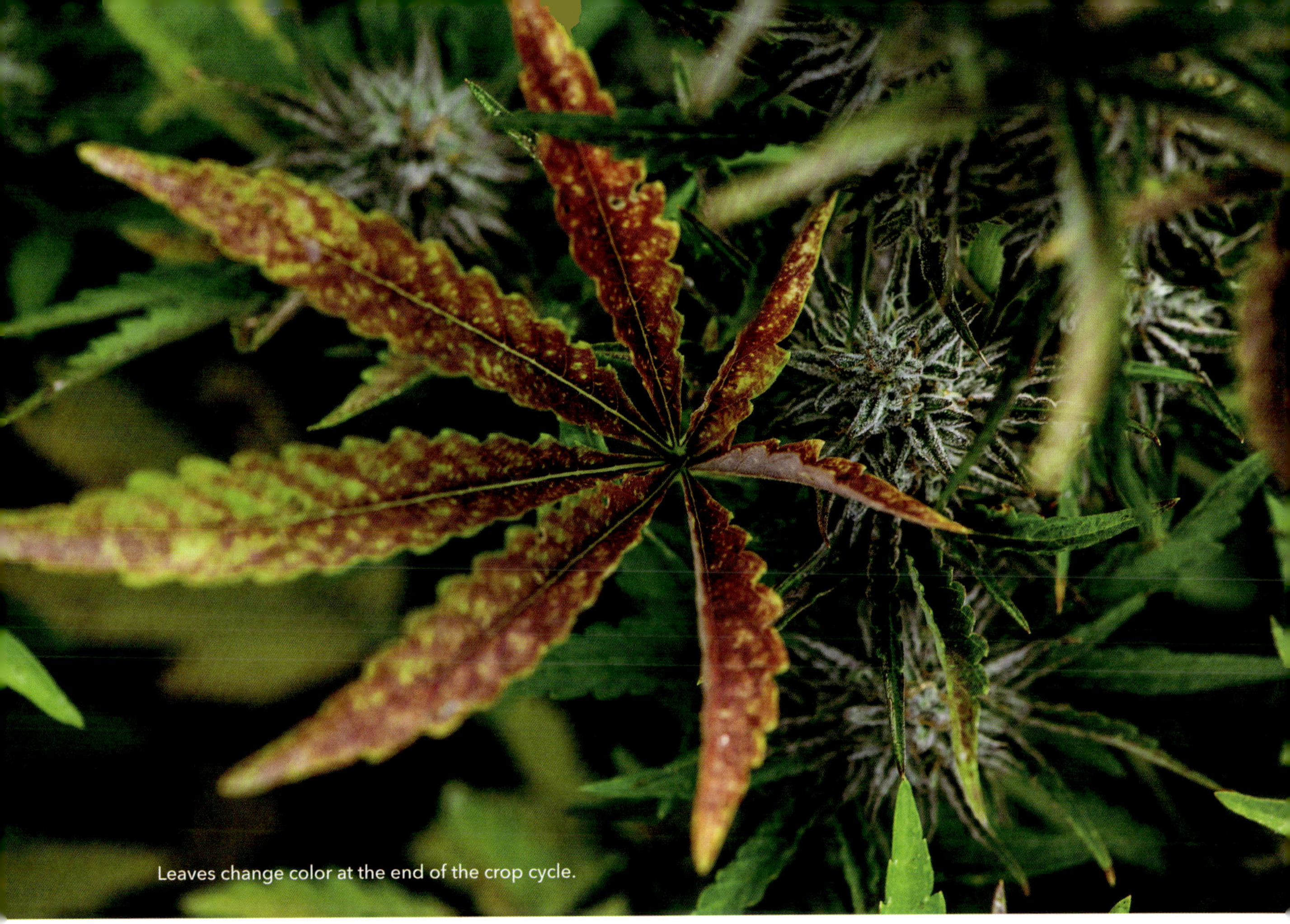

Leaves change color at the end of the crop cycle.

How Does Tissue Analysis Work?

Tissue analysis is used frequently in viticulture (grape growing), but in cannabis its usefulness is not yet proven. The farmer selects leaves from the crop and sends them to a lab for analysis. The tissue analysis can spot nutrient deficiencies before the plants show any obvious signs, so adjustments can be made to keep the crop in optimum growth. If the farmer has the capacity to address deficiencies via fertigation, this allows for in-season adjustments. If they do not have this capacity, then they can take these data sets and apply them to the pre-planting fertility program of the next crop.

Note that the usefulness of these tests is still developing. The labs doing cannabis tissue analysis do not yet have enough years of experience to determine the ideal nutrient needs of the cannabis plant throughout its growth cycle (nor can the analysis be segmented by various light cycle types). If a testing service also provides fertilizers for sale, you might think twice before accepting 100 percent of their advice.

Plant Nutrient Deficiency

It is important to learn to recognize plant nutrient deficiencies visually, although, with proper planning and execution, the signs should rarely present themselves.

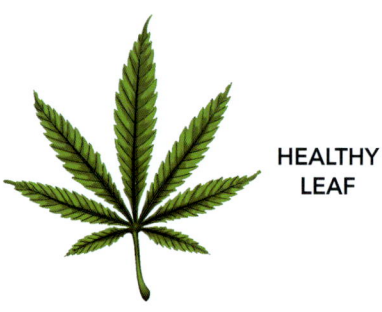

HEALTHY LEAF

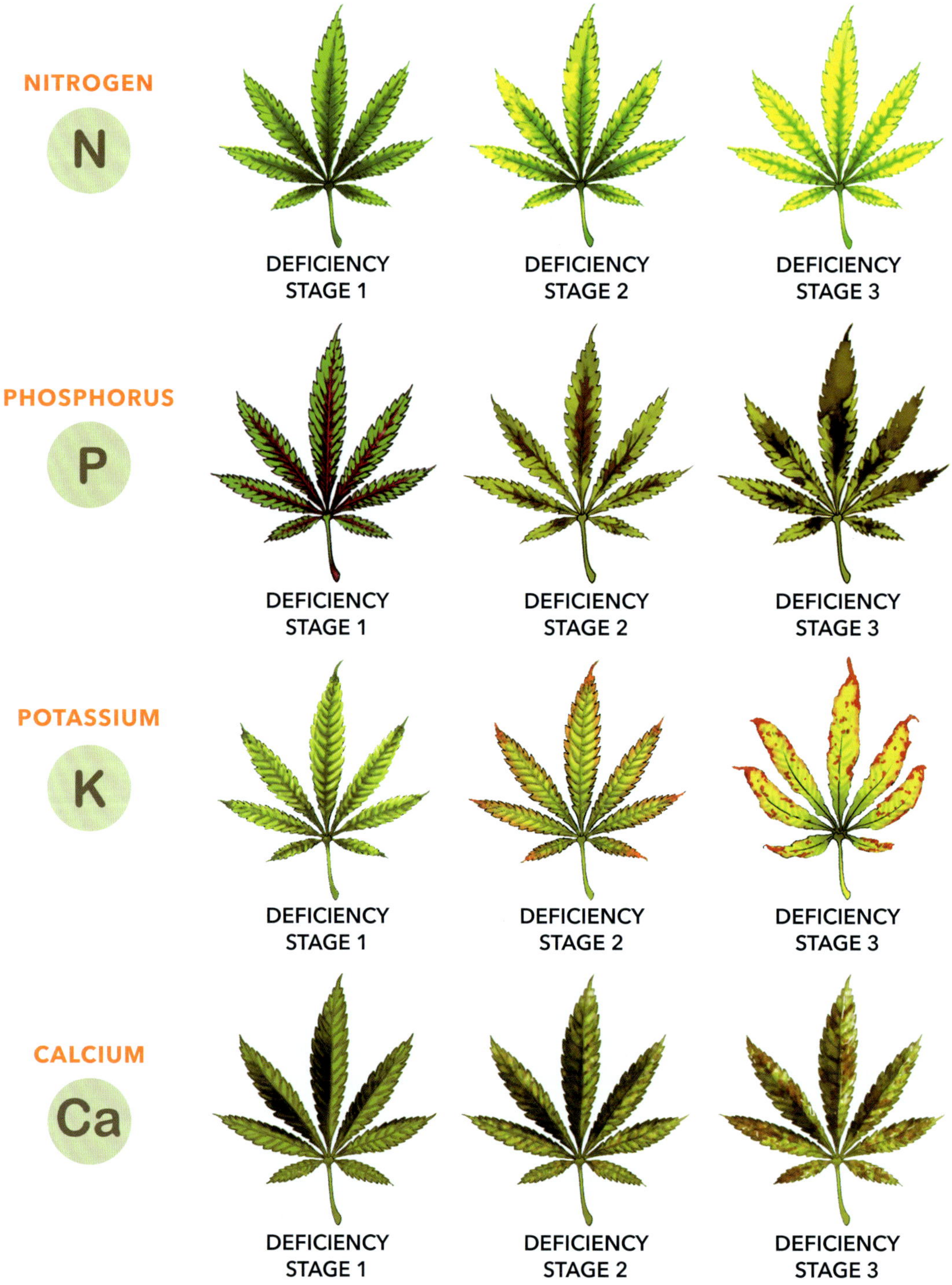

NITROGEN

N

DEFICIENCY STAGE 1	DEFICIENCY STAGE 2	DEFICIENCY STAGE 3

PHOSPHORUS

P

DEFICIENCY STAGE 1	DEFICIENCY STAGE 2	DEFICIENCY STAGE 3

POTASSIUM

K

DEFICIENCY STAGE 1	DEFICIENCY STAGE 2	DEFICIENCY STAGE 3

CALCIUM

Ca

DEFICIENCY STAGE 1	DEFICIENCY STAGE 2	DEFICIENCY STAGE 3

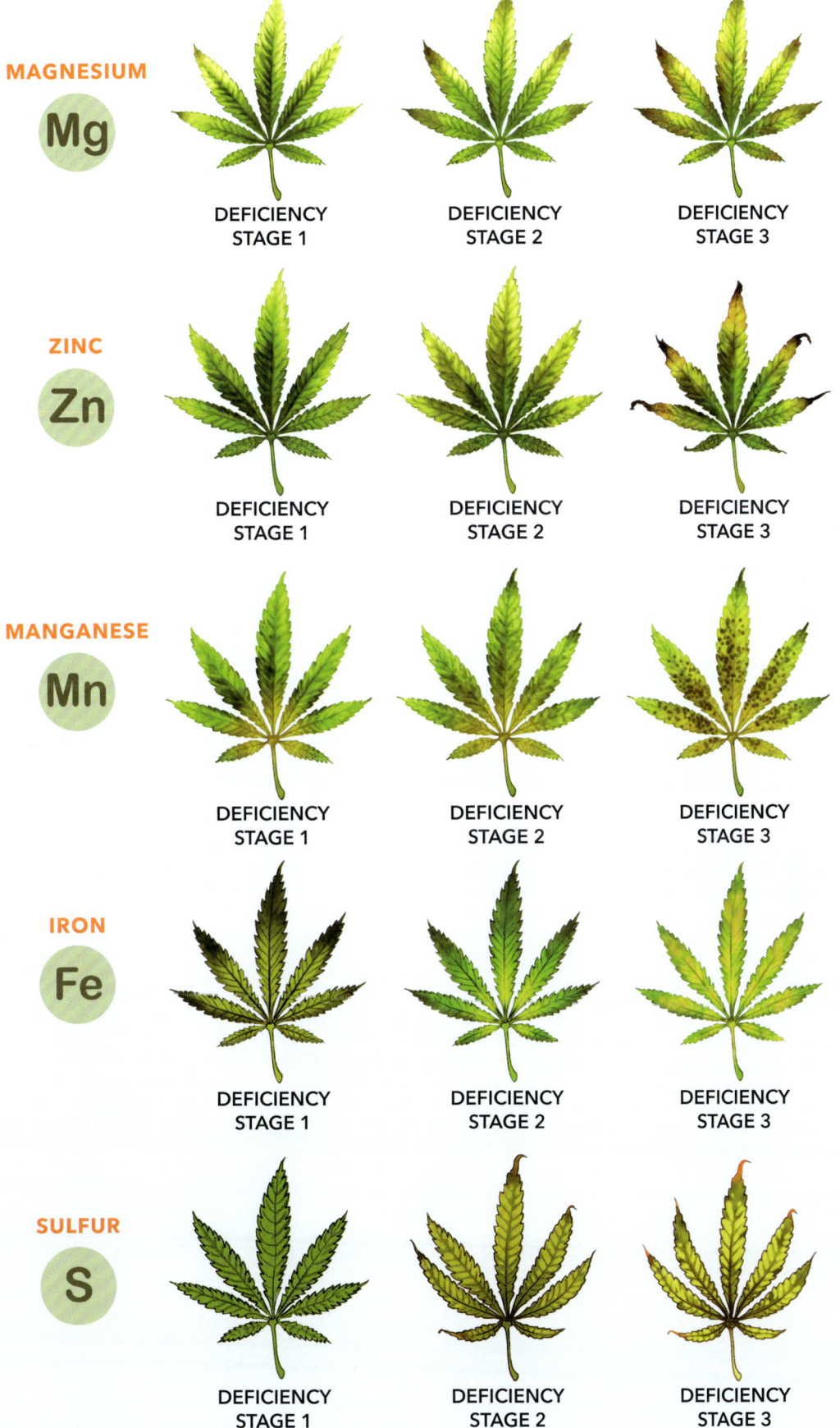

MAGNESIUM

Mg

DEFICIENCY STAGE 1 | DEFICIENCY STAGE 2 | DEFICIENCY STAGE 3

ZINC

Zn

DEFICIENCY STAGE 1 | DEFICIENCY STAGE 2 | DEFICIENCY STAGE 3

MANGANESE

Mn

DEFICIENCY STAGE 1 | DEFICIENCY STAGE 2 | DEFICIENCY STAGE 3

IRON

Fe

DEFICIENCY STAGE 1 | DEFICIENCY STAGE 2 | DEFICIENCY STAGE 3

SULFUR

S

DEFICIENCY STAGE 1 | DEFICIENCY STAGE 2 | DEFICIENCY STAGE 3

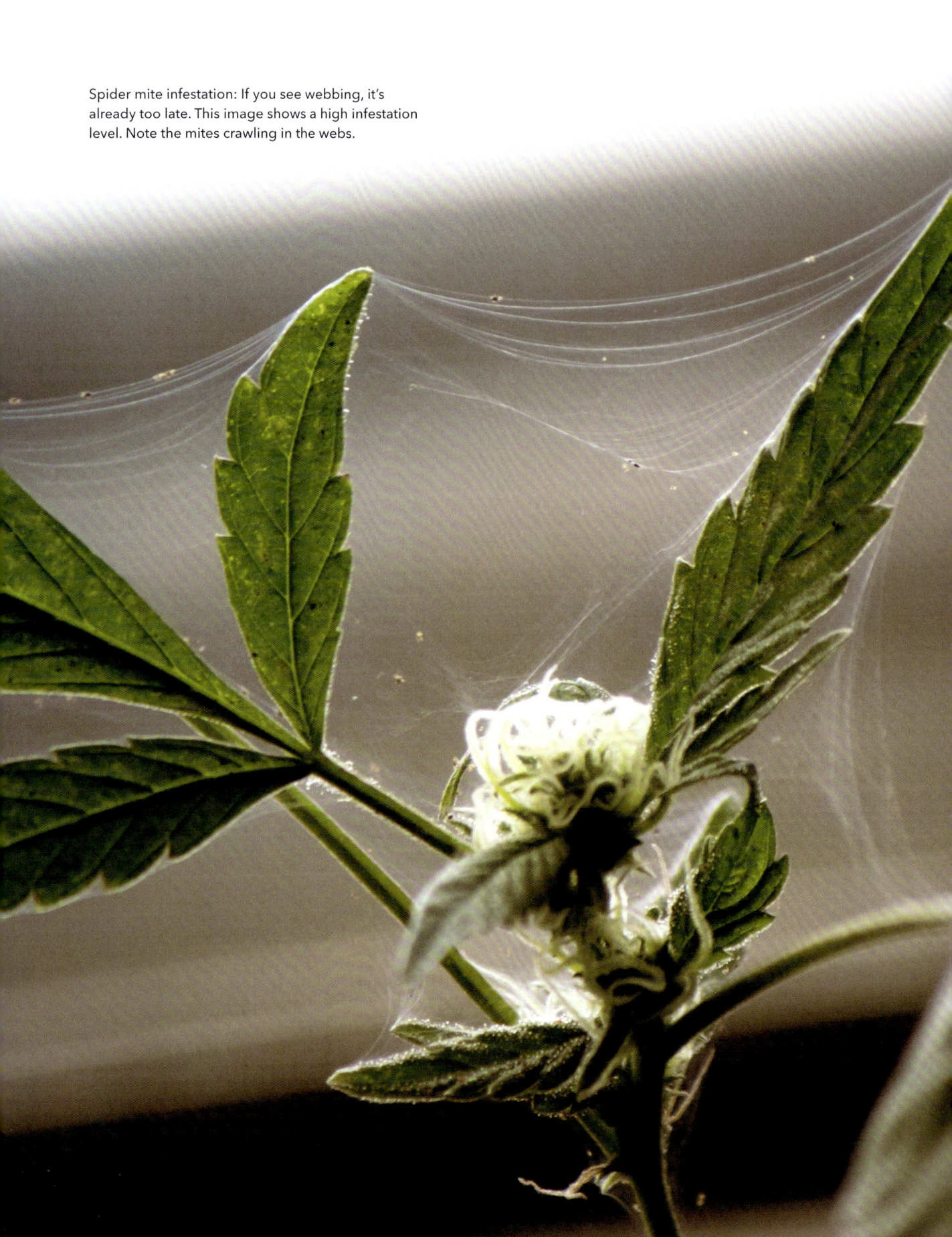

Spider mite infestation: If you see webbing, it's already too late. This image shows a high infestation level. Note the mites crawling in the webs.

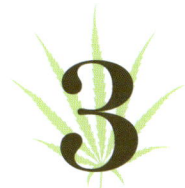

Managing Insects and Fungi

We begin this chapter with an about-face from the conventional view of and approach to the farmer's relationship with the insects and fungi that feed on crop plants. Rather than adopt a war mentality against pests and diseases, an approach that has largely failed in mainstream agriculture, we choose to focus on enhancing the ecosystem itself and apply "systems thinking" to the insects and fungi that may affect our crops.

For simplicity's sake, let us define "pest" as any insect or fungi that feeds on the cannabis plant and *has the potential* to kill or injure it and thus reduce yields. The difference is that rather than view pests as something to be defeated, we see pest pressure as an indication of imbalance, weak or stressed crops, or denuded soil health. As master farmer and author Eliot Coleman puts it in *The New Organic Grower*, "Simply stated, insects and disease are bringing a message that the plant is under stress. That message is incomprehensible as long as we view pests as enemies. In essence, we have been trying to kill the messenger. . . . Plants . . . only become subject to insect and disease problems when they are stressed by unfavorable growing conditions" (Coleman 1989, 173–74).

Let a man profess to have discovered some new Patent Powder Pimperlimplimp, a single pinch of which being thrown into each corner of a field will kill every bug throughout its whole extent, and people will listen to him with attention and respect. But tell them of any simple common-sense plan, based upon correct scientific principles, to check and keep within reasonable bounds the insect foes of the farmer, and they will laugh you to scorn.

—Benjamin Walsh, *The Practical Entomologist* (1866)

An ounce of prevention is worth a pound of cure, as the saying goes, and in large-scale cannabis farming this might translate into something like "An ounce of prevention can save you a million dollars." Besides the obvious step of not importing pests on clones or seedlings purchased off-farm, we will cover preventive strategies before discussing pest mitigation. We divide this approach into three parts, ranked in order of importance: (1) a healthy ecosystem, (2) a plant-positive approach, and (3) appropriate pest mitigation.

A Healthy Ecosystem

Nature maintains an intricate interdependent balance among fungi, plants, and animals. When this balance is intact, we do not see "outbreaks." When something throws off the balance, be it climate change, a natural disaster, or, in the case of farming, tillage, the system will respond and adapt, and we see a proliferation of one or more species and then another in response, again and again, until an intelligent and elegant order is restored. In an agricultural system, of course, we manipulate the environment through tillage and put single crops in places where a diversity of plants would grow naturally. But we can mimic, to the best of our ability, the diverse micro- and macrobiomes that create balance. This includes, but is not limited to, mulching the soil, releasing beneficial insects, planting summer cover crops, putting in beneficial

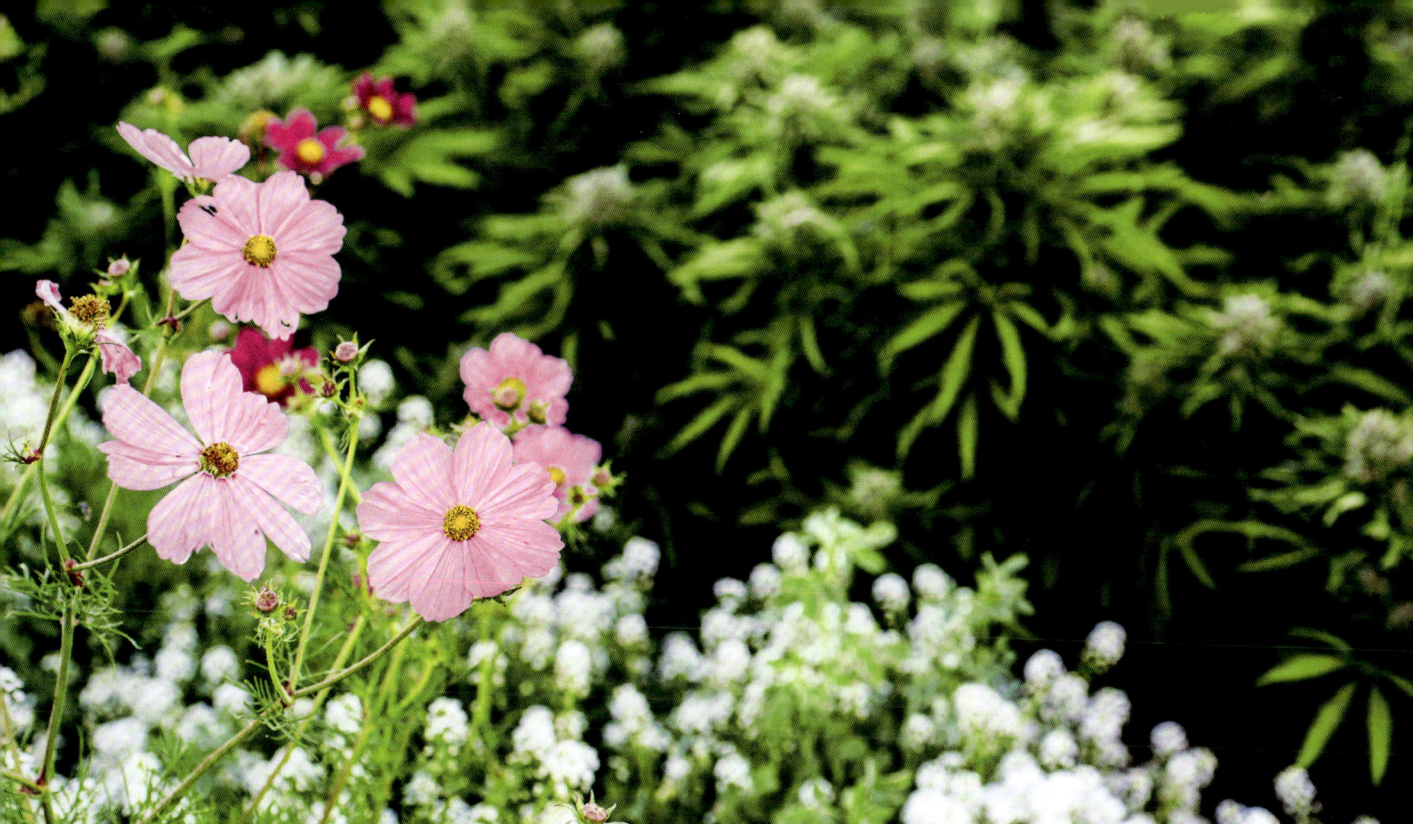

insert–attracting flowers every few beds, planting hedgerows along field edges, using compost and compost teas, paying attention to the wildlands around the farm, and using no-till or reduced-till systems.

Let's begin with examples of practices that actively promote biodiversity to reap the rewards of its beneficial influence on pests and disease.

Using beneficial flowers in crop fields. We plant a mix of beneficial insect–attracting flowers between autoflower beds. This not only fosters diversity but also permits tractor access (our sprayer covers two beds on either side of the tractor) once the autoflowers are too tall to drive over. Check with local nurseries or other growers for what seed blends work well in your area. We use the tractor to spray compost tea, which enhances the microbial diversity present. The open beds allow for a more efficient harvest process as well. In the photoperiod full-term field, we leave an entire bed width between rows of cannabis to provide physical access to perform cultural activities such as weeding, de-leafing, spraying, and harvest. In those fields we use flower seed mixes (available from many commercial seed suppliers) between every two or three rows of cannabis. Using summer cover crops adjacent to or between rows of cannabis is another technique that increases diversity and discourages pest populations.

Planting a mixture of beneficial insect–attracting flowers in between rows of cannabis reduces pest activity significantly.

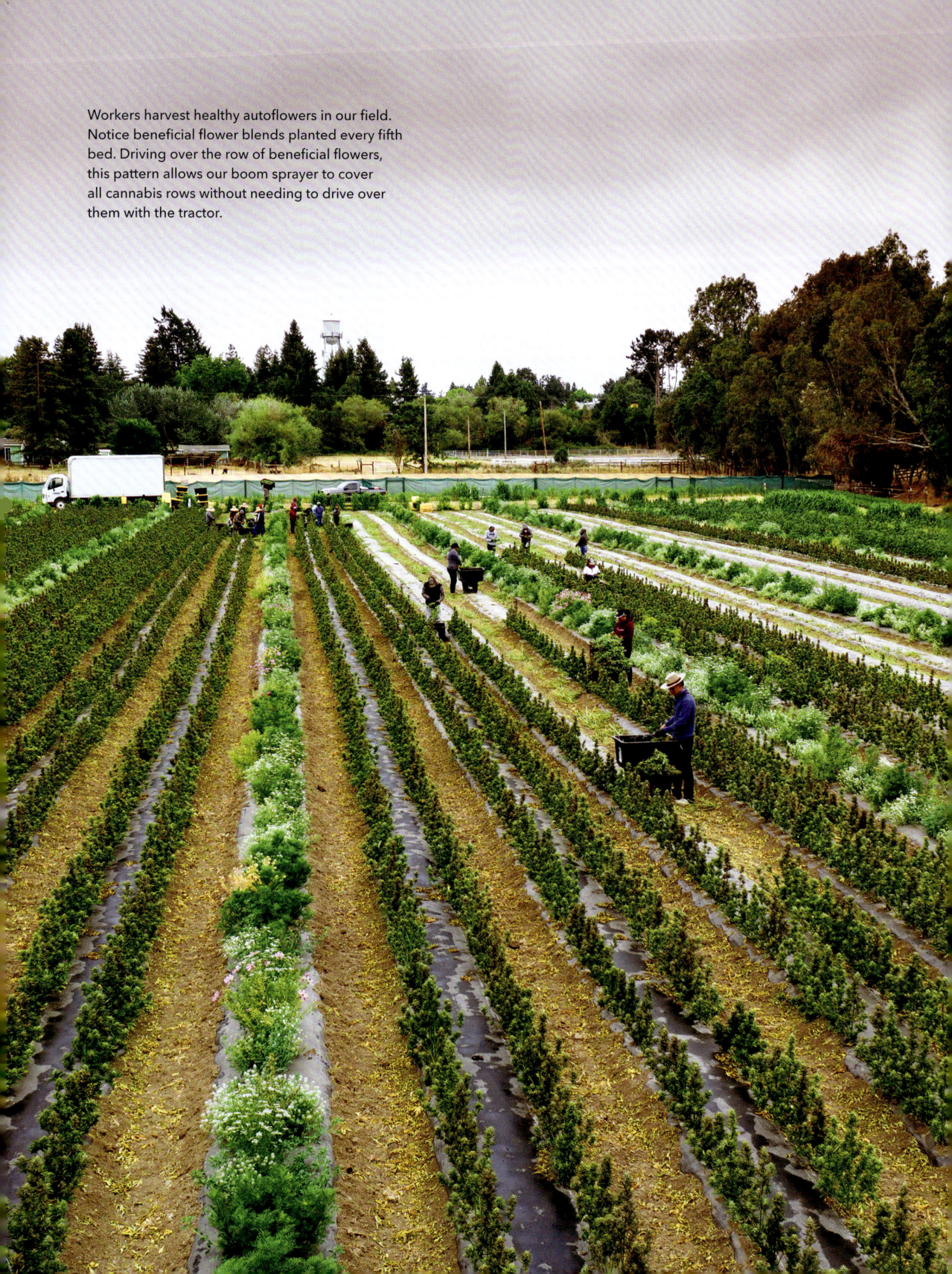

Workers harvest healthy autoflowers in our field. Notice beneficial flower blends planted every fifth bed. Driving over the row of beneficial flowers, this pattern allows our boom sprayer to cover all cannabis rows without needing to drive over them with the tractor.

Establishing perennial hedgerows. We installed perennial hedgerows of beneficial insect habitat around the fields and the farm, creating a diversity of plant life that promotes diverse insect life. Agronomists that we've consulted have noted that pest pressure is significantly reduced in our crops relative to other cannabis farms they have seen. It was nice to hear that. Better still was a simple stroll through the field on a sunny day as our indicator of success: Many thousands of insects buzzed about happily living their lives, and many were known predators of the mites and aphids that attack cannabis.

Attention to the surrounding wildlands, if any exist, is also prudent. Where a field is situated on the property and how adjacent land is managed or left alone can significantly influence insect pest population dynamics. In an ideal agroecosystem, your crop does not represent the majority of plants. Rather, the crop is part of an abundance of biodiversity, whose whole is greater than the sum of its parts when it comes to systemic resilience and buffers against the predominance of any one species.

In an ideal agroecosystem, your crop does not represent the majority of plants. Rather, the crop is part of an abundance of biodiversity.

Nurturing the soil. Proper attention to the soil ecosystem is equally important. The soil is a veritable garden of microorganisms. A single teaspoon (1 gram) of rich garden soil can hold up to one billion bacteria, several yards of fungal filaments, several thousand protozoa, and scores of nematodes. Good soil health has long been known to abate pest pressure.

Green Revolution agronomy, whose tenets still dominate "conventional" agriculture, sees the soil as a medium in which to plant crops and assesses its health based on mineral nutrient levels only. There was a time when farmers thought it was enough to focus entirely on fertilization to provide the best for their crops. We now understand that the soil microbiome health is as or more important. The use of cover crops and the application of compost are two ways growers can improve and maintain soil health and build soil structure, which is especially important in tillage systems. In no till systems, where the soil structure is not disturbed, more stable communities of microorganisms are able to thrive. There are many products containing mycorrhizal fungi and other soil inoculants that claim to improve crop performance. The idea of adding a handful of species to a system that contains billions of bacterial organisms per gram of soil made us wonder. We discovered that studies of these products do demonstrate increased plant growth to a point but also decreased plant tolerance to pest predation. Rather than try to manipulate the species composition of the soil, we prefer to focus on enhancing the soil microbiome that is already present using compost, mulching, and cover crops.

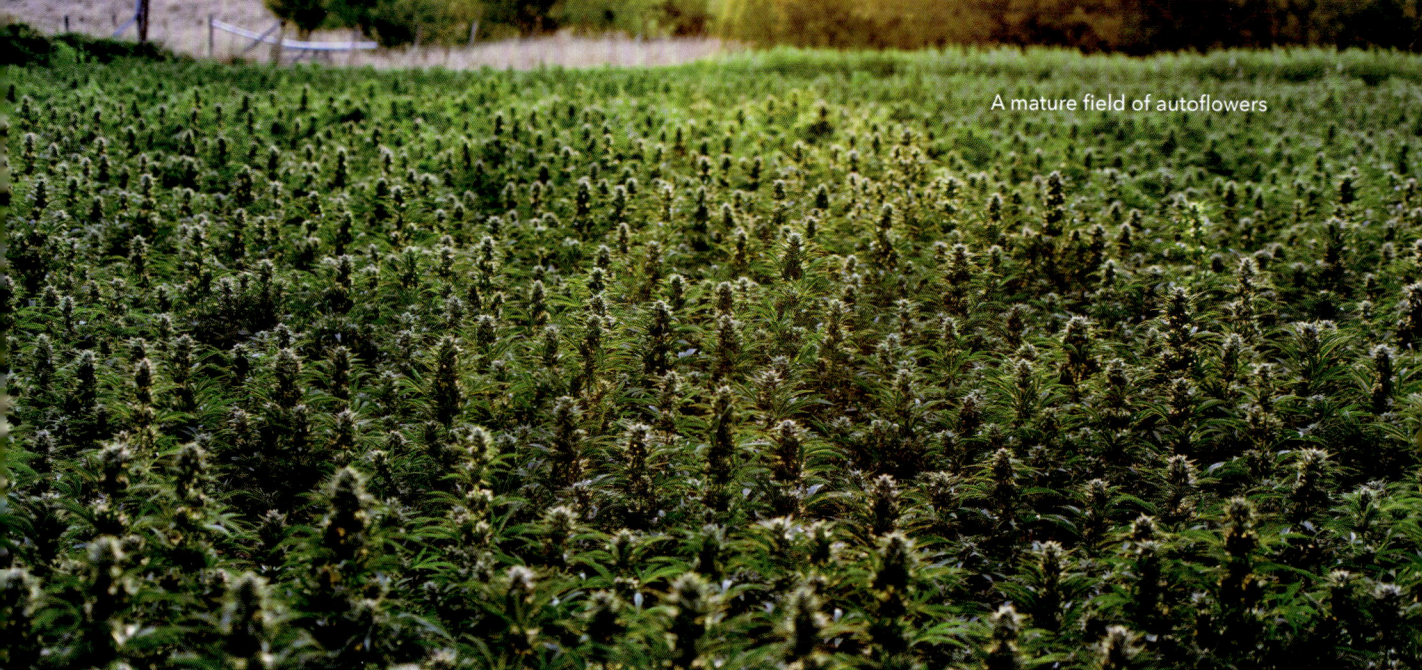
A mature field of autoflowers

A Plant-Positive Approach

In the same vein as promoting a healthy ecosystem to facilitate systemic resistance to pests, the plant-positive approach considers the welfare of the plants as the primary goal so that they become impervious to pest and disease pressure. This concept is not new to cannabis growers: Most farmers can attest to it firsthand. But in cannabis, stress causes a particular problem: A stressed plant will become susceptible not only to pest problems but also to hermaphroditism–called "herming"–whereby a female plant will produce male flowers and seed itself.

First and foremost, we must pay careful attention to each step of propagation to eliminate stress events (see Chapter 5). Once, when discussing the particularly sensitive nature of autoflower seedlings, an experienced grower told us this story: Thousands of seedlings were being delivered to Arizona by refrigerated truck. Each pallet was meticulously labeled and tracked while the seedlings were transplanted. As the crop reached sexual maturity, hermaphroditism developed in a single section of the field, despite identical conditions. The growers considered every conceivable cause, including nutrient deficiencies, irrigation problems, wind stress, heat, a different seed lot, you name it. Eventually they discovered that the affected plants had been situated in front of the reefer unit in the truck and thus had eight or so hours of very cold air blown through them. That was the only time that those seedlings experienced different conditions from the rest.

We have witnessed how stress conditions increase pest pressure and hermaphroditism on numerous occasions. One year we planted autoflowers especially early for our region–early April. We covered the field with floating row cover to protect the seedlings against cold night temperatures and potential frost. One night about a week after transplant, we did get a light frost, but because of the row cover, we remained optimistic that we would not see problems. Later in the crop cycle, small sections of the field displayed decreased vigor and a slight increase in pest pressure. These sections also saw some male flowers produced in the lower part of the plants, where they were difficult to find and remove.

What did these sections of the field have in common? They were all topographically lower than the rest of the field—just soft depressions in the level and an overall very slight slope meant that the colder-temperature air collected there at night during those initial weeks and stressed the seedlings. Furthermore, lower sections tend to receive more irrigation water; in early spring, when soils are still relatively wet, this leads to overly wet conditions that have their own host of problems and stress on the plants.

Countless other examples exist, some of which contain a few obvious stressors, and others for which stress events were small and numerous. As farmers we have always found anecdotal evidence to be the most helpful in understanding broader concepts. So before moving on, let's consider a different story to color in this theme a little more. One year we had a field of photoperiod full-term clones adjacent to a field of direct-sown autoflowers. As we explained in Chapter 1, clones are more finicky than seed, have lower pest and disease resistance, and sometimes come to your farm with pests already on them! Throughout the crop cycle, we dealt with minor populations of hop aphids (*Phorodon humuli*) and some spider mites (*Tetranychus urticae*) by applying oil-based sprays and releasing predatory mites, but the pests continued to pop up. Literally right next to those plants, in the field of autoflowers, we never saw any established insect populations. It was night and day: On the left, constant presence of insect pests; on the right, healthy plants flourishing with no sign of them.

A Note on Genetics

Just as we look to our agroecological environment for natural system resilience, it is important to consider the resilience and natural pest resistance of the genetics. And cannabis is definitely considered a "pesty" crop. This is due to a variety of factors, the main one being that modern breeding has selected away many agronomic traits that support natural plant resistance. Modern Western breeding focuses obsessively on THC and the aesthetics of the flower to the detriment of other important agronomic traits.

In regions of the Middle East or Asia that still grow nonfeminized crops for hashish production, we have observed diverse populations of vigorous plants. Farmers in these areas have nurtured these polyhybrid populations because their genome contains the diversity required to survive a huge range of weather conditions and a variety of pests and boasts enough resilience for some individuals to survive to the next season.

✳ Systemic Crop Health

A Healthy Ecosystem

When nature is in balance, we do not see outbreaks of pests and disease in crops. Rather than adopting a war mentality against pests and disease, support and enhance agroecosystem health to mimic the diverse micro- and macrobiomes that create balance.

A Plant-Positive Approach

This approach considers the welfare of plants the primary goal and understands pests and diseases as messengers. Support plant health throughout propagation to minimize stress and create resilient crop performance.

Appropriate Pest Mitigation

Practice close looking to catch potential problems and make systemic adjustments before spraying becomes necessary. Appropriate use of pesticides can be warranted to save a crop. Note lessons learned and implement them for the next season.

What these examples illustrate is that plant stress obviously initiates problems and increases susceptibility to pest damage. Proper care of your crop leads directly to increased health, vigor, and thus resilience of each individual plant.

However, the predominant attitude around pests is an aggressor vs. defender mindset, focusing mostly on products that eliminate them, however temporarily. In any given crop, the grower will sometimes need to perform forensics to discover the root of the problem and adjust practices accordingly. In many cases, the need to use an elimination product is only due to plant stress events that occurred within the control of the grower. In sum, the enhancement of pest/disease resistance that plant-positive practices have for crops is equal to or greater than the efficacy of spraying.

Close Looking

Plant-positive practices are spelled out throughout the book, starting with and primarily influenced by soil health. We want to introduce the practice of close looking as a segue into the subject of appropriately dealing with insects and fungi. We call it close looking because at every stage of the crop cycle, you go into the greenhouse or out into the field and use your eyes to catch small problems or mistakes that can lead to much larger issues. It sounds basic, but it's the way you notice incompletely filled seedling trays, overly wet soils, or the early stage of a pest outbreak in the prop house.

When we walk into the greenhouse, we don't just look at the tables of seedlings. We pick up individual trays, looking underneath for slugs and feeling the weight of the tray as an indication of how wet the plugs are. We observe how full each tray is with plants to see what kind of germination/emergence percentages we're getting. Are green algae growing on the surface? Are fungus gnats present? Is damping-off prevalent? We created checklists for the most critical steps of close looking that employees use to prevent mistakes and ensure every detail is being covered (see Weekly Pest Check, page 72).

Close looking is a foundation of plant-positive growing. It's essential to catch insect populations or mold/mildew infestations when they are small so that any required actions will be successful. A pest once established in the crop can become challenging to manage. When close looking reveals the presence of pests, we often refer to the UC Statewide Integrated Pest Management Program website, even though the site does not yet include cannabis-specific information.

Elliot assesses the crop. The best fertilizer is the farmers' footsteps.

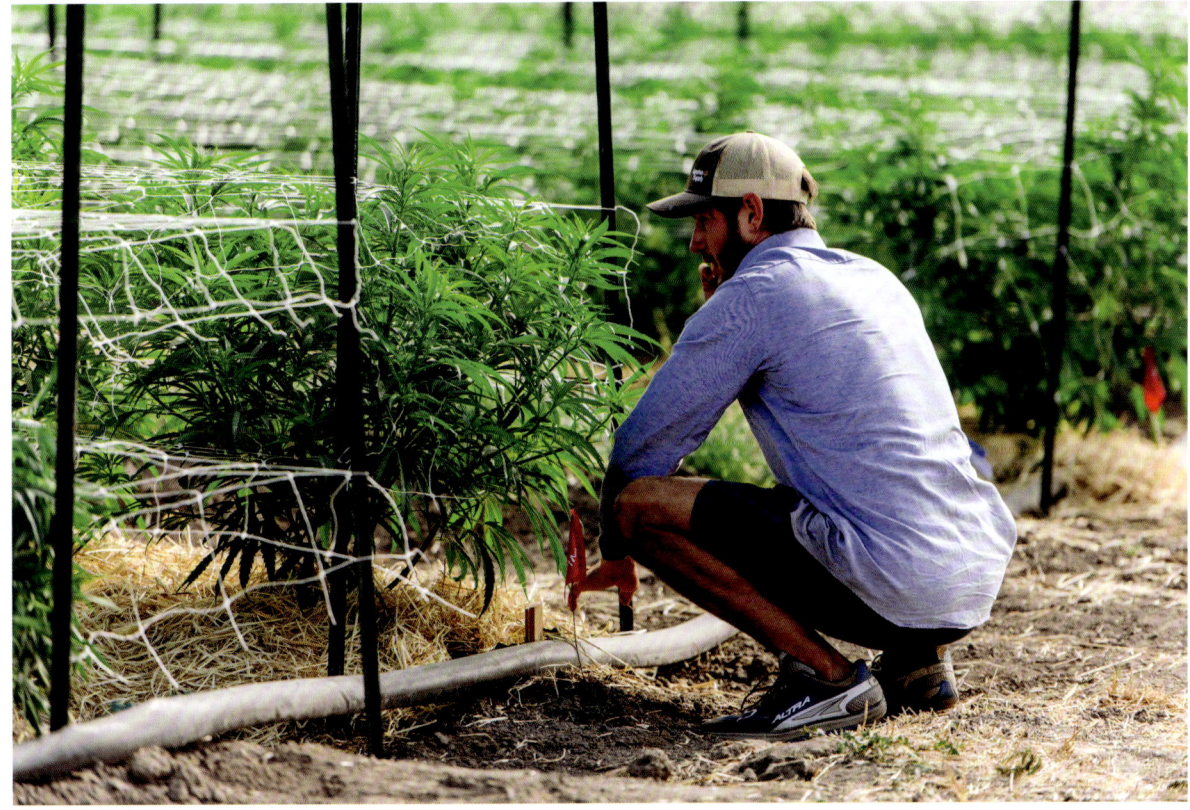

Weekly Pest Check

As the saying goes, the best fertilizer is the farmer's footsteps. If something is off, you will usually notice it by slowly ambling through the fields. Walk four beds per acre up and down, just making general observations.

We stack functions so that when we do our weekly scouting for pests, we also assess general crop health. Our checklist is simple but works for us.

Leaf color and posture. Are leaves dark green and vibrant, reaching upward? Or are they light green and parallel to the ground, or drooping and turning yellow? These are indications of different levels of overall plant health.

Vigor. Are you seeing the growth you would expect, considering the plant genetics, the current weather, and the current crop management practices? If you are seeing less growth than expected, why? Examine weather, fertility, water, virus, pests, etc.

Canopy management. Is there prolific branching? Removing low and redundant branching (covered in Chapter 8) may be necessary to encourage growth of desired colas.

Weed pressure. Weed early and weed often! We perform frequent cultivations when the plants are small and we are still able to drive tractors over the crop. It is almost never economical to cultivate when the weeds are higher than 6 inches.

Soil moisture. Given the projected weather for the coming week, is moisture at acceptable levels? Make an irrigation plan for the week.

Pest scouting. Sample four leaves per bed from four beds per acre. Cover the ends of the fields and the bed. Pick mostly older growth leaves. Use a 60× magnifier to examine each leaf, paying special attention to the petiole margins. You can get inexpensive but effective microscopes that mount to a smartphone camera.

Appropriate Pest Mitigation

We turn now to the most common pest issues we have found with cannabis along with the best practices for their management. Specific details on spraying methods, spray equipment, and spray safety are given in Chapter 10.

Aphids

Compared to other insects, aphids are easy to spot because they are visible to the naked eye (2 to 4 mm) and move slowly. They are sap suckers, and although their damage is not as severe as other pests, it can lead to fungal growth if left unchecked. The cannabis aphid, *Phorodon cannabis*, is similar to the hop aphid and was first identified in the United States in 2016 in Colorado. It is now prevalent in all western states, a testament to the quick spread of pests on live plants and clones. Within a healthy and active ecosystem, aphid populations usually do not get out of hand.

Beneficial wasps, which are attracted by flowers in the Apiaceae family, specifically sweet alyssum, parasitize aphids with brutal effectiveness: Larval wasps hatch from the stomachs of aphids and devour all those around them, like something out of the movie *Alien*. Ladybugs are also well-known predators of aphids, though it is ladybug larvae that primarily feed on and eliminate the highest volumes. We find that beneficial insects generally keep aphids in check.

That said, aphid populations can get out of hand. In 2020 thousands of clones were delivered to us with aphids present on most plants. Despite repeated applications of the multiuse agricultural spray Stylet-Oil, the population was never eradicated, and we had to spray twice during the crop cycle to keep the population under a critical threshold. We have successfully managed aphids using Stylet-Oil, Grandevo (an insecticide that repels insects and is toxic when ingested by the pest), and essential oil–based products that kill on contact and/or smother insects. (Note that oils cannot be used in tandem with sulfur, which is commonly used for mites and fungi, as damage to the plants will occur.) We've also performed extra or early canopy management, such as de-leafing, which both physically removes the aphids from the field and allows for better spray penetration when making applications.

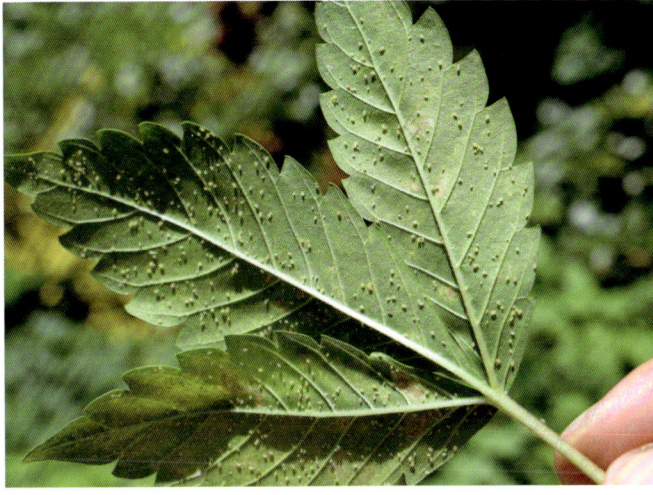

Aphids congregate on the undersides of leaves. They are also typically found on the main stems of the plants.

Mites

The mites that are most common in cannabis are spider mites, russet mites, and broad mites, which are similar in their size, life cycle, and effects on plants. Mites often will come in on clones, but they also exist endemically. They are difficult to spot, especially the broad and russet mites, which require a 10× lens to see. By the time mite damage is apparent, that usually means the infestation has gone too far and is much more difficult to manage. Close looking at the underside of leaves with a microscope mounted on a smartphone camera is critical for mite control.

Spider mites. The two-spotted spider mite is a large, soft-bodied pest that is pervasive and incredibly difficult to eradicate, although control is possible with careful management. Heat stimulates their reproduction and growth, and thus in locations where temperatures are higher, their populations can expand rapidly. They are known to be particularly problematic in greenhouses and other climate-controlled indoor

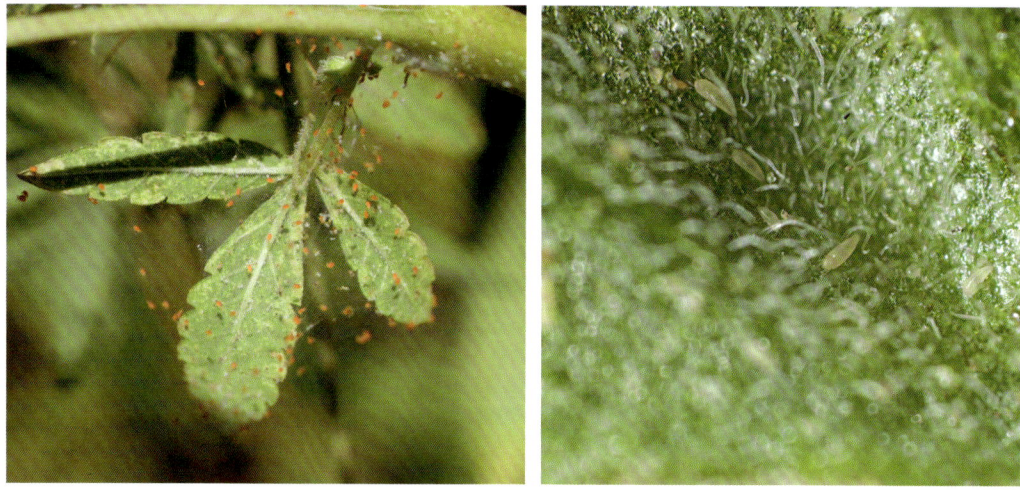

LEFT: Spider mite webbing has gone too far for successful management. RIGHT: Russet mites on the undersides of a leaf can be seen through a 60x scope.

spaces that are less likely to experience nighttime swings in temperatures that can slow growth. Spider mites are also slowed by wind, which means outdoor locations with wind exposure offer natural mitigation. Horticultural oils such as Stylet-Oil or neem oil offer partial control if applied at low or medium population levels.

Broad mites and russet mites are much smaller than spider mites, with a faster overall reproductive cycle. At temperatures around 80°F (27°C), these mites can multiply such that they can severely weaken or decimate a crop within a week or two. Sulfur is incredibly effective against these smaller species, with near or total control achieved with a few applications.

Caterpillars

The corn earworm/tomato fruitworm (*Helicoverpa zea*) is regularly seen on mature flowers. Eggs are laid in developing buds, where the caterpillars hatch and begin feeding. It is not their actual eating that is so damaging to a crop but their excrement (frass), which sullies a flower and leads to mold. A few preventive applications of a *Bacillus thuringiensis* (Bt) product such as Dipel dust works well for these. We typically apply once, a week or two into flowering and again when the flowers are roughly half mature. If we notice any caterpillar activity after that, we do a third application in the final stretch.

Nematodes

These slow-moving microscopic soil organisms thrive in wet and poorly drained areas. It's difficult to completely eradicate them, so the focus becomes population reduction

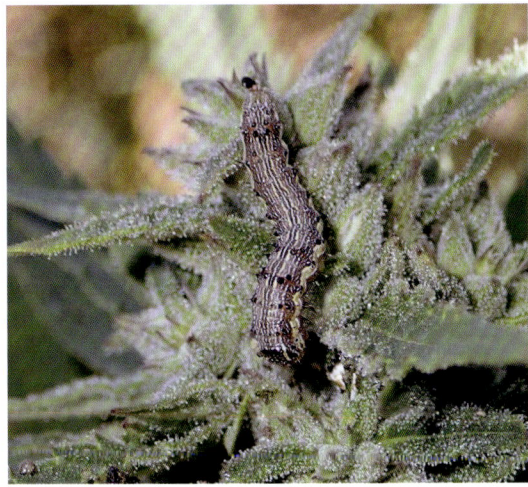
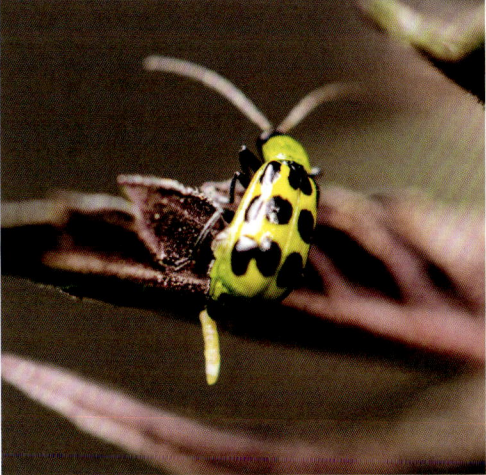

LEFT: Corn earworms are typically found on mature flowers. It isn't the caterpillars that do the damage but their frass, which molds easily. RIGHT: Cucumber beetles are easy to recognize, and their damage is usually not impactful (and we have rarely seen it affect crop outcome).

and improving plant health. We have had issues with nematodes only in newly worked fields or after an application of unfinished compost or manure. Proper soil management should prevent issues. Strategies for population control include avoiding overwatering; improving soil drainage by deep ripping and field grading; applying predatory nematodes or appropriate pesticides to the soil through irrigation lines; planting brassica or legume cover crops; and using a process known as solarization, which involves covering the field with greenhouse plastic for three or four weeks before planting to raise soil temperatures high enough to kill nematodes and weed seeds in the top 5 to 6 inches of soil.

Fungus Gnats

These tiny flies live in propagation areas with small or sensitive seedlings. They cause damage by spreading the fungal spores that they carry on their bodies. Fungus gnats are an issue mostly in manufactured soils and/or in soils that are not properly drying down. To manage fungus gnats, focus on a more thorough dry-down period and irrigate using Gnatrol, a Bt strain that acts as a microbial insecticide, killing fungus gnats in their larval stage.

Cucumber Beetles

Cucumber beetle damage can look extensive because the beetles prefer to feed on the largest and most visible fan leaves, but in most years we just let them do their thing, and the plants grow right through the damage. The beetles are difficult to control using chemicals because they fly away when the spray rigs come rumbling through.

Thrips

Thrip damage looks like tiny dead zones all over lower leaves. These pests can sometimes be difficult to control, but their overall damage is usually limited. We have not seen or heard of thrip damage worth treating.

Root Aphids

Root aphids are a particularly scary pest because they are difficult or impossible to see in plants that are planted in native soil. Luckily, root aphids are most acutely an issue in potting soil. They are easily found by removing a plant from its pot and examining the roots. If you have an outbreak, you could try keeping plants on the dry side or using BotaniGard, which is exceptionally expensive and probably not practical on some scales. Tossing potted plants and starting over is the only option that entirely eliminates the possibility of transmitting root aphids into your field.

Stem or Root Rot

Stem rot is a form of botrytis (see Controlling Fungus on the facing page) that infects the stems and roots almost exclusively in areas where branches have been cut or torn off and/or in overly wet soil conditions. Proper irrigation practices are paramount for avoiding root rot. Cannabis prefers a wet-to-dry swing. We aim for thorough and deep waterings, then let the soil dry down to 40 to 60 percent of capacity, depending on current conditions and soil type. Keeping the soil too wet can severely damage or stunt a crop as well as encourage stem and root rots. When pruning (see Chapter 8), make clean cuts and perform it during dry weather. Once stem rot has set in, it is very difficult or impossible to remove, so plant-positive practices become even more important. A very healthy plant fed compost tea usually grows right through it.

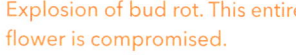

Explosion of bud rot. This entire flower is compromised.

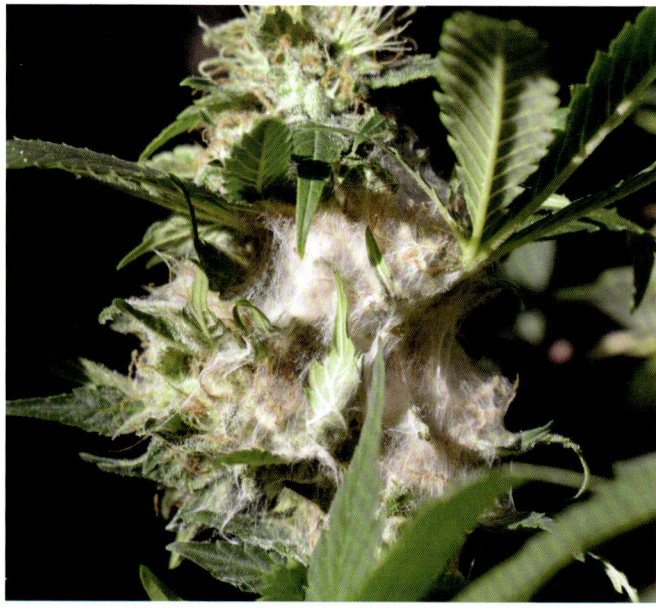

Controlling Fungus

Fungus, in the form of mold and mildew, is the primary yield-reducing pest of cannabis. Bud rot (*Botrytis* spp.) can proliferate in cannabis flowers quickly and cause large reductions in yield combined with huge increases in post-harvest labor. Aside from a crop being pollinated and producing seeds, mold is the number one yield-reducing factor that affects cannabis. Systemic fungicides are unsafe to use for inhalable products and are banned from use on cannabis in most states. Along with the environmental and health externalities, they do not have 100 percent success anyway. Furthermore, tolerance is quickly gained in fungi, and an eradication approach is an expensive merry-go-round that never achieves long-term results. Organic fungicides are mostly ineffective.

As the adage goes, a problem, properly defined, is halfway solved. Let's begin by identifying what molds and mildews need to grow: high humidity and comfortable temperatures. Unfortunately, this describes entire regions of the United States! However, it offers us clues for mitigation of mold pressure. What can we do that decreases relative humidity in the field?

Genetics and Bud Rot

Some genetic features reduce the prevalence of bud rot. These include roomy internodal spacing, terpenes that inhibit mold growth, and flower structures that increase airflow. Nevertheless, a dense, mature cannabis flower will develop bud rot in humid conditions (read: high relative humidity or after precipitation events).

First, a little history and a prediction. The closest relative to the *Cannabis* genus is *Humulus*, or hops. Just like cannabis, hops are grown for their flowers. In the eighteenth and nineteenth centuries in North America, hops were grown predominantly in the humid Northeast, where farmers regularly had issues with mildew. As agriculture practices expanded into the more-arid western states, farmers planting hops had fewer or no problems with mildews. If a region's natural climate conditions eliminate the most common issue for a crop, it will always be more efficient, easier, and less expensive to grow there. Today over 70 percent of domestic hops production takes place in the Yakima Valley of eastern Washington state, where the air is dry and irrigation water is abundant. Over time the industry infrastructure (equipment, supplies, labor and expertise, sales, and distribution) developed there, further entrenching hops cultivation.

It is no leap of logic to assert that future domestic cannabis production will also be concentrated in a few regions of the arid West. Cannabis requires relatively massive equipment and specialized supplies and labor, and it needs post-harvest infrastructure for cultivation, processing, and distribution. It makes sense from a fungi, climate, and logistical perspective that American cannabis agriculture will eventually settle in a handful of geographic regions in the West.

But for now, cannabis's legal status means we cannot ship it across state lines, so technically states must produce their own supply. Therefore, growers in humid regions must adapt to a prevalence of mold in their fields.

Cultural Practices

We advise growers to employ the cultural practices outlined here to decrease relative humidity around the plants or strengthen their natural immunity.

Field Prep and Layout

During and after the potato famine of the 1800s, agricultural researchers studied potato blight (also a fungi or fungilike organism) extensively. They discovered that potatoes planted in hills or raised beds were less susceptible to blight than those planted in flat fields. The reason? The temperature gradient created by the topography of low furrows and raised beds increases airflow where the plant is growing. This simple technique, employed during cannabis field prep, can reduce mold pressure.

Another obvious field prep solution is to increase spacing between plants—fewer plants per acre increases sunlight penetration and airflow into the canopy. Ecological soil management, which fosters microbial diversity, plays a large role, too. Lots of organic matter in the form of compost and/or cover crops is key, as the resulting greater natural diversity of microbial life buffers against the proliferation of any one pest species.

Cover

Many growers in humid regions with summer or fall precipitation use hoop houses to cover their crop. While it may sound obvious, keeping the rain off the flowers makes a huge difference.

Plant-Positive Practices

For mold and mildew abatement, plant-positive thinking entails eliminating unfavorable conditions and giving your crop what it needs to develop natural immunity to fungal outbreaks. Bearing in mind that a very humid environment qualifies as unfavorable conditions, growers can still ensure that their crops are properly propagated, transplanted, irrigated, and fertilized. For fungus specifically, we have found that thickening and strengthening cell walls in plants makes it more difficult for fungal hyphae to pierce and get established. For this, silica and calcium fertilizers are particularly useful.

Preventive Products

Next, a plethora of products exists purporting to increase a plant's natural resistance to mold and mildew. We have experimented with plenty of them. Anything that thickens or strengthens the plants' cell walls (such as calcium and silica, as mentioned previously) will help repel and prevent growth of fungal hyphae. We have noticed a reduction in mold pressure when using Regalia preventively. It creates an immune response within the plants, increasing their resistance to fungal growth.

Many growers spray kill-on-contact products preventively before flowers reach maturity. These include sulfur, essential oil products, potassium bicarbonate, and biofungicides. Before applying any product, learn what can or cannot be used when plants are in flower. Some biofungicides, for example, smell awful and can ruin the scent of the flowers. Sulfur can burn flowers and shrivel the hairs. Sulfur also lingers on plant material and will show up in lab testing, which will deter buyers. (Who wants to smoke sulfur?)

Pruning and Leaf Removal

De-leafing and pruning larger photoperiod plants create more airflow. Growers typically "clean the lowers," removing any leaves or short stems below a certain canopy level (this will be discussed in greater detail in Chapter 8). In our experience this pruning is unnecessary with shorter autoflower plants. As harvest approaches and the flowers reach maturity, removing fan leaves increases airflow and light penetration into the flowers and helps decrease the relative humidity, thus inhibiting fungal growth. Sprays at this point are practically useless.

After rain events, walking the fields with leaf blowers to physically dry off the flowers may be a Hail Mary but is a technique commonly used. Finally, close looking at mold growth in your crop is one of the main factors for choosing when to harvest. If you see some mold, you can bet your bottom dollar there is quite a bit more. Better to harvest early before a mold explosion occurs than to wait for flowers to bulk up a bit more but lose the difference to bud rot. It's a delicate balance.

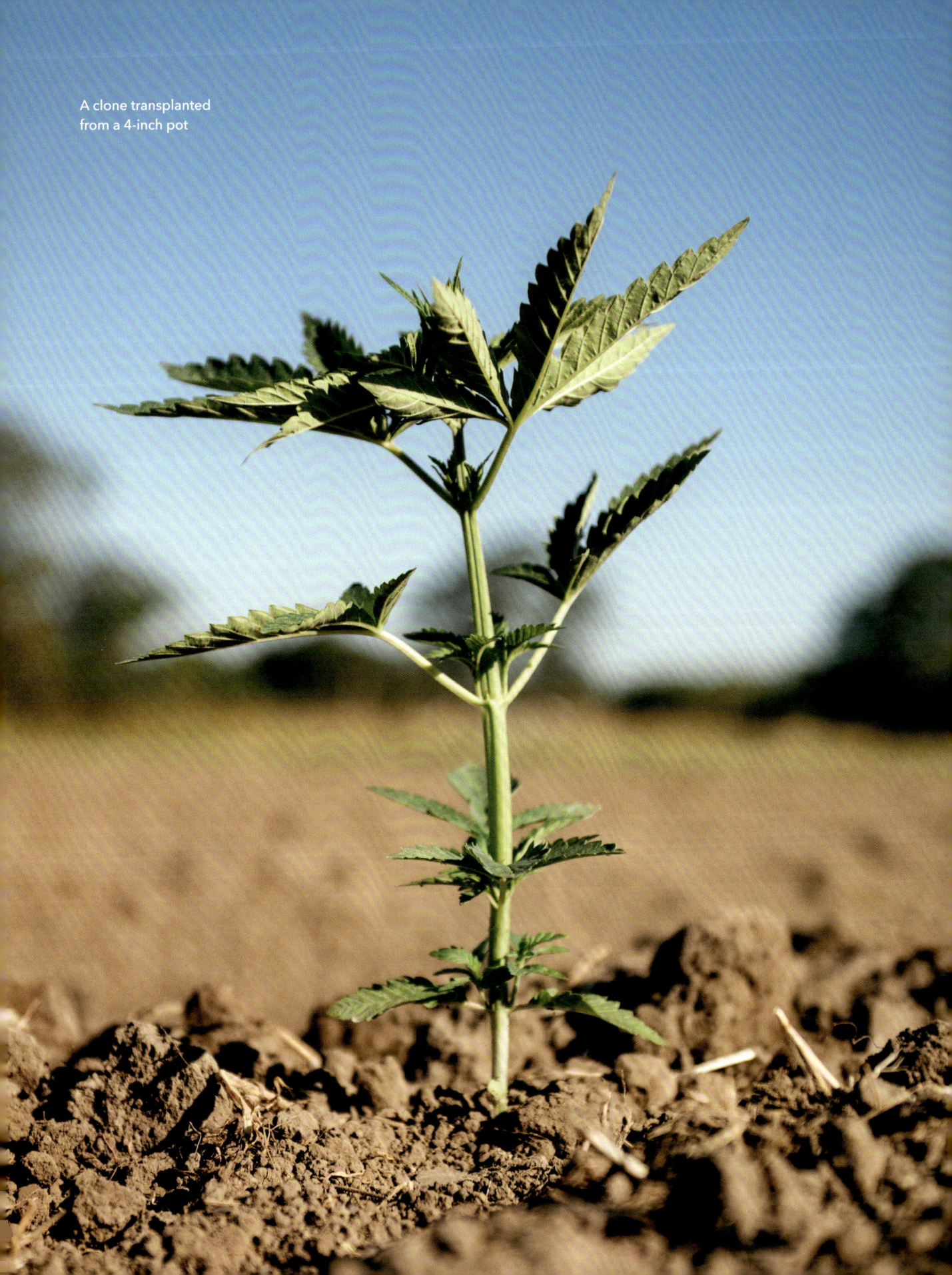

A clone transplanted
from a 4-inch pot

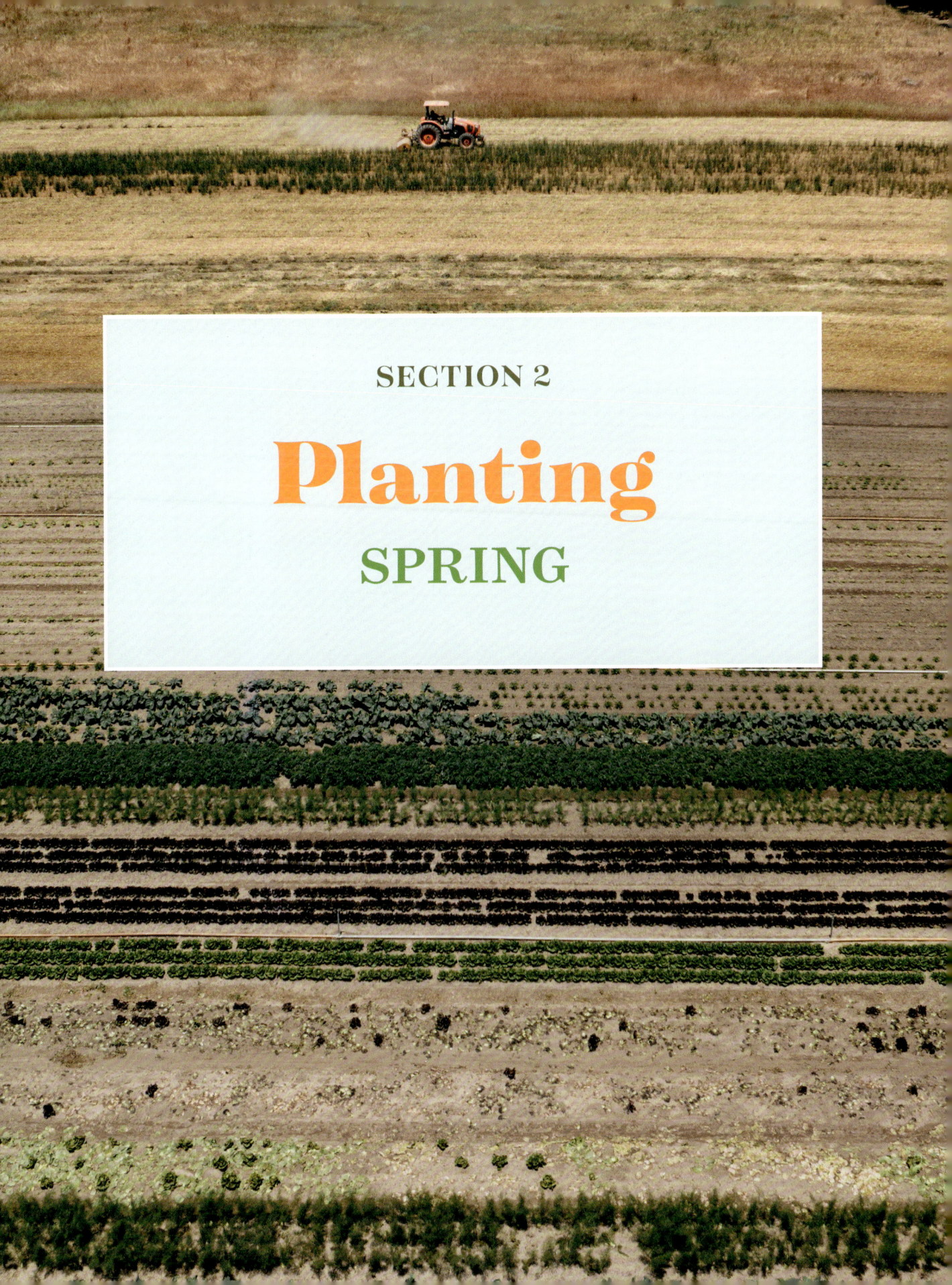

SECTION 2

Planting

SPRING

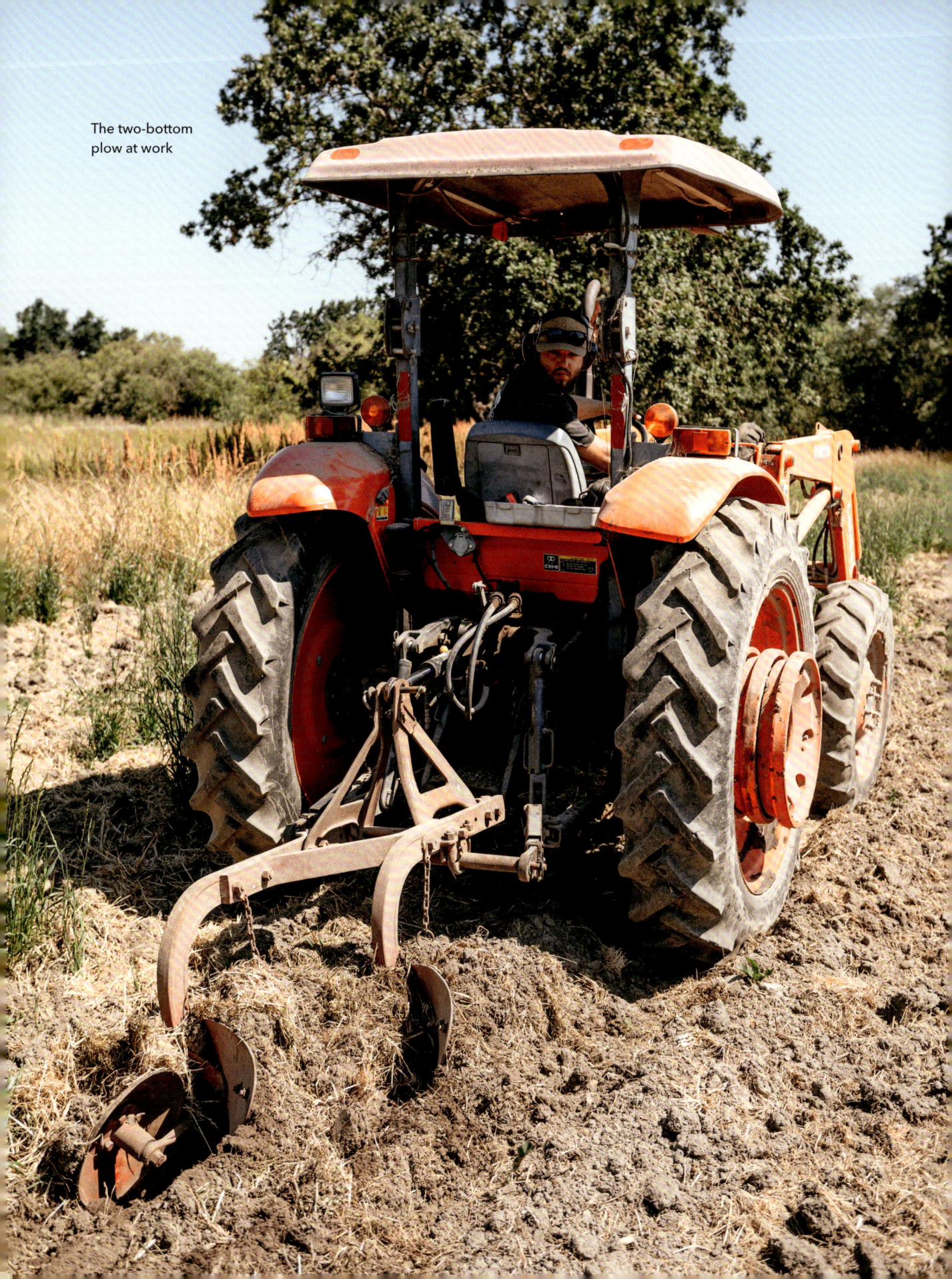

The two-bottom
plow at work

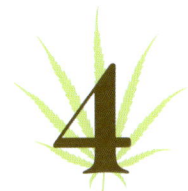

Tillage and Field Prep

The farming season begins with field prep. This step-by-step process forms the foundation for the entire crop cycle, yet it can be easy to overlook its importance. Although the practice of turning soil before planting is an ancient custom, working soil effectively requires a critical eye and a variety of tools. We have tried many tillage approaches—from double-digging beds by hand to a horse-drawn plow to a tractor-mounted mechanical spader. When we started the farm in 2010, we had a walk-behind BCS rototiller. It was a wet spring, and we ran that thing over standing grass so many times we lost count. It never tilled more than a few inches deep, and because the soil was wet and cold, the grass didn't decompose and the field was unplantable even weeks later. In May we finally hired a local guy who showed up in flip-flops with his Italian tractor and spader to work the fields.

That same summer we were given a team of Belgian draft horses named Misty and Quinna. Although we were not excellent horsemen and tilling with horses is slow, we managed to run the farm with those mares for a few seasons. We used a walking plow before eventually upgrading to a riding plow. We had a tiny single-gang disc that would barely sink into the plowed ground. After that we ran a half-busted spring-tooth harrow or a wooden bar-spike harrow to smooth out the field. Bed shaping was often done with chintzy hilling discs mounted on a cart. Since no part of the process was thorough, the bed tops were often littered with clumps of grass and big clods of soil. We ran some climbing rope through a heavy roll of livestock fencing and used the horses to pull that over each bed top to smooth them out.

Moving slowly through the field-prep process over multiple seasons granted us the opportunity to really see and understand how tillage works. It's a massive process. It's no wonder that no-till systems are gaining popularity—why go through the entire tillage process if you don't have to? Furthermore, the soil benefits of the no-till approach are clearly demonstrable. When soil is tilled, the organic carbon locked away underground is oxidized by the atmosphere. What this means is the act of tillage itself produces atmospheric carbon dioxide. You lose fertility just by turning up the ground and emitting CO_2. In contrast, no-till systems result in much less wear and tear on your equipment!

Step-by-Step Field Prep

1. Flail-mow.

2. Apply compost.

3. Spade (tillage), then wait two weeks.

4. Apply pelletized fertilizer.

5. Shape beds or install plastic mulch.

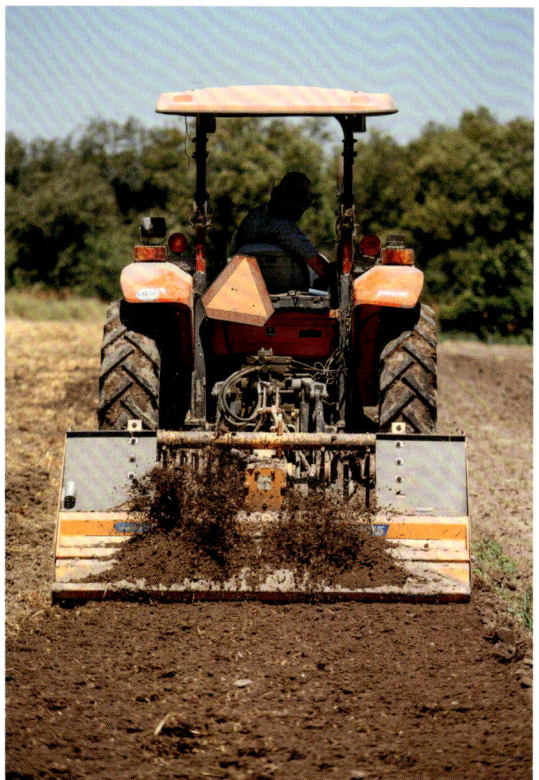

A mechanical spader leaving perfectly lofty soil

Effective Tillage Techniques

Although we are actively experimenting with no-till systems, we still make judicious use of tillage to prepare our fields for cannabis planting. There are a variety of factors to consider when choosing equipment, but the best combination of tools we have found over the years is a flail mower and a mechanical spader. For operations on our scale, mowing with a flail mower and then tilling with the spader produces the best results. The flail mower chops cover crops or crop residue into tiny pieces that are easily incorporated into the soil during spading and that decompose rapidly. For very large-scale operations, this setup is too slow. But small is beautiful—and it allows you to do the best job possible.

A mechanical spader, which is the equivalent of several shovels working simultaneously, is the most advanced but least affordable method of soil preparation for planting. It is run by the power take-off (PTO) device behind a tractor. The spader operates like a rototiller but with reciprocating spades. It is a superior method of soil preparation for planting, because unlike a rototiller, it improves the soil structure without creating a hardpan underneath the tilling layer. Moreover, the spader is capable of deeper tilling. The drawbacks to the spader are its slow speed and its many moving parts.

In clay soils, where spaders often will not leave perfect tilth, a rototiller or power harrow may need to be used in the top few inches of the bed. Spaders must be greased constantly and can break, leaving you in a pinch. Not only are you unable to use it, but you also have to fix it, which requires some advanced mechanical skills and sometimes esoteric parts. That's why we also have a drag disc on hand. The disc is heavy and requires multiple passes but gets the job done—albeit by really chewing up the soil structure and, if the soil is at all dry, producing massive dust clouds. It is the standard tool used in large-scale operations, as you can drive pretty fast with it and it tills a very wide swath per horsepower compared to PTO equipment.

When we open new ground, or in particularly difficult conditions, after mowing we occasionally use a two-bottom plow, which is extremely effective in turning over very well-established sod and unearthing bindweed taproots. We follow plowing with the drag disc or the spader to pulverize chunks and improve tilth. In new ground this often takes many passes. Finally, we use a deep ripper every few seasons to break up any hardpan and create softer soil for crop roots to penetrate.

Achieving good success during tillage requires working the soil at the appropriate soil

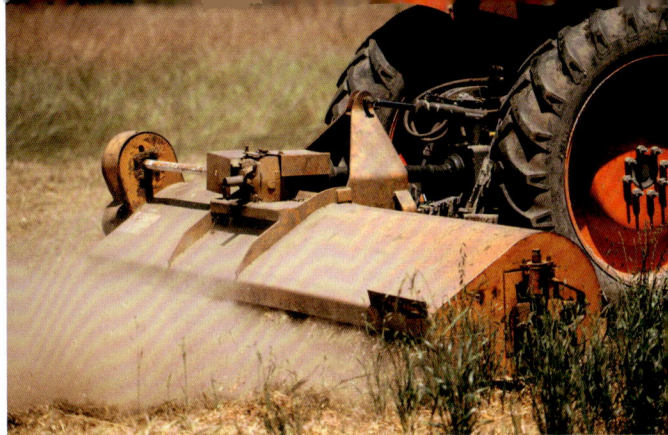

A flail mower is useful for pulverizing vegetation prior to incorporation through tillage.

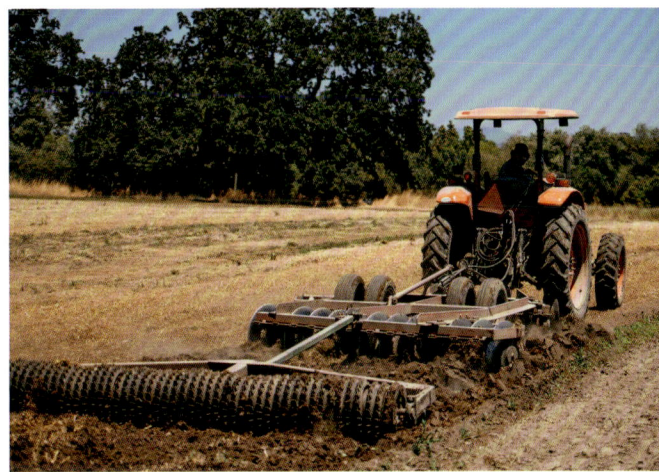

A drag disc is a ten-foot-wide disc with a roller behind to help break clods and smooth the soil.

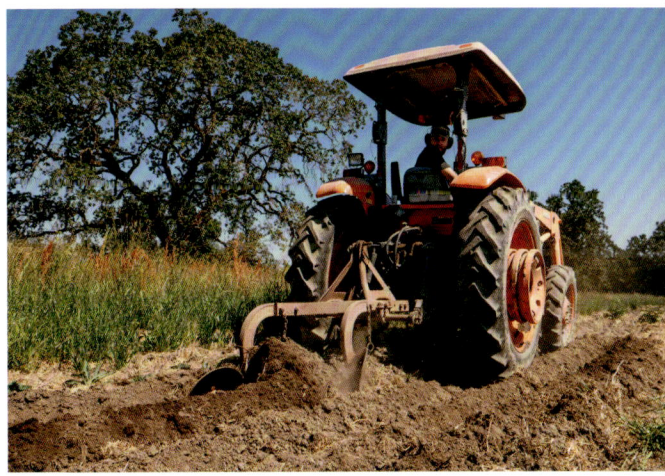

The two-bottom plow is the oldest tillage implement in agriculture and still has its uses.

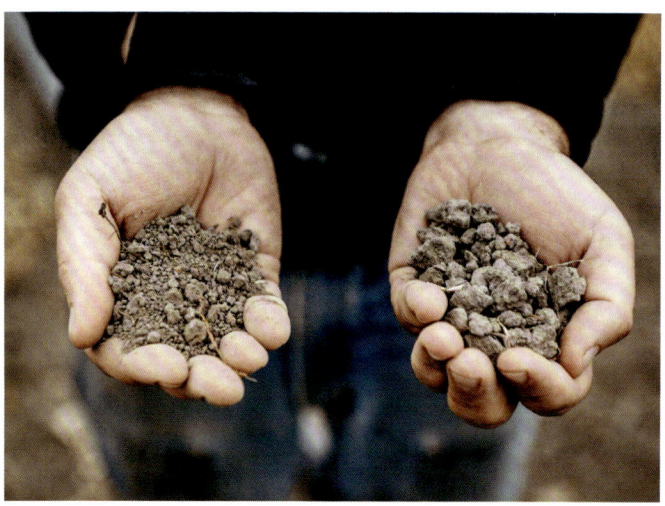

Performing tillage at the perfect soil moisture with the right tool creates the best tilth. Adam holds an example of well-worked soil (left) vs. micro-clods (right), which make direct sowing or setting transplants very difficult. Clumped soils like this also do not retain water well.

moisture level. "Appropriate" soil moisture describes a range of soil moistures that, tillage equipment depending, allow you to work your soil to a fine aggregate with as few passes as possible and minimal soil loss to wind. Ultimately, experience with tillage in your specific soil-type growing region is the most helpful tool and cannot be understated. If you are new to the area, we recommend talking to as many experienced local farmers as possible to get clued in to the specificities of the region. If you are unsure that soil moistures fall within these parameters, do a few trial passes and observe. Don't be afraid to stop and wait another week. If the soil is too wet, tillage will only need to be repeated, and soil compaction is a risk.

Before we move on, a word on tillage in fallow fields or virgin fields: It never ceases to amaze us how much tillage, and time, is required to properly prepare fallow fields. It takes two to six times more tillage passes and, depending on species (perennial or annual), may take an additional three months of decomposition before the field is ready for planting. As a rule, any fallow or virgin field should be worked thoroughly and cover cropped in fall, then worked again in spring prior to planting.

Achieving soil with plantable tilth, depth, and structure usually requires tilling, taking a break, then tilling one or two more times. In our fields we spade once or disc three or four times, wait two or three weeks, spade again or disc again one or two times, and finally shape beds. Regardless, the soil should be well worked and uniform with good particle size prior to planting. If you have large aggregate, effective transplanting can be difficult or even impossible. Look closely and pick up handfuls or shovelfuls of soil in various parts of the field to ensure that the soil is appropriate for planting. When clay soil clods dry out, they are usually impossible to break down further. Sometimes additional passes during primary tillage are required to reduce aggregate size, especially if warm and dry days are expected that will rapidly dry the soil.

Initial Application of Fertilizer

After primary tillage comes single-crop fertilizer application. We typically apply compost and other stable amendments such as rock dust, gypsum, or lime before breaking ground. This reduces compaction, because you avoid driving heavy and fully loaded equipment over tilled soil. However, if the field was not turned properly the year before or there are extensive divots and imperfections, it can make for quite the bumpy ride and cause additional wear and tear on equipment. When using a pelleted fertilizer, apply it just before planting, otherwise the nutrients could leach out of the soil before the crop has a chance to use them. We use a spreader cone and a tow-behind spreader to apply pelletized fertilizer before planting.

Leveling the Field

The last tillage tool we acquired, in hindsight, should have been one of the first: a pull-behind grader. This hydraulically raised and lowered scraping box flattens the field and fills in any dips or sinks. Over the years we lost plenty of crops by skipping this step. When there is too much topography in a field, irrigation water collects in the low points, and crops in those areas can be stunted by too much water. The tractor tire may sink during bed prep or cultivation, exacerbating the problem. Over time salts collect in low points, too. We have done soil testing in native low points in some of our wetter fields and found a four times higher concentration of salts there relative to higher points less than 10 feet away and only inches higher. As grading a field needs to be done only once, owning a grader is not necessary if you can hire a local operator to do the work.

Adam and Max inspect a recently shaped field for plantability.

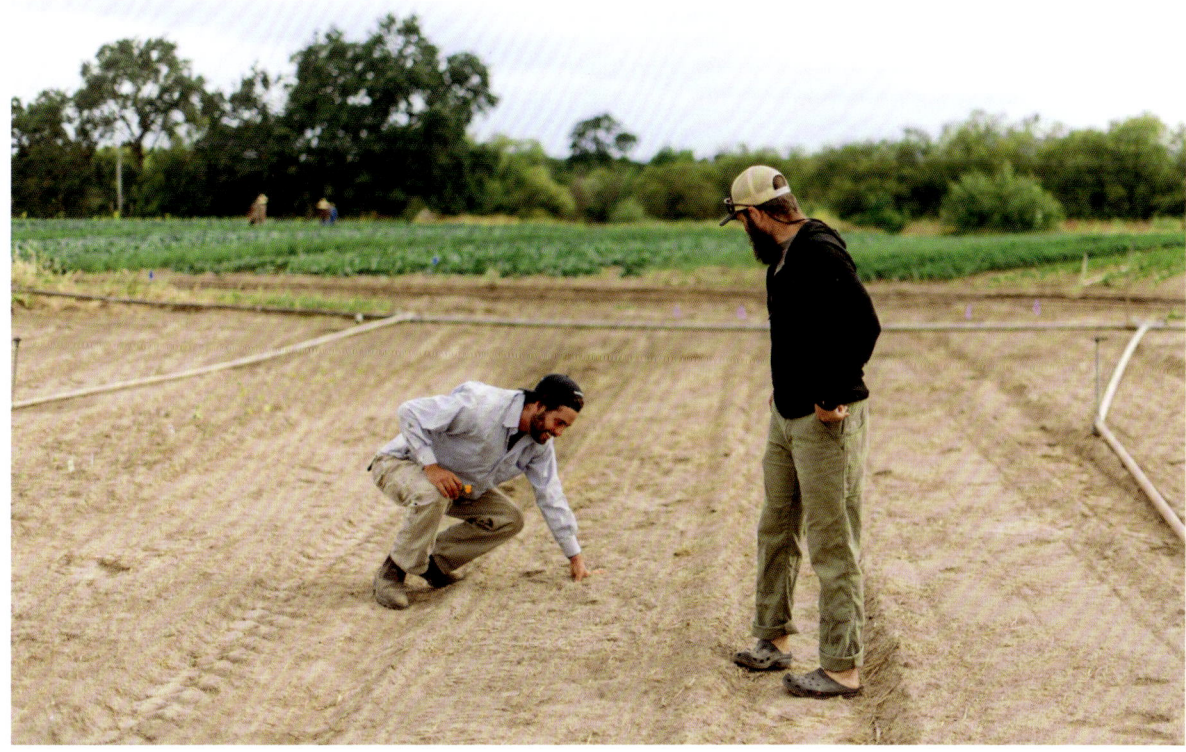

Shaping Beds

There are many reasons for having shaped beds, but the main advantage is that it allows you to provide conditions that encourage optimal plant health. With shaped beds, farmers can navigate their fields in defined furrows, thus confining compaction from foot traffic or tractors to specific areas. Limiting compaction assists with dry down and drainage in root zones, which gives ideal soil conditions to the crop. Defined beds also create a more technical layout for transplanting efficiency and quality. And finally, weed management and cultivation are streamlined in well-shaped beds.

We use a variety of equipment to shape beds, depending on the soil conditions, the time of year, and the size of the plants.

Rototiller shaper. This implement begins with a rototiller that has simple shaping discs and a leveling bar behind it. We do not like rototillers in general because they burn up organic matter, destroy soil structure, and leave a till pan, which can be especially detrimental to the crop. However, many farmers use tiller/shapers and still have success.

Pan shaper. These implements are steel welded into the shape of a bed. As you drive the tractor, soil is pulled into the pan (usually by gathering discs or shanks) and compressed within it, leaving a perfect contour. Your tillage needs to be exceptional before using a pan shaper. Our plastic mulch layer has a pan shaper, and we have used only the plan shaper component on occasion (without laying plastic).

Cultimulcher. This has a very small tiller that works only the top 2 to 4 inches of soil as well as a pan shaper. It combines gentle tillage with a very sturdy pan to produce an exceptional bed. This class of equipment produces an excellent seed bed for direct sowing or for putting in small transplants. However, as it creates the seed bed, it also tightly packs the soil, which makes planting large plants more challenging.

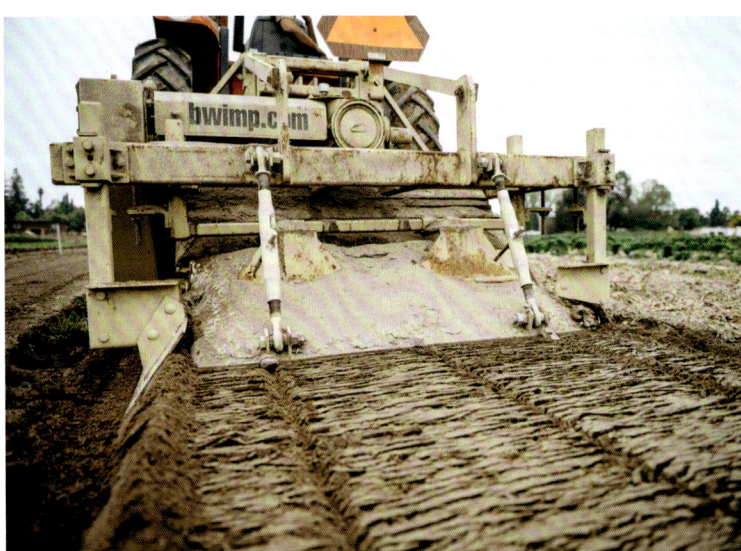

After trying almost every cheaper option available we finally settled on the cultimulcher for making beds, and we never looked back. Notice the three evenly spaced lines behind the tool—we added bolts to the pan to mark beds as we make them.

Tractor tires. If your primary tillage leaves you with great loft (we find the spader does an amazing job of this), then you have the option of "shaping beds" by simply driving your tractor in straight rows down the field. We have used this approach more frequently in recent years when primary tillage has gone smoothly, because it reduces a tillage step, which is better for the soil and results in less wear and tear on our equipment.

Homemade bed shapers. We fabricated a bed shaper using a thick toolbar, a Perfecta roller, hilling discs, and a section of spike-tooth harrow. This bed shaper creates a tall, well-drained, and lofty bed. We use this bed shaper regularly.

Plastic Mulch Considerations

There is a philosophical and ethical decision to make when preparing beds with plastic mulch. Plastic trash and microtrash are pervasive, and we prefer when reasonably possible not to use plastic mulch. However, it does have resource conservation benefits: It significantly decreases water usage and eliminates cultivation passes with the tractor, thus reducing overall diesel use per crop cycle.

Plastic mulch is primarily used with high-value crops such as strawberries, tomatoes, and peppers, or with long-day crops such as onions that require lots of weeding. The added cost of materials plus additional labor to lay the plastic, remove it, and throw it away contribute to plastic mulch being used only in specific situations. Although it costs more and is generally used on high-value crops, plastic mulch has a whole range of potential benefits.

There are a wide variety of plastic mulch layers on the market. Make sure you choose one that is thoroughly vetted, in person by you, in the conditions or soil type that you will be laying plastic mulch in. We went through three models before finding one that really worked—the Rain-Flo 2570. You really do get what you pay for. If you are oscillating between options, we recommend looking at the weights of the models and choosing the heaviest option.

Benefits to Using Plastic Mulch

In some cases, plastic mulch is the best option to aid in conserving water, suppressing weed growth, and keeping roots warm during cooler seasons.

Regulates water usage. Plastic mulch limits soil dry down, significantly reducing water use and increasing water efficiency. In spring and early-summer field trials, we found that using plastic mulch reduced water use by 50 to 70 percent. This can be a double-edged sword, depending on your fertility management program. Because we water only once or twice a week for about 40 minutes at a time, we have fewer opportunities to fertilize. Consequently, we focus heavily on soil health and front-loading our soil with fertility. If your program is centered around a heavy and very frequent liquid fertility program, using plastic mulch could be challenging. Humidity, wind, temperature, and soil type are all factors in dry down and need to be thoughtfully considered in deciding whether to use plastic mulch.

Note that water wheel transplanters come with water tanks for watering in at transplant time. Many growers include some fertilizer or compost tea for this initial watering to help kick-start the crop. We have observed decreased transplant shock and more explosive growth when using this strategy.

In regions where rainfall is plentiful or excessive during the growing season, plastic mulch may be used for water exclusion. Cannabis plants want a regular dry-down period during most parts of their life cycle at or less than 50 percent of soil moisture capacity. With plastic mulch, only a small percentage of rainfall enters the hole where the plant is. The rest of the water is shed off the plastic, and thus the root zone stays drier.

It is very satisfying when the plastic mulch layer works correctly, though it rarely does. The first row must be perfectly straight, as any imperfections are magnified as more beds are laid.

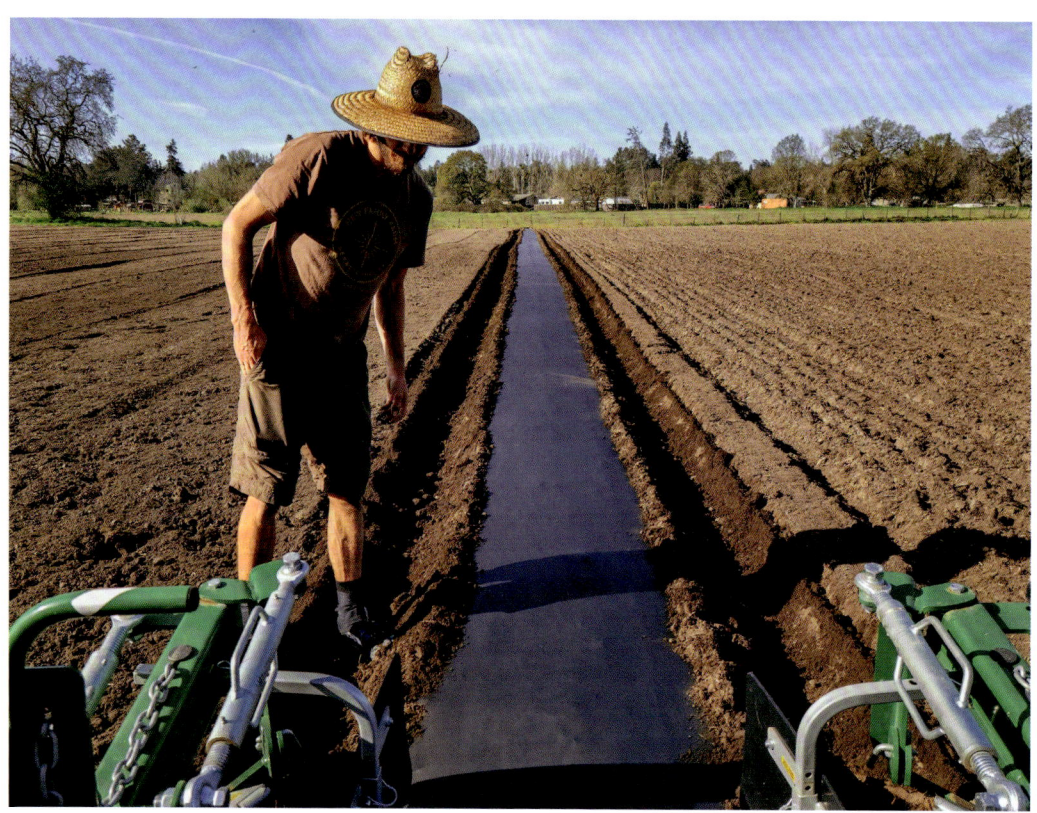

Planting

Suppresses weeds. For longer crops such as onions or photoperiod cannabis, plastic mulch may save a farmer from the labor of five or more weeding passes both by hand and mechanically. Depending on the weed seed bank, weeds may sprout and still need to be maintained in the walkways between the beds, on the shoulder of the bed where dirt holds the plastic in place, and in the holes where the crop is planted. Plastic mulch saves money by reducing cultivation costs, but there is another benefit. Anytime a farmer performs a cultivation activity around a standing crop, shallow feeder roots are killed. Depending on the cultivation tools being used and the operator, a substantial and meaningful number of roots may be disturbed or killed. For shallow and/or weakly rooted crops such as new transplants or just clones in general, cultivation practices slow down plant growth.

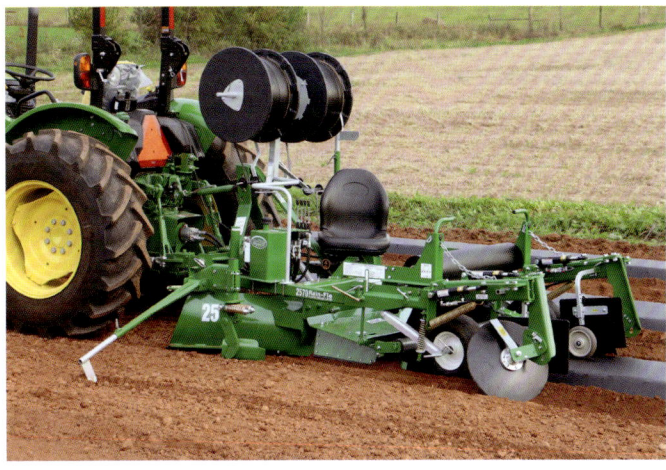

When selecting mulch layers, the heavier the better. We use the largest Rain-Flo model. Photograph courtesy of Rain-Flo

Warms root zones. Cannabis plants thrive with warm soil, and on a sunny day temperatures under plastic mulch can be up to 30°F warmer than ambient temperatures. This can be especially helpful in spring or fall for season extension or in a region where the primary growing season does not have temperatures in ideal ranges for cannabis.

Potentially increases yield. Plastic mulch use with tomatoes has been shown to increase yields by up to 20 percent. The red spectrum worked the best. More research is needed to determine if a specific color of plastic is more beneficial for cannabis.

Difficulties in Using Plastic Mulch

Working with plastic mulch can sometimes create more problems than it solves, so it's important to consider the challenges before deciding if it's right for your setup.

Requires exacting soil preparation. The main challenge with plastic mulch is that every step before you lay the mulch must be perfect. The soil must be worked with great tilth and little to no aggregate. Fist-size chunks of soil or partially decomposed cover crop are absolute no-nos; having even fingernail-size aggregate can make the job challenging. In addition to minimal aggregate, the soil needs to be worked deeply. We recommend a deep rip or plow in conjunction with a spader or a disc.

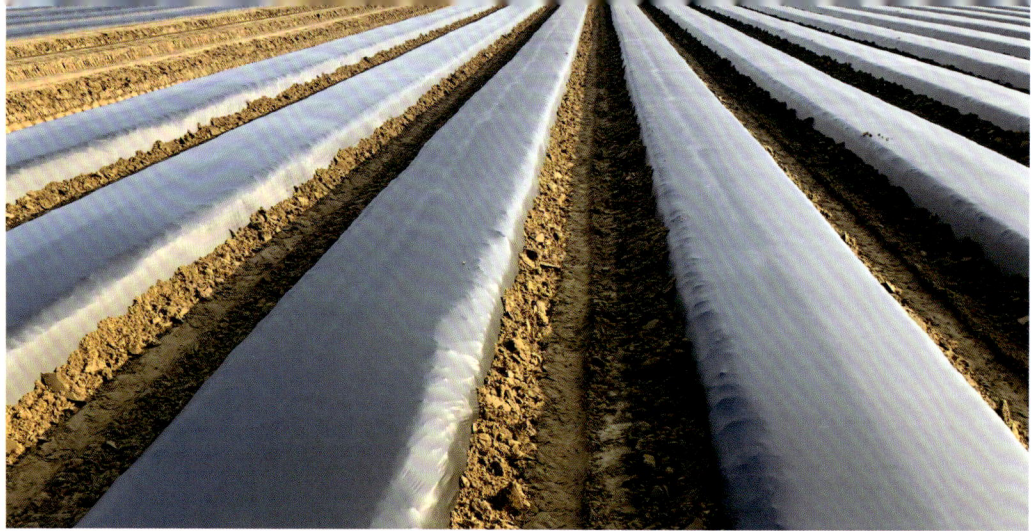

After primary tillage and before laying plastic, we recommend listing or rough shaping. You can do this with a variety of tools, including hilling discs or a pan shaper. This process delineates where the bed will be located, and it helps avoid air gaps when laying the plastic. Finally, the process of laying plastic mulch requires a talented and patient team. Getting it set up and working correctly takes time and many micro-adjustments. Do not attempt it on a windy day!

If you are planting on a large acreage in an agricultural hub, consider hiring someone who does custom ag work and has extensive experience laying plastic.

Can come loose. If the plastic isn't laid perfectly, you will end up with loose or flapping sections of plastic. Flapping plastic mulch, which we refer to as FPM, can lead to other problems. First, FPM traps hot air, which escapes through the holes where the plants are planted, potentially frying tender seedlings. Second, FPM can create a parachute effect that swallows transplants and kills whole sections. And finally, FPM builds on itself like a snowball rolling down a hill, eventually coming off entirely and covering any remaining living seedlings.

Hides soil from view. This makes it difficult to see damage from gophers, moles, rats, mice, and other pests working at or below the soil level. It also makes it hard to find irrigation leaks or places where lines are clogged. In general, irrigating thoroughly and effectively is more difficult, although it does not necessarily take more time overall because most people irrigate less or use fewer cycles with plastic mulch.

Complicates end-of-season cleanup. On our farm, at the end of a crop cycle, we hitch the flail mower and mow all the stocks to a pulp and then use the disc to incorporate the stubble into the soil. When you have plastic mulch, there is an extra labor step of pulling it out or using another specialized removal tool. The mulch is then bundled and brought to the landfill. Regardless of how you remove the mulch, there will inevitably be a certain amount of microplastic left in your field.

Planting into Plastic Mulch

If you choose to go the plastic mulch route, you will also need a planter designed to work through plastic mulch. If you want to direct seed into plastic, you will need a specialized seeder. If you choose to transplant, we have found success with the Rain-Flo water wheel transplanter. We like it so much that we even use it to plant fields that aren't mulched in plastic.

Just as laying plastic mulch is a specialized skill, planting into plastic takes practice. First, we've calculated that planting through plastic mulch is roughly half as fast as transplanting into well-worked native soil. Operators may have to make regular adjustments including:

- Adjusting the flow of the water

- Positioning the seats if they start tearing the plastic

- Positioning the wheels to avoid damaging the drip lines, which are under the plastic

- De-mudding the transplant wheel, depending on water flow and soil conditions

- Stopping to wash off muddy hands to continue planting quickly and accurately

Another consideration with plastic mulch is how to appropriately harden off plants. Regardless of the degree of FPM you might encounter, a certain amount of air that is much hotter than ambient temperature escapes from under the mulch, which can stress or even kill seedlings. If the forecast is calling for very hot days, the seedlings may need a few extra days of hardening off to make sure their stems and leaves are ready for the shock.

This is especially tricky when planting autoflowering crops. These plants prefer uninterrupted growth, which is especially challenging in spring with variable conditions that may leave you limited in capacity to thoroughly harden off plants. There needs to be a balance between utilizing the lush conditions of the greenhouse to get the vigorous growth we all want to see and getting the plants properly acclimated. We recommend that you take these situations on a case-by-case basis.

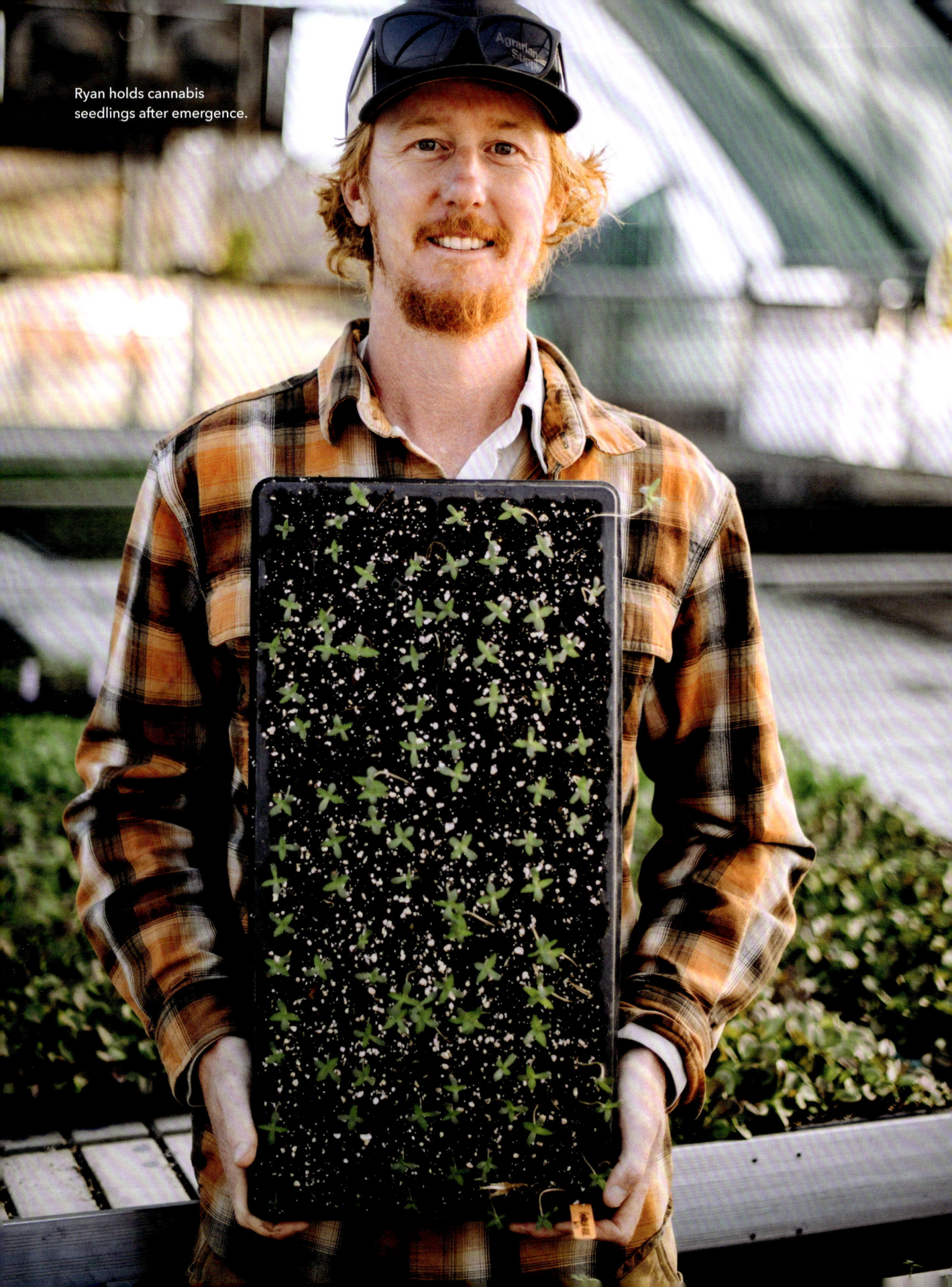

Ryan holds cannabis
seedlings after emergence.

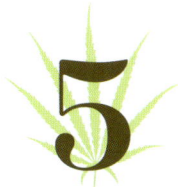

Propagation

Propagation is the process of germinating seeds and preparing them for transplant. Good farmers know that the first steps in the crop cycle are the most important: Tillage/bed prep→ healthy transplants→ appropriate irrigation→ first cultivation. Mistakes made at the beginning of the season jeopardize the success of the entire crop. This chapter focuses on the requirements for producing healthy transplants. Autoflowers present their own difficulties: They are extremely finicky and have a low tolerance for stress or mistreatment. Therefore, we address each category of plants separately.

Starting Autoflower Seeds

Autoflowers perform best when directly seeded into the soil, so if direct seeding is practical, we recommend this approach. We talk about direct sowing more extensively in Chapter 6. Unfortunately, direct seeding isn't practical for many farmers. This means that farmers are forced to go through a gauntlet of challenges to successfully propagate and transplant autoflower seedlings. Most important, achieving good yields is dependent on uninterrupted root growth and minimizing shock or stress to the young plants.

Autoflowers need to be transplanted somewhere between day 8 and 15 from seeding. This is an extremely early transplant date relative to other commonly transplanted annuals, such as broccoli or tomatoes. This necessitates the need for what's called a floating medium.

Choosing a Floating Medium

There are three main approaches to floating mediums.

Peat plugs or stone wool cubes are most often used for cloning, though many home or hobby growers use them for starting seeds. We don't generally recommend them because they are unnecessarily expensive, require more careful fertility management during the propagation phase (since they contain no fertility), and do not decompose.

Growcoons are biodegradable, perforated plastic inserts (they look like small, rigid nets) that you manually put into 10 × 20-cell trays. There are some logistics associated with pairing the Growcoons correctly with different tray manufacturers, so be sure to try combinations before purchasing. After the Growcoons are inserted into your 10 × 20 trays, you fill them with your choice of potting soil. With Growcoons you must utilize a high-quality, vetted, and trusted source of potting soil. We have made the mistake of using subpar potting soils either to save money or because we weren't sure what would work best. Doing so netted us a whole bunch of problems: fungus gnats, fertility-starved plants, seedlings that stayed too wet or dried down too fast.

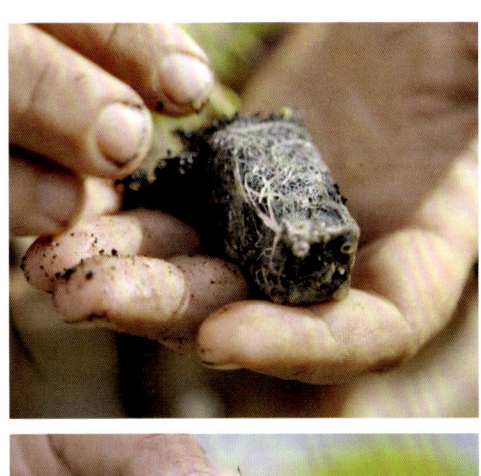

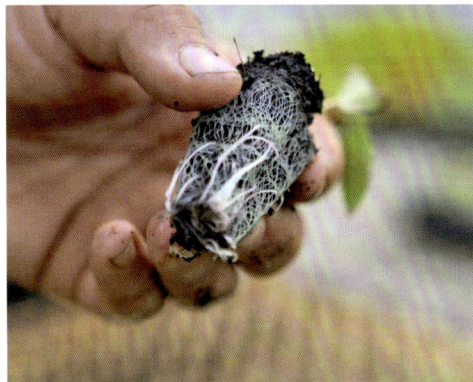

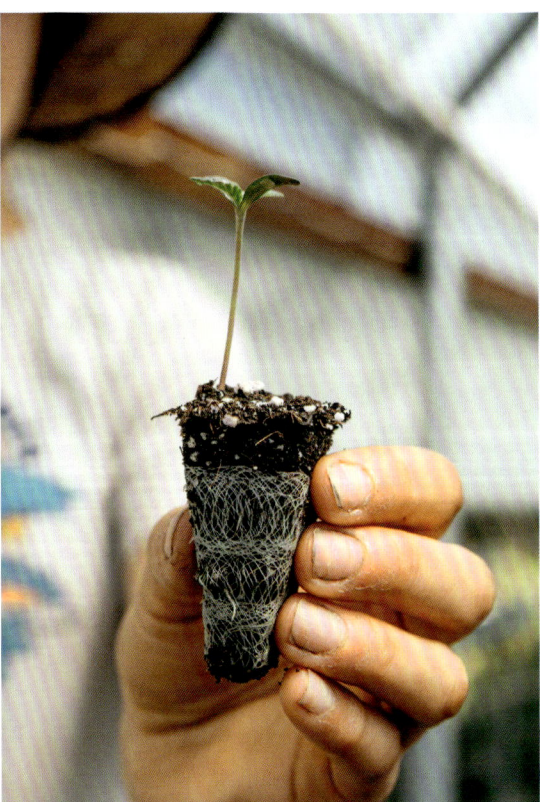

The advantage of Growcoons is the ability to pull transplants long before they are rootbound. These are perfectly rooted transplants at day 12 from sowing. This additional cost and process is only warranted with autoflowers.

Ellepots are made with a proprietary paper that holds a custom blend of potting soil and is formed into a cylinder that fits inside the cell of a 10 × 20 tray. We like Ellepots because they are part of a simple and streamlined system. The Ellepot trays come prefilled with the Ellepots, which minimizes labor. We pull the trays off the pallets they come stacked on and insert them right into our seeding line. The main drawback is that roots have some difficulty penetrating the paper membrane, so we see decreased root growth relative to the Growcoon or in straight soil.

Choosing the Right Tray Size

Factors that influence tray size choice include availability of greenhouse space and crew, transplant timing flexibility, and desired plant size. For available greenhouse space, the considerations are simple: You need to be able to fit all the trays in the greenhouse. In terms of the crew, make sure you have enough people to plant and water in the number of starts available on a given day. There is no point to starting 10,000 seeds in one day if you do not have the equipment and crew sufficient for transplanting all the seedlings in the correct time frame of 8 to 15 days.

We have found success with anywhere from 50- to 128-cell trays. Keep in mind that a bigger cell size can net you a bigger plant and gives you a larger window to transplant and still avoid root binding or plant stress. It's also important to note that 128-cell trays are two and a half times more space efficient than 50-cell trays.

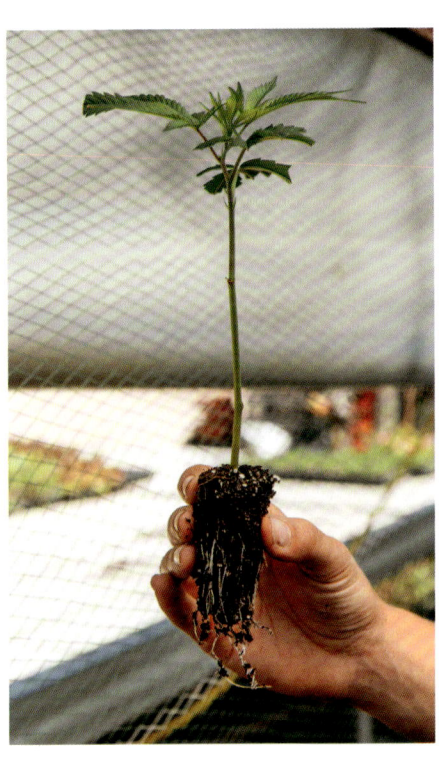

Full term seedling in a 72-cell tray plug

 ## Damping-Off

Damping-off is a fungal infection on the stems of newly germinated plants that causes the tiny babies to just fall over and die. It is commonly spread by fungus gnats but can be present without them. At times we have seen our greenhouse swarming with fungus gnats that rest on the surface of the soil, but when we pass our hand over the seedling trays, the insects fly up in a cloud. Some soil mixes are sterilized for this reason.

Applying pesticides in propagation is not ideal at all and weakens the seedlings, which can lead to issues throughout the crop cycle. We take a biological approach and use the product RootShield to prevent damping-off or other fungal diseases.

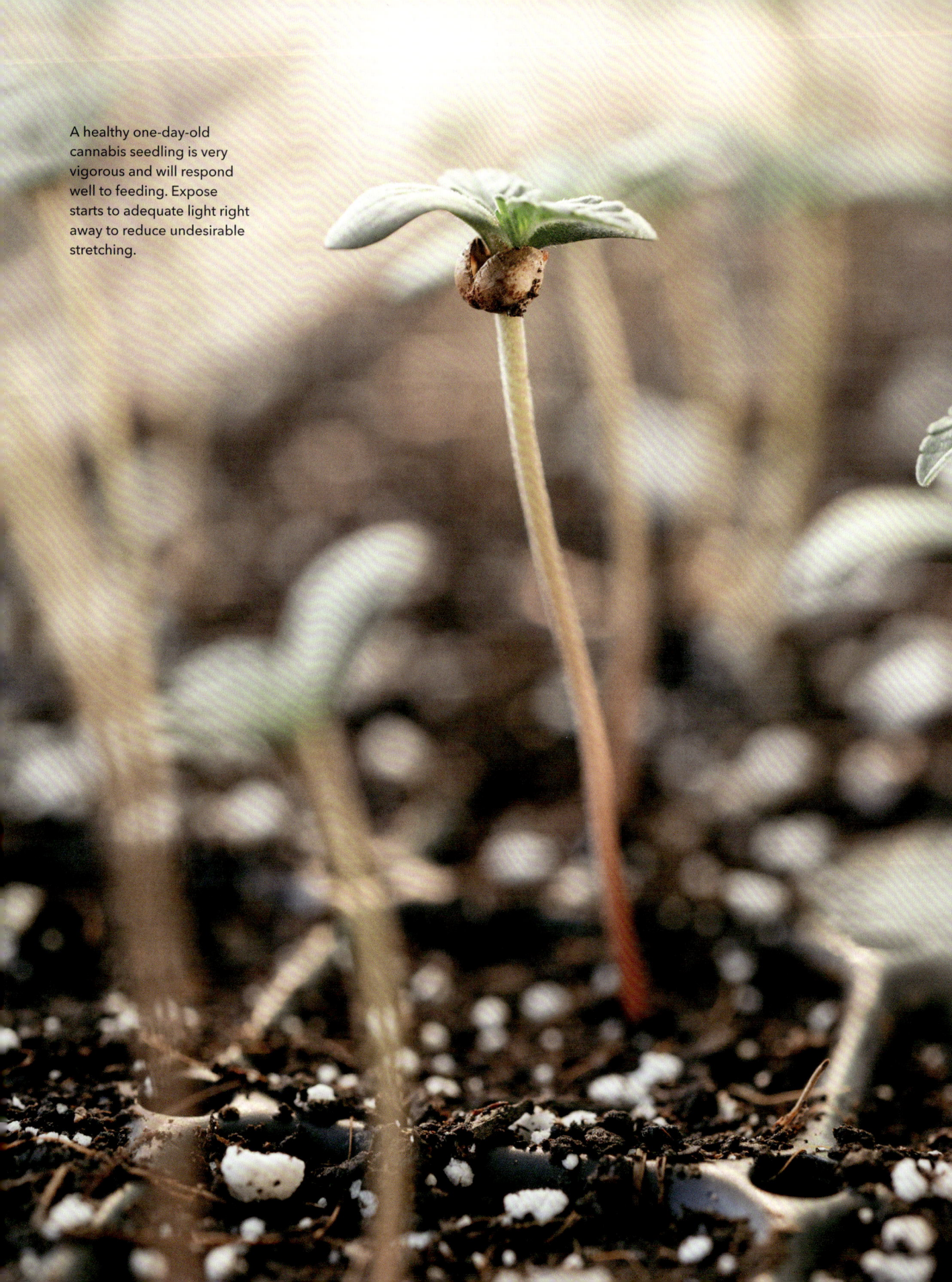

A healthy one-day-old cannabis seedling is very vigorous and will respond well to feeding. Expose starts to adequate light right away to reduce undesirable stretching.

Starting Full-Term and Semi-Full-Term Seeds

Full-term and semi-full-term seeds are not usually sensitive to root binding or stress in the propagation phase. For this reason, and for the fact that full-term seed is usually much more expensive than auto seed, we only recommend direct seeding for those who have extensive experience and excellent soil preparation.

Because seeds in this class are hearty and vigorous in the propagation phase, they do not require a floating medium. Depending on available greenhouse space, we prefer using bigger cell trays. Be sure to choose a high-quality potting soil and/or a proper fertigation plan during this early phase of growth.

Full-term plants can tolerate being rootbound and are *much* more resilient than autoflowering plants. (Being rootbound can slow or stunt plants, but it makes seedlings easier to remove from the cells.) Seedlings can be up-potted into larger containers depending on scale, weather conditions, field conditions, and availability of labor. Anything larger than a seedling tray cannot be mechanically transplanted. For operations larger than 5 acres, we do not think up-potting is economical in terms of additional soil or labor. For hand-scale transplanting, we regularly up-pot in 3- or 4-inch pots so the plants are well established, larger, and more resilient for transplant. Anything larger than that becomes impractical very quickly.

Always Have Extra Plants

When ordering seed, order 25 percent extra. When ordering transplants from a nursery, order 5 percent extra (usually they will give you extras as part of their internal calculations). It's always better to have plants or seed left over at the end of a planting cycle rather than find yourself short. Some seed will not germinate, some will not emerge, some will grow poorly or lack vigor, and some plants get broken during transplanting. Make sure to account for realistic losses at each step.

Also, have a plan for a complete crop loss in propagation. Rats, mice, birds, an employee who "forgot" to water or open the greenhouse, a malfunctioning automatic watering system, a sneaky heavy frost: We've seen it all, and most growers will experience at least one of these setbacks. Do you have reliable and quick access to more plants or more seed? It's best to have a backup option in mind going into the season.

Seeding

There is a certain scale, or a certain number of transplants produced annually, at which seeding by hand is overly laborious and starts to feel ridiculous. For seeding more than a few acres, we recommend a vacuum seeder. There are many different vacuum seeders, and it's important to identify the one that is appropriate for your scale.

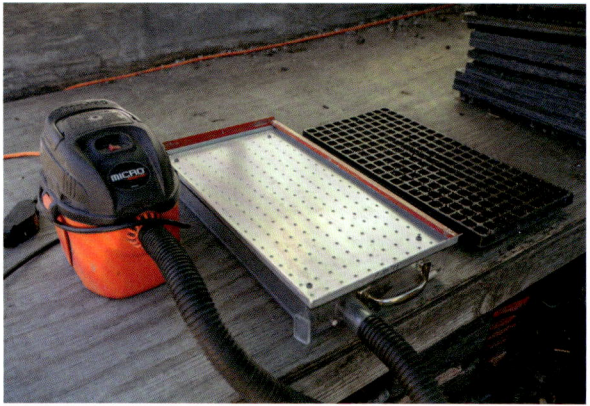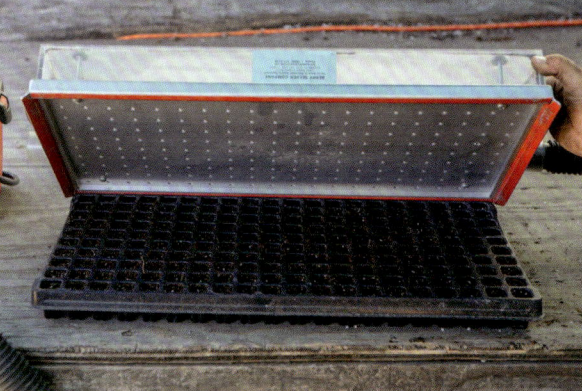

The vacuum seeder is a very efficient way to sow trays quickly and accurately. Tray sizes sometimes vary, so check that your tray and the plate for the seeder are matched. Much more expensive and sophisticated models are available for larger operations.

We have a Berry vacuum seeder (readily available online) that utilizes a small household vacuum plugged into a chambered tray that fits over a 10 × 20 tray. The top of the chamber is a removable plate that can accommodate different tray sizes.

Using it is simple, at least in theory. Dump some seed onto the plate and swirl it around until it lands in the holes, turn the vacuum on, then flip the chambered tray upside down onto your fully prepped 10 × 20 tray. Turn the vacuum off to let the seed fall into the tray and you're done. Admittedly, there is some trial and error to get the system working well, but we love the adaptability and cost (around $1,000) for a piece of equipment that makes the job go four to eight times faster than seeding by hand. For small lots of seed, say less than a thousand seeds, we recommend hand seeding. The process of "seeding by hand" literally means dropping each individual seed one by one into each cell of your 10 × 20 tray.

Planting Depth
Plant autos and photos roughly ¼ inch deep, and gently cover the seeds with soil.

Watering
After planting either autos or photos, water them heavily, though not to the point of leaving standing water in the cell tray. Keep them on the spectrum from moist to wet (not soaked or soggy!) prior to emergence. In mild or cool conditions, trays may not need water for 24 hours or longer, whereas on hot, dry, or windy days, they may need water five times a day or more. Allowing trays to dry down in cool conditions—though never bone dry—may be helpful in avoiding algal growth on the top layer of soil, which is a common sight in overwatered, poorly ventilated, or just generally cool spaces. After seedling emergence, water anywhere from one to three times a day, depending

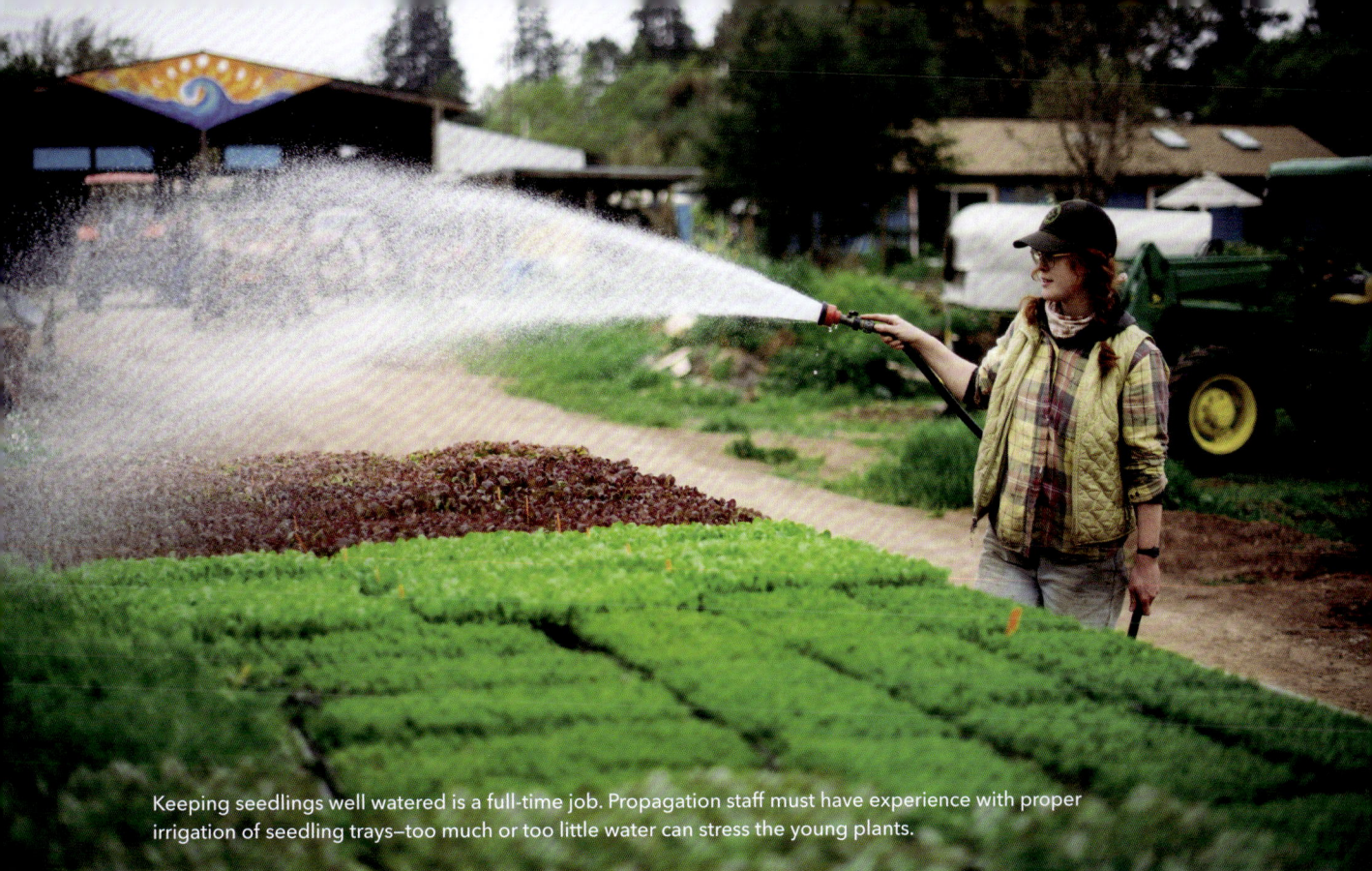

Keeping seedlings well watered is a full-time job. Propagation staff must have experience with proper irrigation of seedling trays—too much or too little water can stress the young plants.

on your medium and temperatures. The seedlings enjoy a wet-to-dry swing, so do not keep them always wet. Conversely, never allow them to dry down completely.

Days to Emergence

Germination refers to moment when the first root, called a radicle, emerges underground from the seed itself. *Emergence* refers to the point when the first leaves break through the soil into the light.

When autos and photos are kept in the optimum temperature range, seeds should germinate in 48 to 72 hours and should be finished emerging after six days.

Ideal Germination Temperature

For both autos and photos, the ideal germination temperature range is 75 to 80°F (24 to 27°C) and greater than or equal to 70 percent relative humidity. We recommend using a germination chamber, heat mats, or a climate-controlled greenhouse to aid in thorough, quick, and even emergence. After experimenting with many different setups, we settled on using a germination chamber. This is a small, enclosed space with racks for seedling trays and a heating/humidity system that maintains the interior at the perfect condition. This is the most space-efficient and reliable way to achieve the best germination rates.

There are fancy germ chambers available for purchase through greenhouse supply companies, but it is quite simple to build one yourself. The internet is full of examples and do-it-yourself guides.

We typically leave trays in the chamber until we see the first few seedlings emerging, then we bring them all into the greenhouse. Because the chamber does not have lighting, there is a danger of overly stretchy seedlings that make for poor transplanters. This makes the timing of the move especially important.

Light Requirements

For autos and photos seedlings, there is no need for supplemental light. In some instances, however, supplemental light may play multiple functions (serving as both heat and light), so if it's in the flow, let them glow. It is the easiest time in the life cycle of the plant to give them the highest-quality care, so take this into consideration. Note that clones do need supplemental light in early spring before the natural light cycle is at 15 hours, otherwise they could flip into their flowering cycle earlier than desired.

Be careful when weaning plants off supplemental light before planting them in the field. We recommend a gradual reduction, say 15 to 30 minutes a day until the natural light cycle is met, rather than dropping from 18 total hours per day to 15 hours a day. Some genetics are more sensitive than others to the number of hours of sunlight needed to maintain vegetative growth and/or sudden and drastic changes in the hours of light per day. Regardless, a well-planned transition from supplemental lighting to natural light is key to maintaining vegetative growth in spring as the plants move from propagation to the field.

Soil Fertility

For autos and photos, a pre-transplant fertility program is highly dependent on the type of potting soil used and the size of the tray. We always recommend using more expensive and higher-quality potting soil rather than a cheaper one. Sometimes the ingredients list on the bag paints an incomplete picture of the fertilizers contained, so we recommend calling the potting soil company directly to speak with someone who deals with commercial growers to get more information. Regardless of the type of potting soil, we advise watering transplants with compost tea and mostly nitrogen fertilizers immediately after emergence and continuing every one to three days, depending on conditions.

Days to Transplant

With autos, transplant as early as your equipment, labor, and the plants' physical condition allow. If you let the plants sit in their containers too long, it will stress them and trigger early flowering, which can significantly reduce yields. Depending on the size

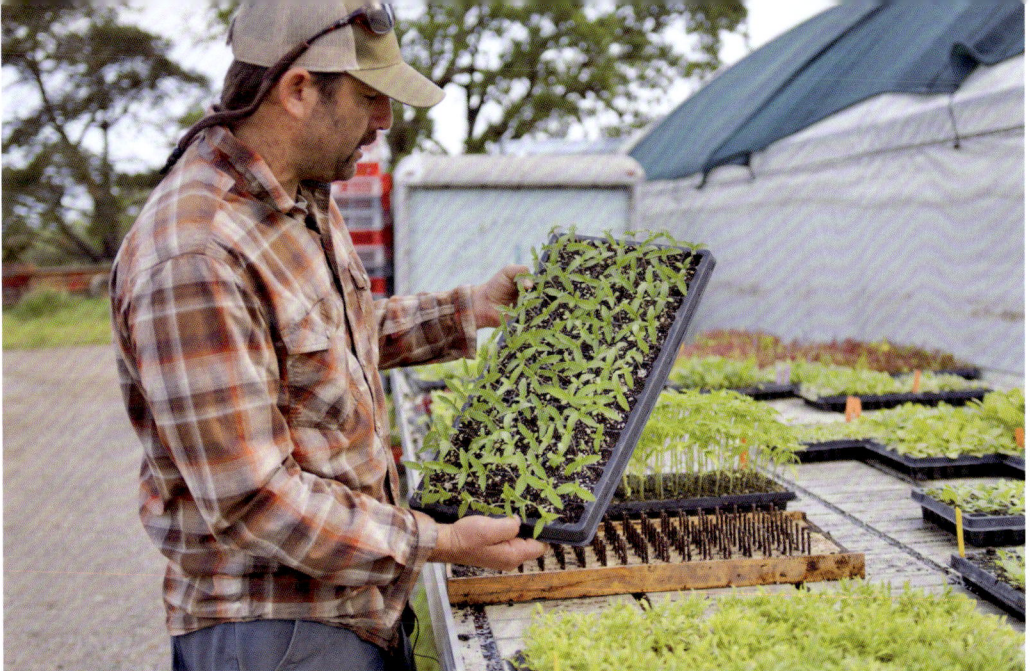

Adam inspects a tray of autoflowers ready for transplant.

of your container and your propagation conditions, we recommend planting at 8 to 15 days from sowing. If you have to let the plants sit in trays for longer than is ideal, make sure they are getting watered and fertilized appropriately.

With photos, since these plants are more resilient and will not initiate flowering quickly like autos, we recommend transplanting sometime between day 15 and 25. You don't need to take special precautions with full-term and semi-full-term crops when transplanting. Use common sense and they will be fine.

With autos, however, try to avoid shocking them at all costs. Here are a few tips.

To Avoid Shock, Do Not:

- Over-water or under-water.

- Over-fertilize or under-fertilize.

- Let them get too cold or too hot. Be especially vigilant with black seedling trays: If the floating medium is not firmly pressed against the side of the tray, little pockets of air can heat up and bake and kill tiny roots. Use shade cloth in hot climates.

- Let transplants get rootbound.

- Handle them roughly at transplanting.

- Transplant too late in the day in sunny or hot conditions.

- Expose roots to light for longer than necessary.

- Sneeze within 30 feet of them or speak of politics within earshot. (Okay, we're overexaggerating now, but you get the point: Autoflower transplants are sensitive.)

Hardening Off

Hardening off refers to the process of moving seedlings from the protected conditions of the greenhouse and into conditions closer to those they will be exposed to in the field. The best time to perform the initial move is in the late afternoon so plants will get a gentle introduction to direct sunlight. Hardening off is an important step to reduce the risk of transplant shock, but when improperly executed can induce shock of its own.

Since autos are more delicate and younger when transplanted, extra care must be taken with hardening off. Pay attention to the weather forecast, and do not remove trays from the greenhouse when temperatures are at or below 40°F (4°C) at night. Do not set trays into direct sunlight when temperatures are above 85°F (29°C). Meticulously check trays to ensure that they have proper moisture, as they will dry down quicker in direct sun. In conditions unfavorable for hardening off, a middle ground can be achieved by setting trays somewhere with partial shade, or outside but covered with floating row cover at night. Sometimes, due to unfavorable weather, we have been forced to skip hardening off altogether. In such cases pay close attention to conditions and proceed with care.

Once the plants have left the greenhouse to harden off, extra care must be taken if night temperatures get near freezing.

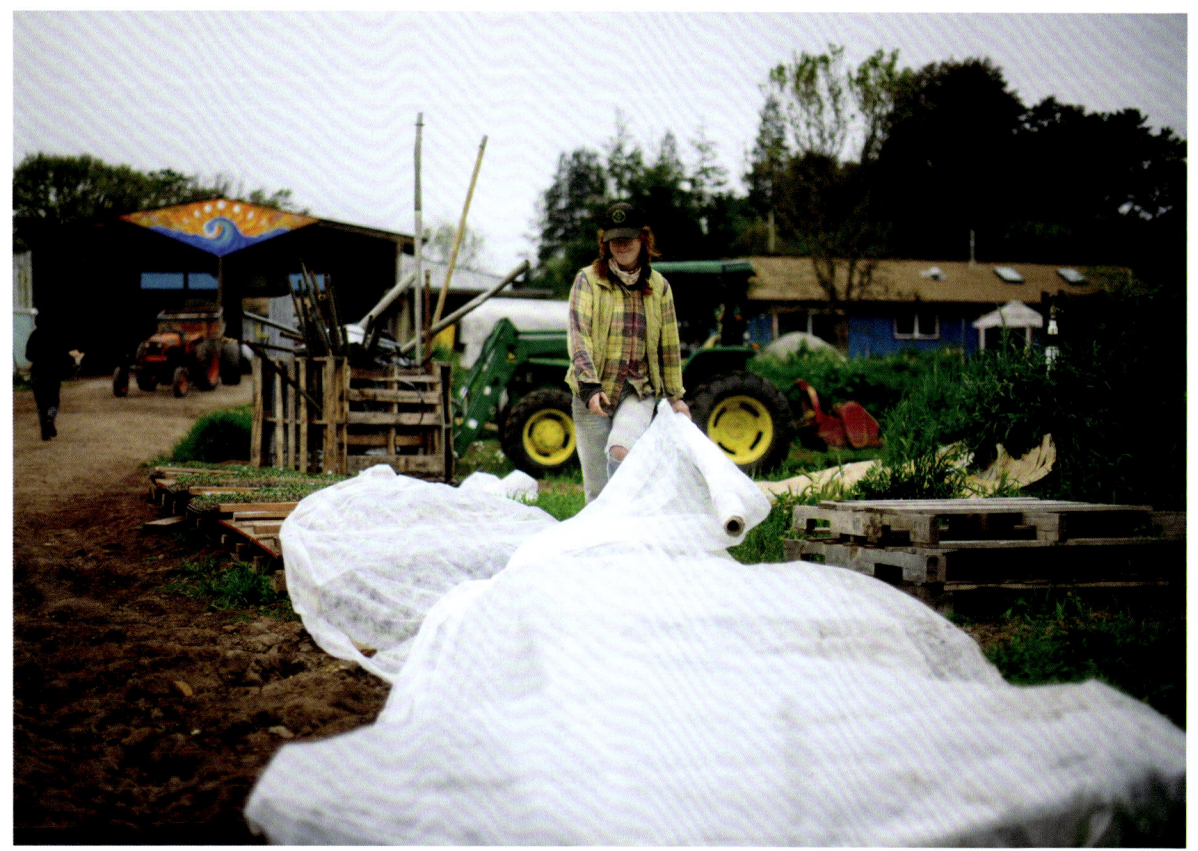

How to Navigate Commercial Nurseries

As the industry matures, more and more professional nurseries offer clones and seedlings. There are definite advantages to outsourcing propagation in a cultivation system, as well as some disadvantages. We prefer to propagate in-house so that we can nail exact timing for precision planting schedules. Due to the sensitive nature of autoflower starts, we like to do it ourselves, so we are sure that no stress events occurred and we know we are planting a well-tended seedling. That said, we have come across expert nursery operations that we would trust to perform this function.

When it comes to clones, we outsource. We have done our own cloning in the past but always found that it requires too much specific infrastructure, is slow and awkward, and has a steep learning curve. However, sourcing clones from outside your farm opens you up to pest and disease transmission. It happens all the time.

We have identified a few themes that help us choose which nursery to work with. First and foremost, visit the nursery and see their operation for yourself. Once there, look at their mother stock—do the plants appear healthy? Are pests present? Ask about their pest- and disease-mitigation protocols. To address the hop latent viroid, some nurseries have gone to extremes—utilizing tissue culture, keeping super-clean mother stock in a separate room from the production stock, etc. Ask the nursery if they bring in clones from other nurseries to fill orders when their production is insufficient. Use your inner lie detector to judge their answer. We're not kidding. Ask the nursery for grower references if you do not have any already. Ask around—it will be time well spent.

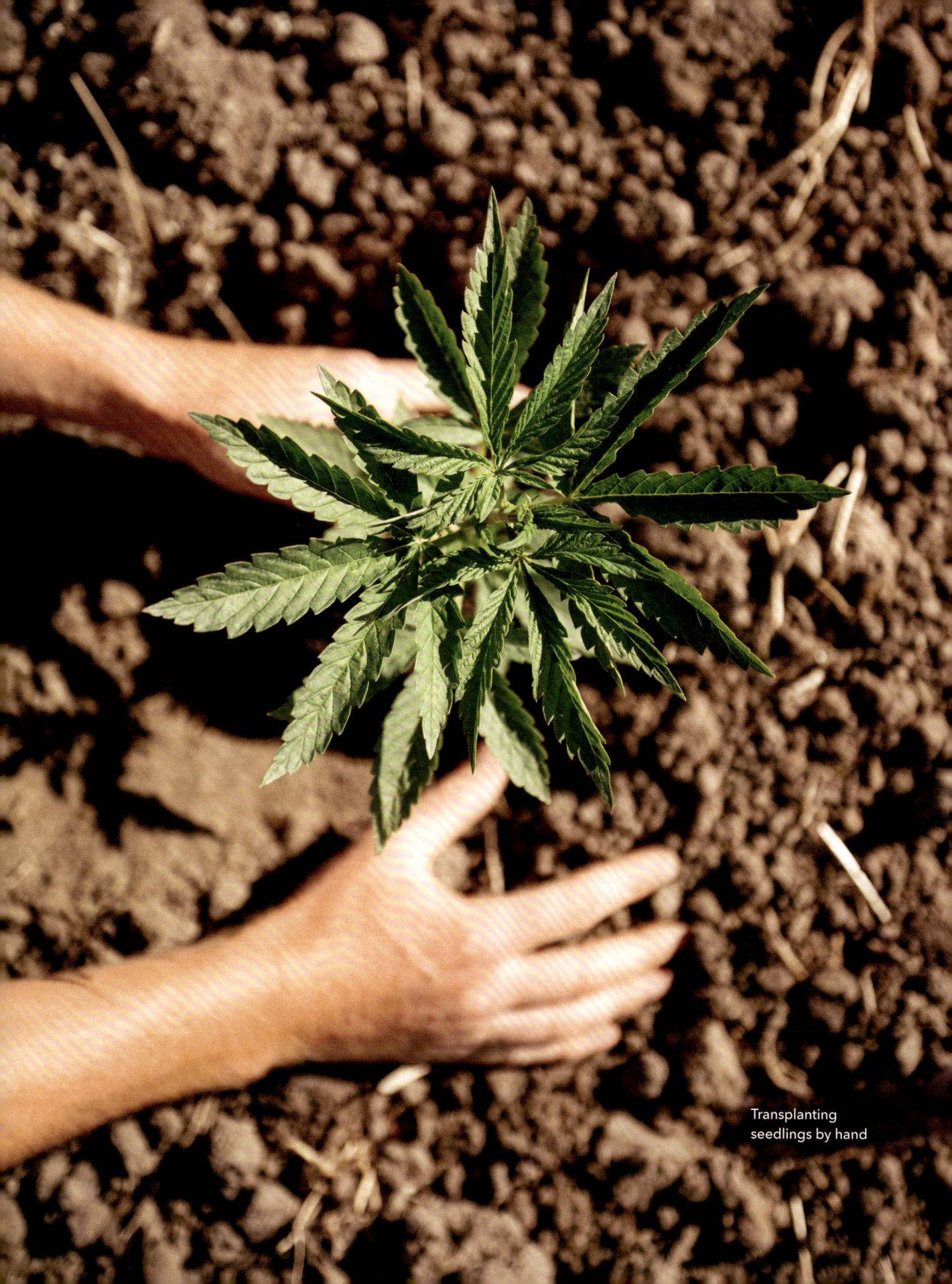

Transplanting
seedlings by hand

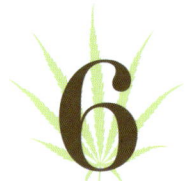

Planting Your Crop

When the field is ready and the plants are ready to leave the greenhouse, the first phase of the crop cycle is complete. The next phase, putting the plants into the ground, accounts for most stress events and crop problems. It's a critical point when your crop transitions to growing in the field. Planting truly reflects the skill and experience of the grower. It is very time sensitive, and, like pouring cement, once you begin, you cannot just stop and start over. Preparing beds properly, choosing the best time to plant, and starting extras in case the first planting fails—the work you've done so far all leads up to the day of planting, and that has to go smoothly, or the entire crop suffers.

Transplanting

Transplanting is the process of setting out seedlings in the field. By starting the seeds in trays in the greenhouse, you get a short jump on the season. This is particularly important in regions with short growing seasons or when quick turnarounds are needed to plant multiple successions in a season.

There are three main ways to transplant: by hand, with a water wheel transplanter, or by a mechanical/carousel transplanter. As with so many other things in farming, choosing which method to use depends on many factors. Availability and cost of labor, soil type, existing equipment, and access to capital are the primary considerations. Another is whether you need to plant in perfectly straight lines to accommodate mechanical cultivation. If you do not have the tools or the intention of doing mechanical cultivation, straight lines are much less important.

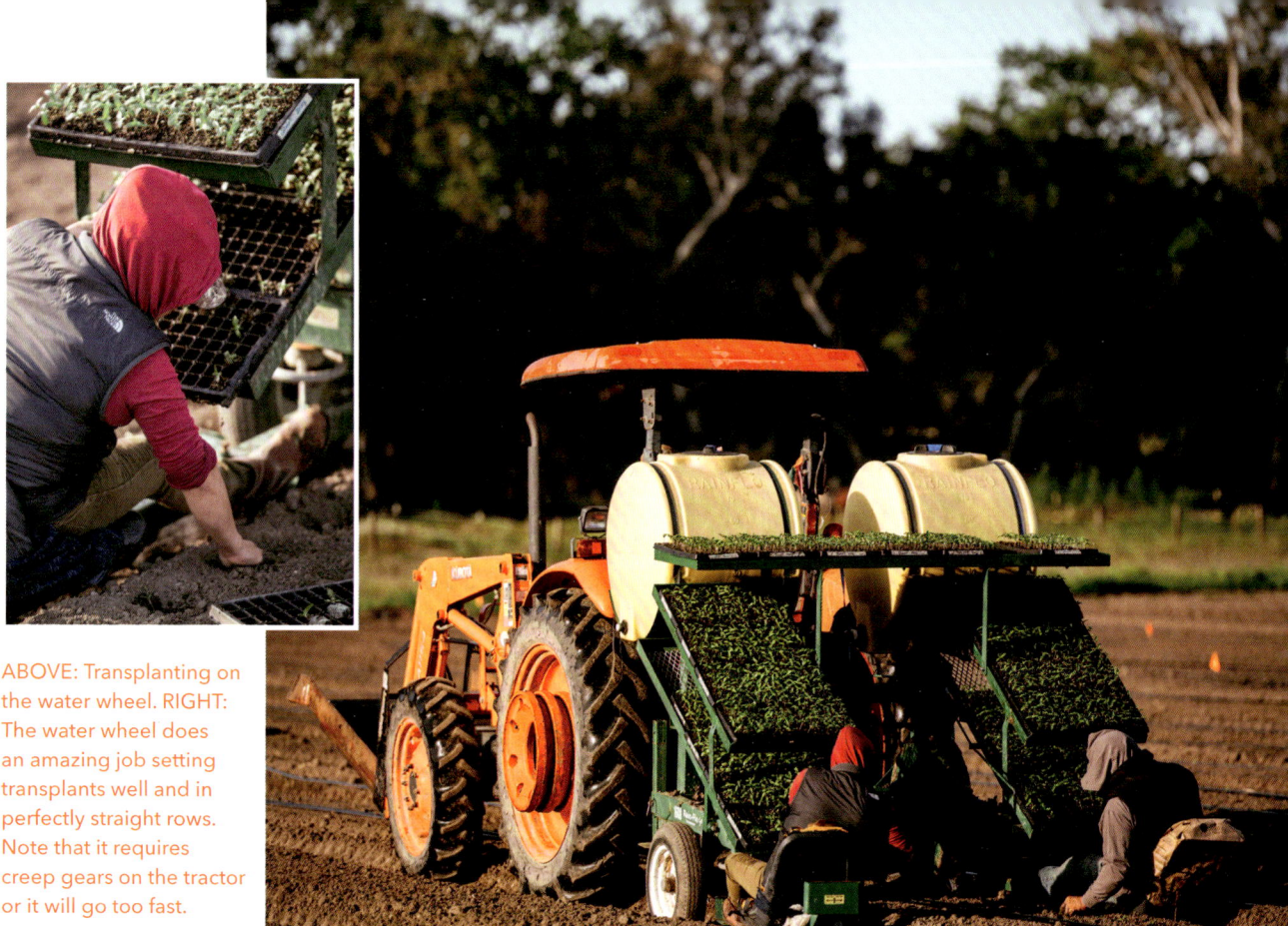

ABOVE: Transplanting on the water wheel. RIGHT: The water wheel does an amazing job setting transplants well and in perfectly straight rows. Note that it requires creep gears on the tractor or it will go too fast.

Planting by hand does not require any specialized equipment, and it gets the job done. If you want to plant by hand and still have laser-straight lines, there are a few options. The easiest and most effective is to use a hand or tractor-mounted dibbler and mark the lines for planting holes. Another technique is to set a stringline and plant along the line.

The water wheel transplanter is a great tool for intermediate-scale growers. Although not necessarily faster than planting by hand, it is certainly much easier, and it waters in the transplants immediately. We recommend adding fertilizer or compost tea. If the water flow is set high enough, transplants can sit all day and overnight without any additional irrigation. A water wheel transplanter allows growers to plant in perfectly straight lines to accommodate mechanical cultivation. It also provides flexibility by offering the option of planting into either bare soil or plastic mulch.

Water wheel transplanters come with a variety of configurations and seat setups, with anywhere from one to six workers simultaneously handling plants. On an efficient and experienced team, each crew member can put up to 20,000 transplants per day in the ground.

Mechanical transplanters, also known as carousel transplanters, are the most efficient type of transplanters in terms of both labor required and actual ground speed. But they are also the most expensive and difficult to use. They require level fields, extremely high-quality and consistent bed prep, and highly proficient operators. We recommend these types of transplanters only for larger operators. Also of note, these transplanters do not handle young or poorly rooted plants well, and we haven't had any success using them to transplant autoflowers.

Each brand and type of transplanter is designed only for a certain range of transplant plug size. Large pot sizes, such as 3- or 4-inch pots, and 50-cell trays may not be compatible with many models, so make sure your planting equipment and pot sizes work together.

How Big a Crew Do You Need?

Being prepared for every aspect of planting is essential, and that includes being sure you have enough people for the task at hand. Five people can easily plant an acre in a day (possibly up to 2 or 3 acres), and depending on the soil type and irrigation setup, it may be possible to do it with four people. For an acre, you will need two planters, a tractor operator, a floater who walks the beds to do quality control checks, and an irrigator. A mechanical transplanter would allow for 10 to 20 acres per day of planting with four people, though, once again, this number would flex depending on the irrigation setup.

Transplant Shock

All transplanting involves shocking the seedlings to some degree. Transplants are handled physically; their roots are briefly exposed to light; they are removed from the controlled conditions of the greenhouse and thrust into an entirely new environment with inclement weather and a different soil type. A primary goal of transplanting is to minimize the inevitable shock. Handle seedlings with care (especially autoflowers) and be sure to keep them evenly moist before setting them out in the field. During a long day of transplanting, this means watering the seedlings as you load up your transplanting equipment each time.

It is easy to make mistakes on transplant day. Many times we've seen beds of wilting transplants even in mild conditions. Various factors can cause transplants to wilt or get stressed. The most common is hot, dry soil, which will wick moisture from transplant plugs surprisingly fast. The easiest way to address this is to irrigate your soil before transplant. Additionally, large soil particle size can create large air gaps in the soil that can fry transplant roots; control this with good tilth and proper particle size.

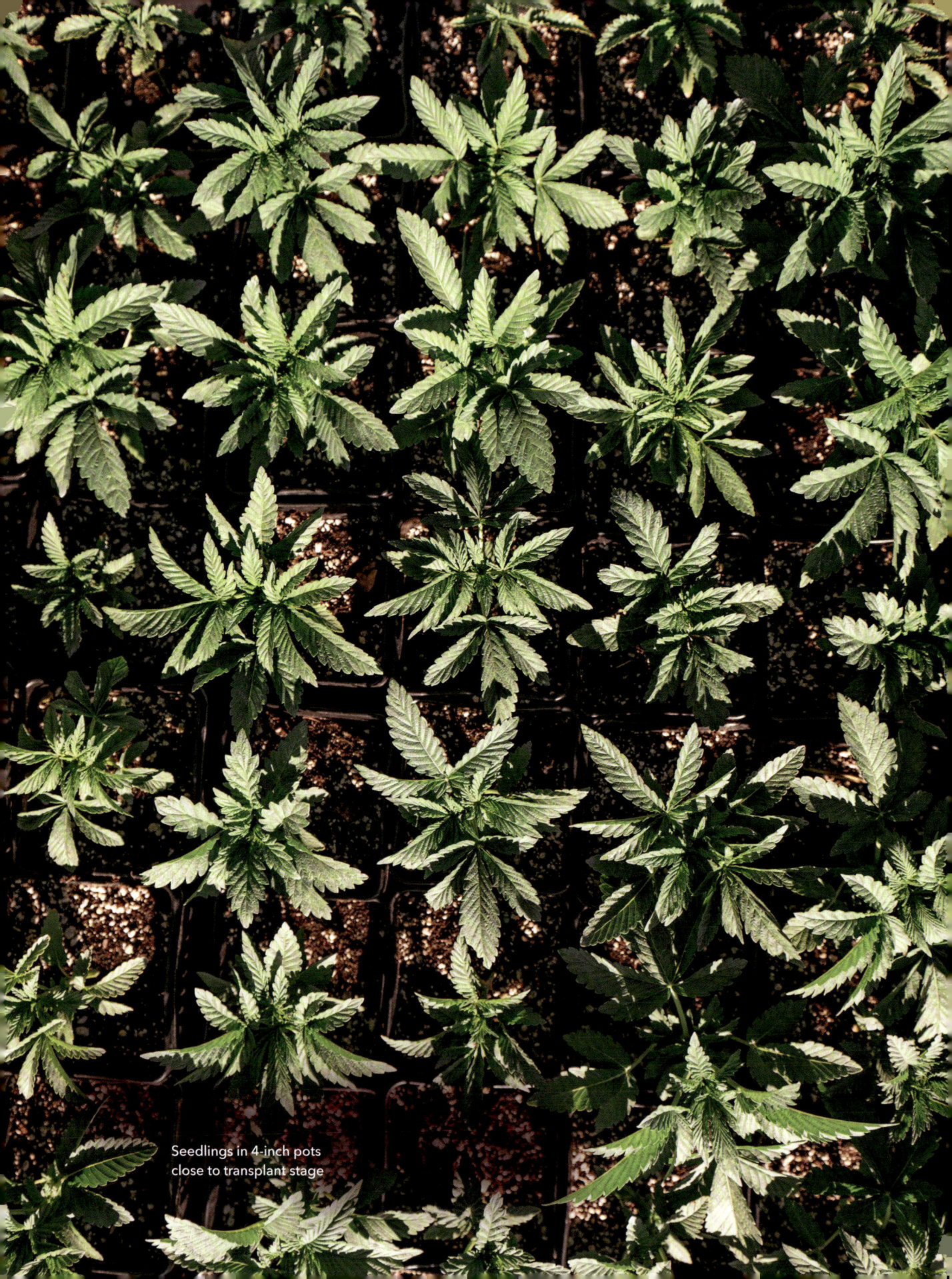

Seedlings in 4-inch pots
close to transplant stage

Plants need extra support during their transition into the field. Cool temperatures and plenty of water help ease that transition. Choose the mildest day of the week, if possible, and start transplanting at or before first light. If using drip irrigation, lay the lines on the bed as soon as it is planted. Start irrigating immediately; as the transplant crew moves through the field, the irrigation crew follows right behind. That way none of the transplants sit in dry soil longer than any others.

Planting Full-Terms and Clones

Although some clones are sold as "field ready" and full-term seedlings can be set out from trays, another option is to up-pot them into 3- or 4-inch pots. This system has the benefit of allowing you to plant later in the season with larger, more robust plants that will still fill in the desired canopy. Larger plants are less susceptible to transplant shock. Depending on the ambient conditions and vigor of genetics, up-potted seedlings can hang out for up to an additional four weeks before getting rootbound.

Up-potting requires significantly more potting soil, labor, and space. Additionally, the transplanting must be done by hand. It is not practical on a very large scale, but we have done up to 5 acres smoothly. Very good tilth and lofty beds are recommended so that workers can dig the holes by hand easily when planting.

Transplanting Checklist

The afternoon before transplanting, look at the forecast to make a final decision about when to transplant. It is ideal to begin planting at or before first light. Other tasks to do the day before include:

- ❏ Check the transplants for ease of pull and make any final decisions regarding what is going to get planted.

- ❏ Check the weather forecast and soil temperature to determine if pre-irrigation is warranted.

- ❏ Soak all transplants the night before transplanting.

- ❏ Confirm location(s) of transplanting.

- ❏ Communicate start time, locations, and any areas of concern to managers and crew members.

- ❏ Confirm that the transplanter is hitched and spacing is correct.

- ❏ Check that all necessary tools or supplies are loaded on the tractor: extra spikes if using a water wheel, impact driver, sockets, any tools needed for adjustments, etc.

The morning of transplanting, load transplants according to what is being planted first and where.

Managing Transplants

For the first week, transplants are delicate little things. They are not yet rooted into the surrounding soil and can therefore dry down much more quickly than expected. They are also more susceptible to herbivory by insects, and even a little damage at this stage can stunt the crop. Be extra careful to maintain proper moisture at the top few inches of soil alongside the row of plants. This sounds obvious, but it is not uncommon for driplines to drift, and problems can occur even when the lines are 4 to 6 inches away from the plants. If a plant is overly stressed during the transplant stage, it will never reach its full potential. Our ideal is to set plants using overhead irrigation and then, after the first few cultivations, lay drip. This is not always possible, however, due to availability of water or other factors.

Wait until the plants are thoroughly set—usually seven days—before cultivating or disturbing the soil in any way.

Direct Sowing

The decision to run a direct-sow program involves many variables that should be carefully considered up front. In the transplant stage, autoflowers are particularly sensitive to root stress, including from root binding, rough handling, dry down, and heat. We have observed large yield increases with autoflowers, 20 to 40 percent, when direct sowing instead of transplanting them. The process of planting an acre is also much faster. With a tractor-mounted tool, a single operator can plant an acre in an hour or less. For these reasons we believe direct seeding will constitute a meaningful portion of crops in the future.

Photoperiod cannabis thrives when direct sown. The taproot can go straight down from the very start. Direct-sown plants have great resilience, and you skip the whole transplant phase with its associated shock, not to mention higher labor costs. As with all management practices in farming, there are trade-offs.

Comparing Direct Sowing and Transplanting

DIRECT SOWN	TRANSPLANTED
• More resilient plants	• Far less seed used
• No transplant shock	• Uniform plant count per bed
• Higher yields	• Earlier start possible
• No propagation infrastructure needed	• One fewer weedings needed
• Much faster	• Easier to weed
• Only one person needed	

Drawbacks with Direct Seeding

Direct-sown crops require exceptional weed control. Whether by flame weeding or by hand, an extra weeding pass must be done when the plants are smaller than transplants. The crop must usually be thinned as well at the second weeding pass.

When transplanting, the cycle is plant, then weed between 7 and 14 days later. When direct sowing, the cycle is plant, then flame weed or hand weed, then weed 7 to 10 days after emergence, then weed and thin 14 to 21 days later.

Additionally, successfully direct-sowing crops requires extra attention and effort in the field-prep and tillage phase. It requires exceptional tilth and small aggregate size to achieve optimal levels of emergence and uniform growth, especially in the early growth stages.

Transplant Timeline

AUTOFLOWERS

DAYS 1-3	DAYS 4-6	DAYS 7-9	DAYS 10-14
Seed Germination	**Seed Emergence**	**Continue Fertilizing**	**Prepare for Transplant**
• Seeds should germinate between 48 and 72 hours. • Be sure to keep trays warm (77°F/25°C) and provide supplemental light if needed. • Plants need 16 hours of light until transplanting.	• Seeds should finish emerging after 6 days. • As soon as seeds have emerged, begin feeding with mycorrhizae. • Allow a wet-to-dry swing with your daily watering.	• Continue fertilizing the seedlings with mycorrhizae, increasing strength daily. • Consider transplanting if conditions allow (equipment, labor, weather, seedling health, etc.).	• Fertilize with mycorrhizae again before transplanting. • Be sure to get your plants in the ground ASAP for best results with vegetative stage of growth.

PHOTOPERIOD

DAYS 1-3	DAYS 4-6	DAYS 7-19	DAYS 20-28
Seed Germination	**Seed Emergence**	**Continue Fertilizing**	**Prepare for Transplant**
• Seeds should germinate between 48 and 72 hours. • Be sure to keep trays warm (77°F/25°C) and provide supplemental light if needed. • Plants need 16 hours of light until transplanting.	• Seeds should finish emerging after 6 days. • As soon as seeds have emerged, begin feeding with mycorrhizae. • Allow a wet-to-dry swing with your daily watering.	• Continue fertilizing the seedlings with mycorrhizae, increasing strength daily. • Consider transplanting if conditions allow (equipment, labor, weather, seedling health, etc.).	• Fertilize with mycorrhizae again before transplanting. • Transplant as soon as seedlings are ready and field conditions allow.

Direct seeding autoflowers means that the crop is growing in the field for roughly two weeks longer than normal autoflowering crops. If your system is built for quick turnover or you are planting multiple successions in the same ground, direct seeding may not be the best choice for you.

Equipment for Direct Sowing

There are two main types of seeders: mechanical and vacuum.

Mechanical seeders are affordable ($750 to $1,000) and can be pushed by hand or mounted on a tractor toolbar and stacked to allow for multiple rows on a bed. Cole Planet Jr. and Jang seeders are two of the more popular seeders on the market. These work great with a variety of seed sizes and shapes, though they are not particularly accurate with seed placement or seed counts per foot.

Vacuum seeders are much more expensive ($5,000 to $15,000) for the complete setup and must operate on a tractor. However, these are precise tools, and seed use per acre as well as subsequent tasks such as thinning and weeding are minimized. Monosem is a commonly used tractor-operated unit. We have seen a walk-behind vacuum seeder demonstrated but have not tried it, although it looks promising.

Depending on the seeder type and seed emergence percentage, we recommend using a multiplier based on the required number of plants to decide how much seed to put down for a direct-sown crop. Use a multiplier between 1.25 and 5. For example, a standard acre using 60-inch centers with two rows on the bed at 1-foot spacing in row is 17,424 plants per acre. If you were transplanting, you would want to have at least this many healthy and viable transplants. For direct sowing, if you were to use 2 as a multiplier, you would attempt to put down 17,424 seeds × 2 = 34,848 seeds/acre.

Planting densities of photoperiod cannabis are somewhere between a third and an eighth of that of autoflowers, thus we do not generally recommend direct sowing this class of plants without a vacuum seeder. Since the number of plants per acre is less than for autoflowers, it is well within the realm of reasonable to do it by hand. We always put in at least two seeds per hole. Obviously, this decision is influenced by the current market price of seed. If seed is cheap, then purchasing extra seed for direct sowing will more than offset savings in labor. However, if seed is expensive, it may be more cost effective to germinate under ideal conditions in the greenhouse and transplant into the field.

Plant Spacing

When it comes to laying out your field or deciding what densities to plant, there are three distinct plant-spacing metrics: bed spacing, row spacing, and in-row spacing.

Bed spacing refers to the distance, from center to center, between the beds. In a tractor system this is also the distance from center of tire to center of tire (see illustration on facing page).

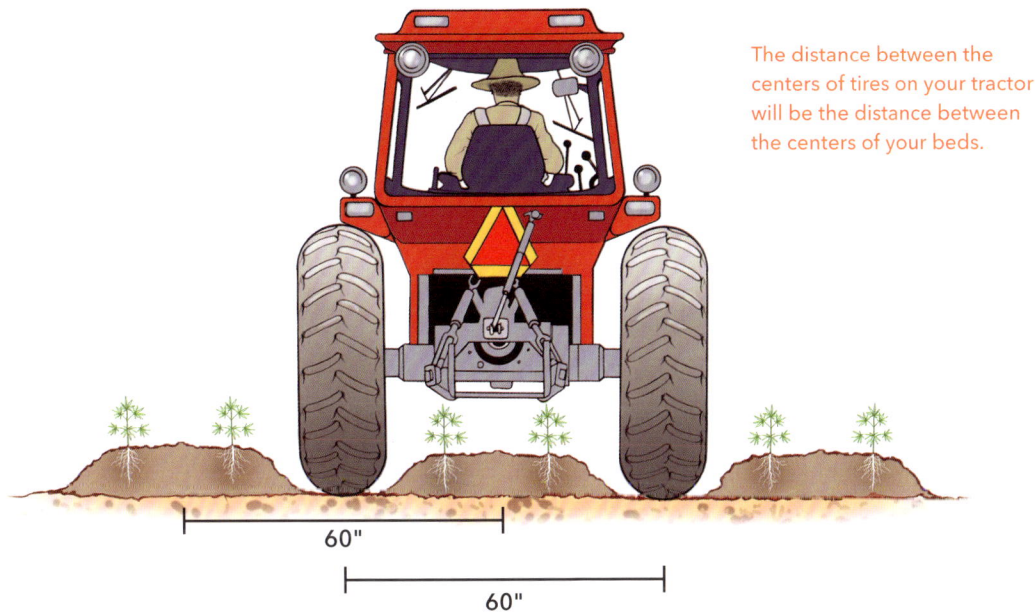

The distance between the centers of tires on your tractor will be the distance between the centers of your beds.

60"

60"

Row spacing refers to the distance between rows on the bed. (When only one row is present, we call it single-row spacing.)

In-row spacing refers to the distance between plants within the actual row. So both bed and row spacing are measured along one axis, and in-row spacing is measured along the perpendicular axis. More spacing provides easier access for all the cultural activities such as weeding, spraying, and harvesting. In an ideal world, just the right amount of space would be given to easily cultivate a crop. However, rules and regulations and some climate considerations come into play that necessitate less-than-ideal plant-spacing modifications.

When total acreage is constricted by regulations, growers must squeeze in as much canopy as possible to make ends meet. Even absent regulations, the total space available may be too low to allow the farmer to achieve desired yields without dense plantings. That said, in areas with high humidity, giving the plants space to ensure air flow and sunlight penetration is crucial to reduce the likelihood of mold.

It is also necessary to properly space beds to allow access for spraying. Depending on the scale, a hand or backpack sprayer can suffice, but if using a tractor, some beds must be skipped to allow access. To allow for sprayer access, we leave every fifth bed open for autoflowers and every other or every third bed for full-term. (We'll discuss this more in Chapter 10.)

Our tractors and equipment are all set up on 60-inch centers (60 inches measured from the center of one back tire to the center of the other), with narrow-profile tires on both the front and back of the tractor. Planting densities and schematics can be adjusted to meet the needs of your equipment and system.

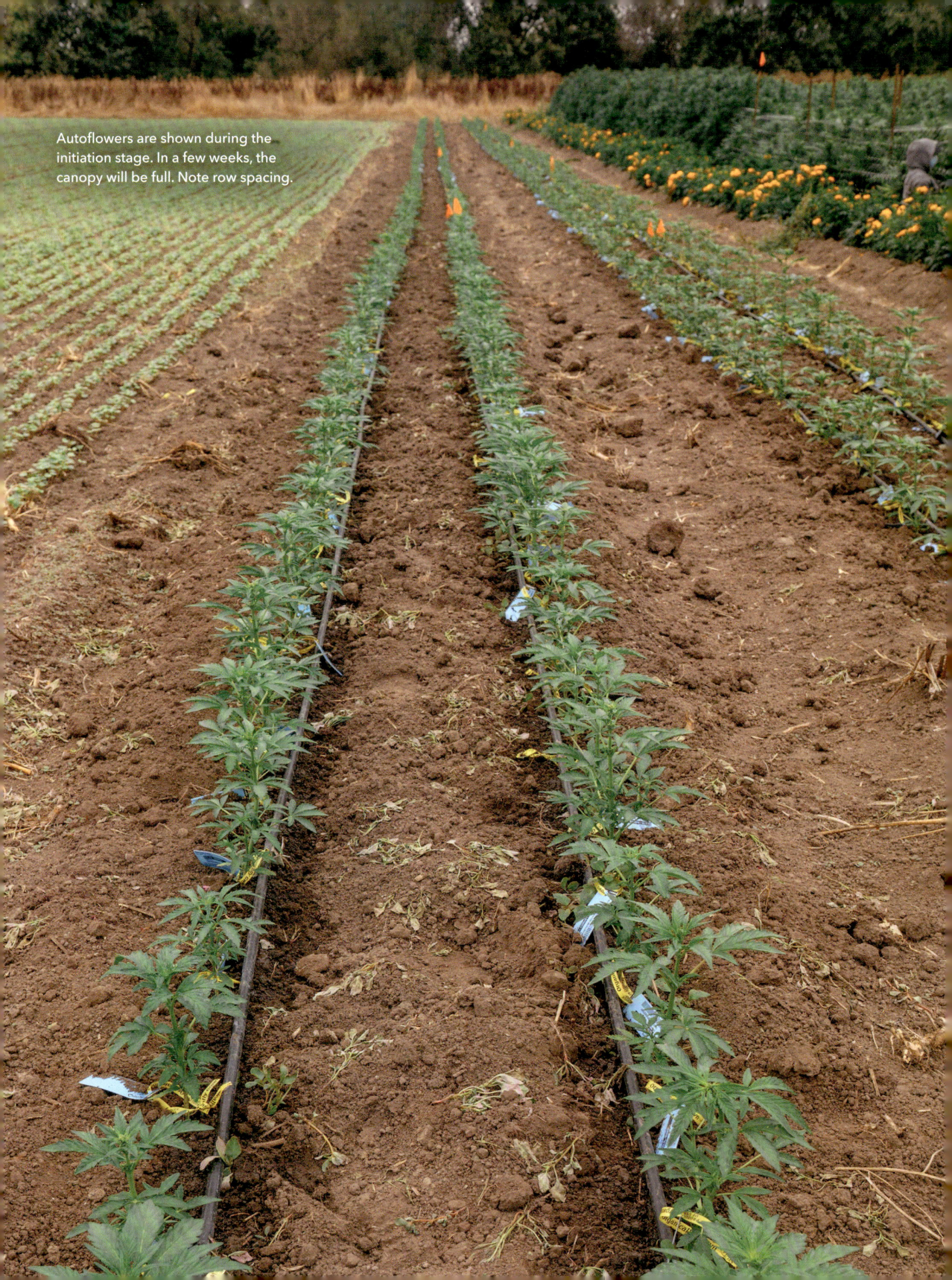

Autoflowers are shown during the initiation stage. In a few weeks, the canopy will be full. Note row spacing.

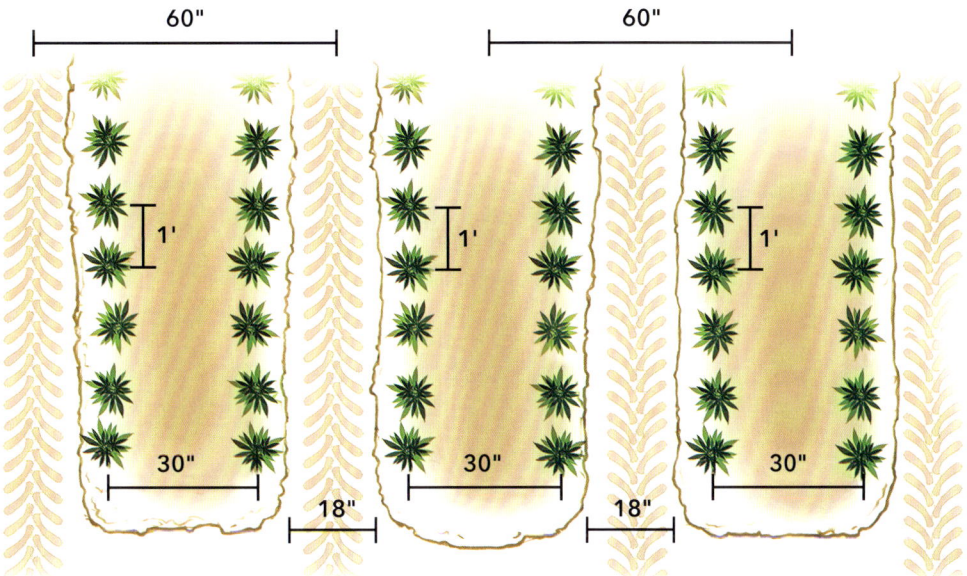

This illustration shows autoflower spacing on a 60-inch bed system. Plants needed per acre will depend on these measurements. Calculators are available online to help growers determine how many plants to start.

Spacing Autoflowers

In a 60-inch tractor-base system, we recommend spacing plants 1 foot apart in the row ("in row") with two rows, 30 inches apart underneath the tractor. This means that all the rows in the field end up 30 inches apart. This amounts to 17,424 plants per acre. This scheme allows for good sunlight penetration and limits or eliminates the need for trellising because the plants support each other. As a range we recommend anywhere from 8,000 to 21,000 plants per acre.

Spacing Semi-Full-Term and Full-Term

Semi-full-term and full-term grown from seed are given more space than autoflowers. On the same 60-inch tractor-base system, we generally plant one row at 3 feet (2,904 plants per acre) or 4 feet (2,178). Some growers may opt to open the spacing to 6 feet in row, or for later plantings increase densities to two rows.

For later plantings or for those farmers with limited plantable ground, higher densities may be appropriate, although we do not recommend densities greater than two rows planted at 2 feet, which amounts to 8,747 plants per acre.

Clones are significantly less vigorous than seeds. For this reason many growers plant clones more densely than seeds, with planting date factoring in strongly. We've heard of growers attempting to sneak in a late-season succession of clones and planting up to 10,000 per acre, though more common plant densities are 2,500 to 4,000 per acre. When planting in July, we typically space clones 2½ to 3 feet on a single row per bed.

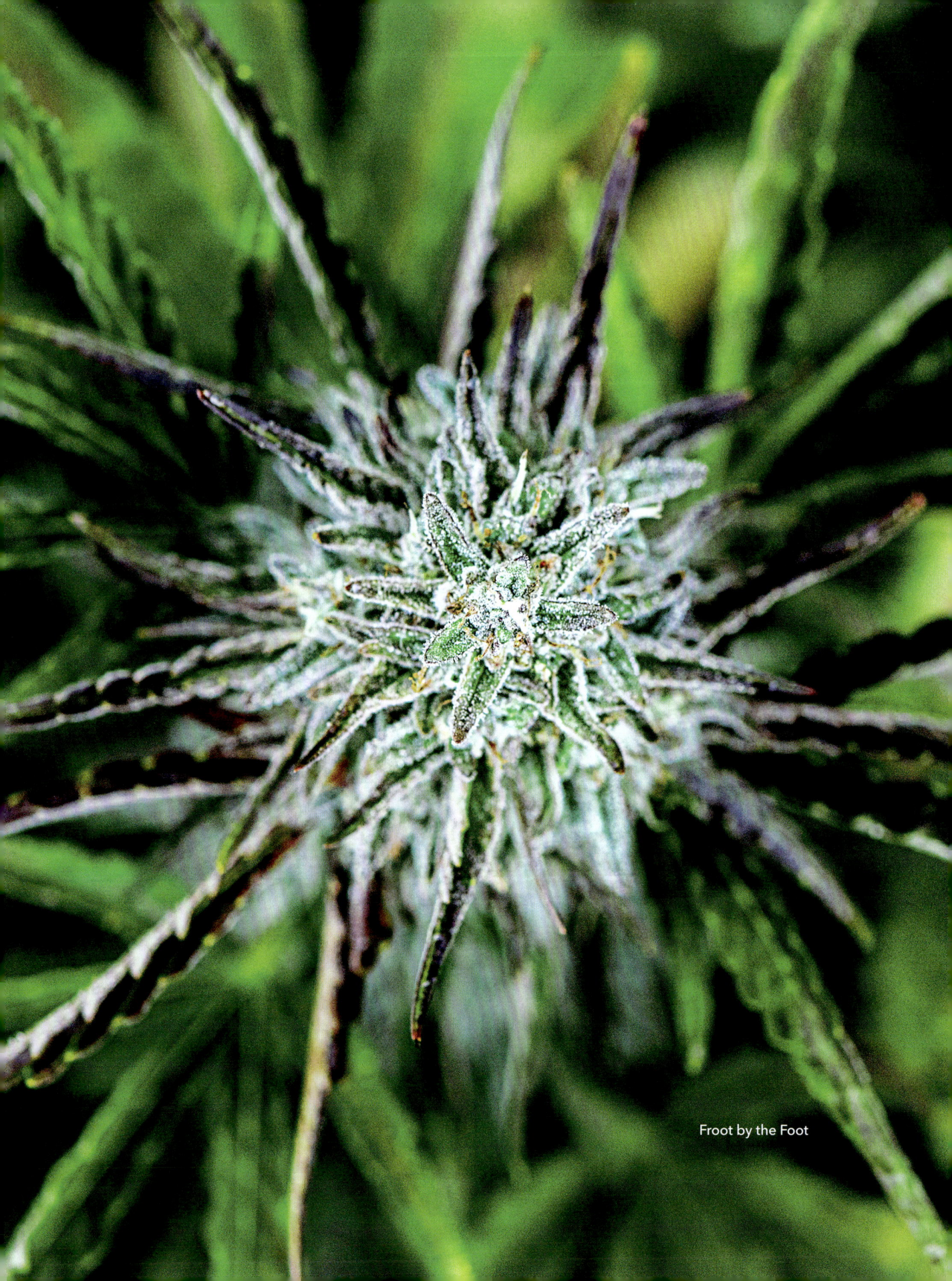

Froot by the Foot

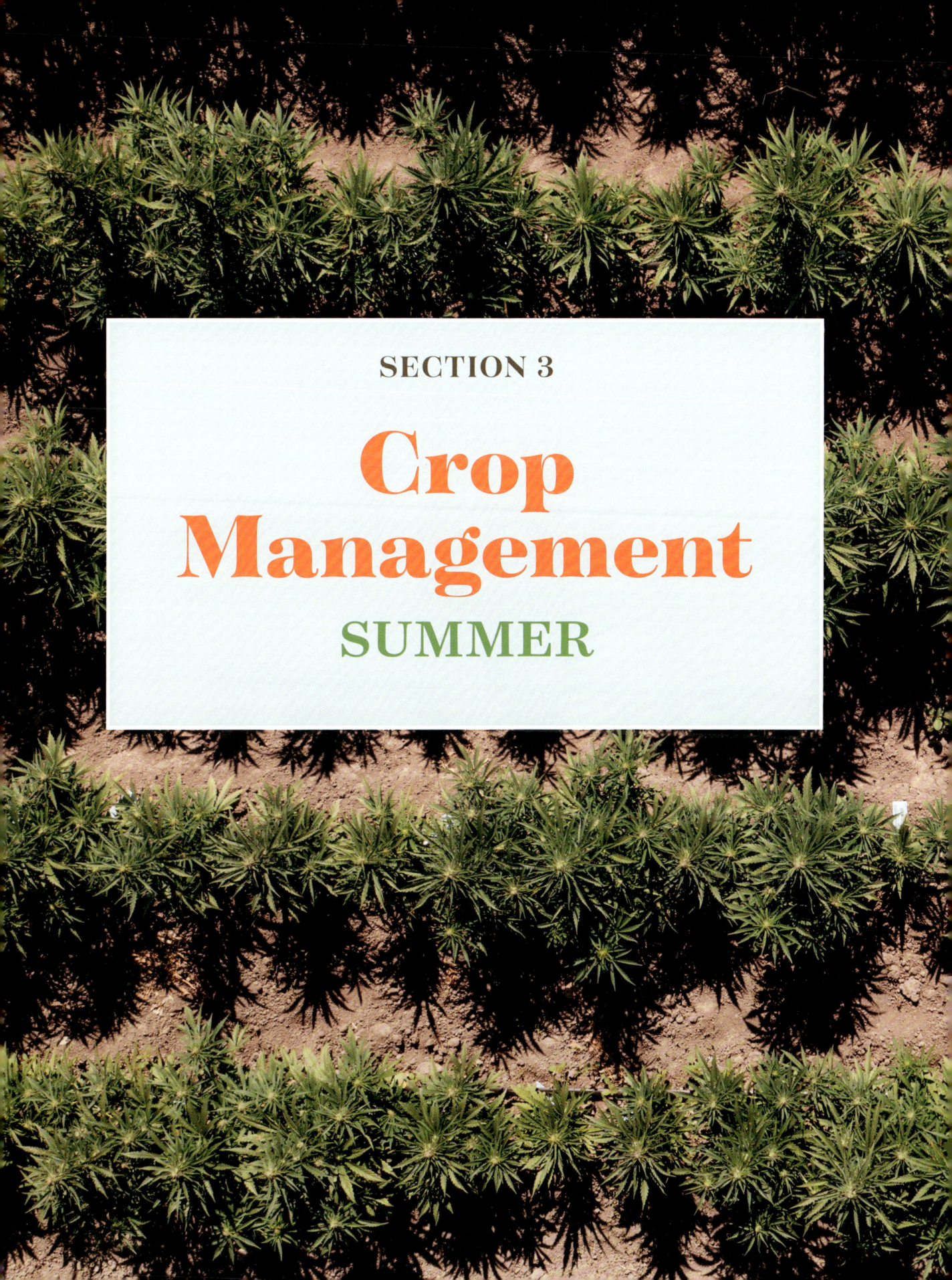

SECTION 3

Crop Management

SUMMER

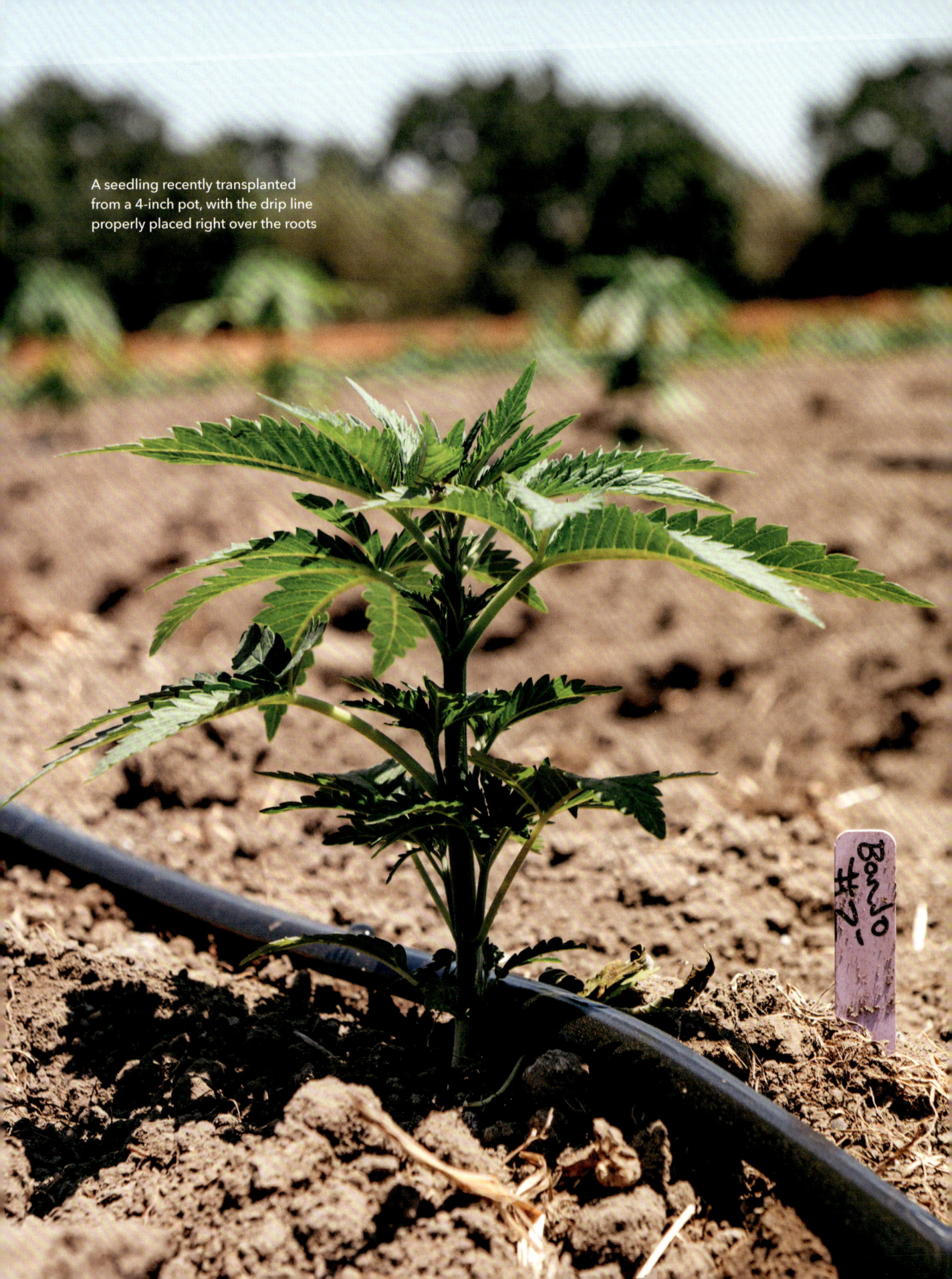

A seedling recently transplanted from a 4-inch pot, with the drip line properly placed right over the roots

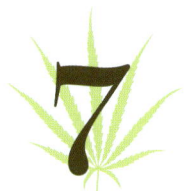

Watering and Weeding

A lthough watering and weeding are very different activities, we combine them here because of how much they influence each other. Where and for how long you water directly affects where weeds grow and how much weeding you ultimately must do. In fields with drip irrigation, most of the weeds grow in the band of water put down by the drip tape, roughly 2 to 4 inches across. In fields with overhead irrigation, the weeds grow roughly uniformly all over the field. Thus the cultivation frequency and equipment needed from one type of irrigation system to another vary.

Determining Watering Needs

Deciding when and how to irrigate your cannabis crop, as with other management decisions, is highly dependent on the conditions in the field, the anticipated weather in your region, and the seasonal availability of water. In our soil conditions, depending on the size of the plants, we generally water two or three times per week for an hour. However, friends who farm just 1½ miles away in a hotter and drier microclimate with very well-drained soils water for an hour every single day.

Some agricultural institutions have developed all manner of irrigation metrics, from crop evapotranspiration to percent capacity. Some growers use a computerized combination of soil-moisture probes, weather stations, and forecasts to decide when to water. In our view, these systems may be helpful on very large operations, but for smaller scale (less than 50 acres), an intuitive combination of basic conceptual understanding and crop observation is more than sufficient.

Soil moisture is measured in *percent capacity*. Capacity refers to the total amount of water the soil can hold before it starts puddling. Soil types vary in how much water they can hold and in how quickly they drain. Sandy soils are the fastest- and best-draining soils, but this is not always a good thing. Sandy loams are the gold standard within the agricultural community, as they drain well but also contain higher soil organic matter, which aids in water retention. There are other reasons why soils may drain well, including large aggregate or particle size, which means that larger air pockets allow water to move quickly. Clay is the smallest particle size and gets very wet and sticky, taking longer to drain. Silt is in the middle. Developing a sense for your soil requires frequent observation and plenty of trial and error.

Cannabis prefers a wet-to-dry swing in soil moisture. In percent capacity terms for mature plants, we let the soil dry down below 50 percent capacity and then irrigate enough to bring it up between 80 and 90 percent.

Tools for Measuring Water Needs

A variety of tools help determine when to irrigate. The first "tool" is looking for visual cues as you inspect your crop. Are there signs of wilting or limpness? Are the leaves turgid? The idea is to develop the visual acuity to notice when plants are beginning to droop but are not yet wilting. Over time you will notice the moisture swing the plants go through between waterings and learn when the ideal time to irrigate is. The tools discussed here help develop this skill.

A simple but effective method is checking the soil's percent capacity by using the ball test. Take a handful of soil from about 6 inches down in the root zone. Roll the soil into a ball roughly the size of a golf ball. If it won't even form a ball, the soil too dry. If it does, bounce the ball firmly in your hand until it begins to break apart. Depending on your soil type, how quickly the ball breaks tells you the percent capacity. For sandy soil, if the ball breaks apart in less than three bounces, your soil is below 50 percent capacity, and it is likely time to water. If it holds together, then the soil is still wet.

Moisture probes and weather forecasts provide other means of assessing the best timing for watering. A moisture probe is a little metal rod, somewhat like a meat thermometer, that measures soil moisture via electrical conductivity. As water is a great conductor of electricity, wet soils hold higher currents than dry ones do. In large operations, moisture probe data may be aggregated with weather station data and software to make irrigation recommendations. These systems are commonly used in vineyards or large-scale field crops but will take time for more scale adaptation in cannabis farming.

For medium- and small-scale farms we recommend a combination of crop presentation, soil ball tests, moisture probe, weather forecasts, and your own experience to make your irrigation decisions and to develop an appropriate watering schedule.

Watering During Vegetative Growth

Cannabis plants need to swing from higher to lower moisture to thrive. Your plants will stagnate in overly moist soil. Use a moisture probe or visual cues to determine the proper percentage of moisture (which may be different for different soil types) to produce healthy, praying plants. "Praying" refers to perky plants with turgid or firm leaves with a slight reach toward the sky.

Once the transplants have set, let them dry down a bit to ensure the roots have to reach down for water. There should be plenty of moisture around the roots, since you've watered regularly up to this point. As the moisture in the root zone evens out and dries, the leaves should perk up, going from a downward arc to extending out and above the horizontal.

LEFT: A droopy plant that is either over- or under-watered. RIGHT: A properly watered plant praying.

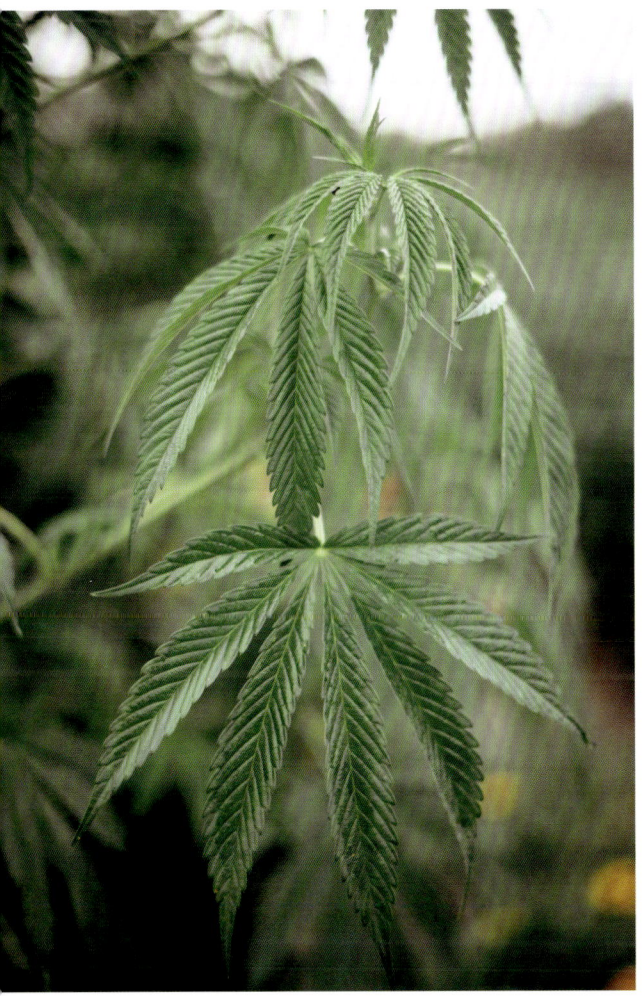
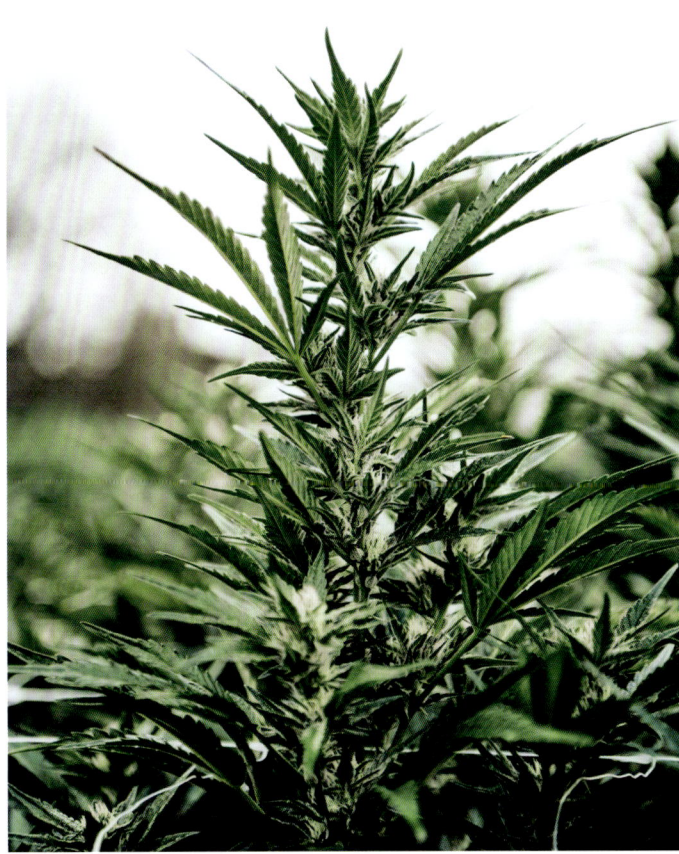

Continue to water as conditions indicate. Waterings need to saturate at least 3 feet around the base of each plant. Surface moisture encourages the growth of lateral roots, and deep moisture encourages penetrating, mining roots. The rootballs will grow wider and deeper as the plants age, so let your waterings become wider and deeper accordingly. Depending on how your soil drains, you may need to do an occasional long watering to get water down deep and shorter waterings in between to put water nearer the surface. Know your soil and check how it holds subsurface water by occasionally digging down at least 18 inches. Heavy clay soil, for example, may hold subsurface water too well, meaning you should do more frequent, shorter waterings to keep the surface moist without drowning the vertical mining roots.

Overhead Irrigation

Many farmers choose overhead irrigation when setting a crop. This system uniformly wets the soil profile, ensuring exceptional root-to-soil contact. It completely avoids the dreaded scenario of "the drip line wiggled off the row and a 10-foot section of plants died." However, setting crops with overhead irrigation can create a couple of significant problems.

Cannabis transplants need a dry down within a few days after transplant to avoid shock and ensure they set properly and continue growing.

The first relates to field dry down. Some fields drain poorly because of soil type or slope and may take days (or even weeks!) longer to dry down than other fields. In our home farm we have two fields that are 800 feet apart with a 20-foot difference in elevation. The higher field is crowned and slopes down very slightly on each side, and the soil is sandy loam. In spring this field is ready for field work three weeks before the bottom. The lower field is perfectly flat with heavy clay soil and can take up to three days longer to dry down after receiving an equal amount of water.

Why is knowing this so important? Because cannabis transplants need a dry down within a few days after transplant to avoid shock and ensure they set properly and continue growing. Plants that are attempting to set and grow in saturated soils develop lazy roots, which is exactly what it sounds like: roots that do not want to grow. Plants with underdeveloped roots will never reach their potential yield. For that reason, we replaced the tricky-to-regulate overhead irrigation in our lower field with a precise drip system. This allows us to water for periods as brief as 15 minutes when indicated.

The other main challenge with overhead irrigation is that it germinates a ton of weeds, and this can create a significant amount of extra work.

Drip Tape Irrigation

Using drip tape involves some trade-offs. On the plus side, it can save on water use substantially—up to 50 percent. It allows you to water any time of day, which is beneficial in windy conditions. It provides quick delivery of water to the root zone, which can help plants on transplant day or in the first few weeks while the plants are still settling in. It also minimizes weed growth because water is applied only to a percentage of the exposed soil.

On the flip side, using drip tape means committing to more plastic use. Some farmers claim to get multiple crop cycles out of drip tape, and although we have tried, we have never been successful in this effort. In a world full of plastic, we do our best to be thoughtful and limit its use. Drip tape also makes mechanical cultivation more difficult or more work or both. Some farmers choose to move drip tape out of the way on cultivation days, while others have systems or tools that allow them to cultivate underneath the tape without damaging it. Finally, drip tape requires regular maintenance, because small and large holes seem to appear regularly. Birds, gophers, and rabbits, just to name a few, bite the lines to access the water, and sometimes the lines just rubbing against large-aggregate soil causes lots of little leaks.

Irrigation water moves differently through different soil types. The number of drip lines and the emitter spacing on them must be chosen according to soil type as well as crop spacing.

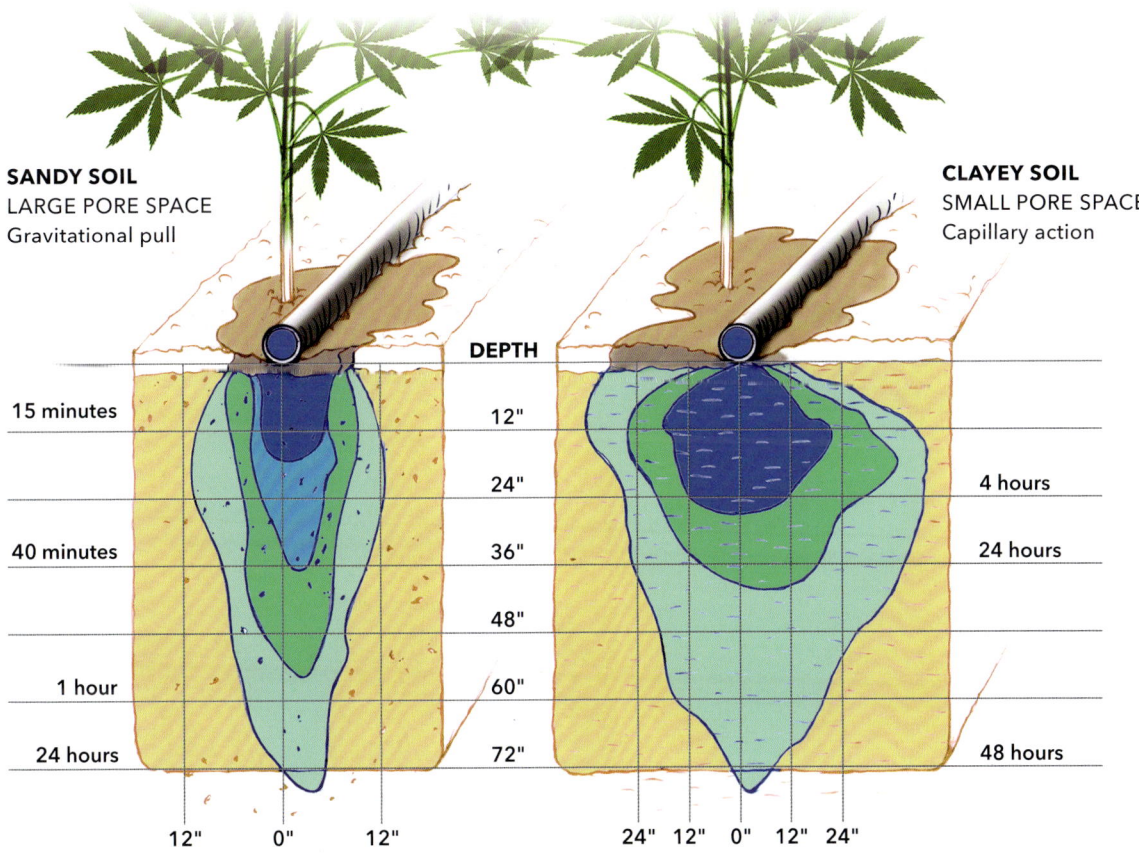

SANDY SOIL
LARGE PORE SPACE
Gravitational pull

CLAYEY SOIL
SMALL PORE SPACE
Capillary action

DEPTH

Sandy	Depth	Clayey
15 minutes	12"	
	24"	4 hours
40 minutes	36"	24 hours
	48"	
1 hour	60"	
24 hours	72"	48 hours

12" 0" 12"   24" 12" 0" 12" 24"

Installing Drip Tape

Drip tape comes with many options. The most common variables are tape thickness, usually 5 to 10 millimeters, and emitter spacing, generally 4 to 12 inches. Pressure-compensating drip tape can be especially helpful in ensuring that liquid fertilizers are distributed evenly throughout the crop.

For autoflowering crops, we use one line of drip tape per line of plants. Two lines of drip may be appropriate (that is, not a waste of money or time or plastic) in some climates and soil types, but we have found that in our conditions one line is more than sufficient. We prefer 4- or 8-inch emitter spacing because it quickly puts down a uniform band of water. With 12-inch spacing, it takes a longer irrigation cycle to achieve the same uniformity.

For semi-full and full-term crops, either from clone or seedling, we recommend two lines of drip tape per one row of plants, again at 4- or 8-inch emitter spacing. This is

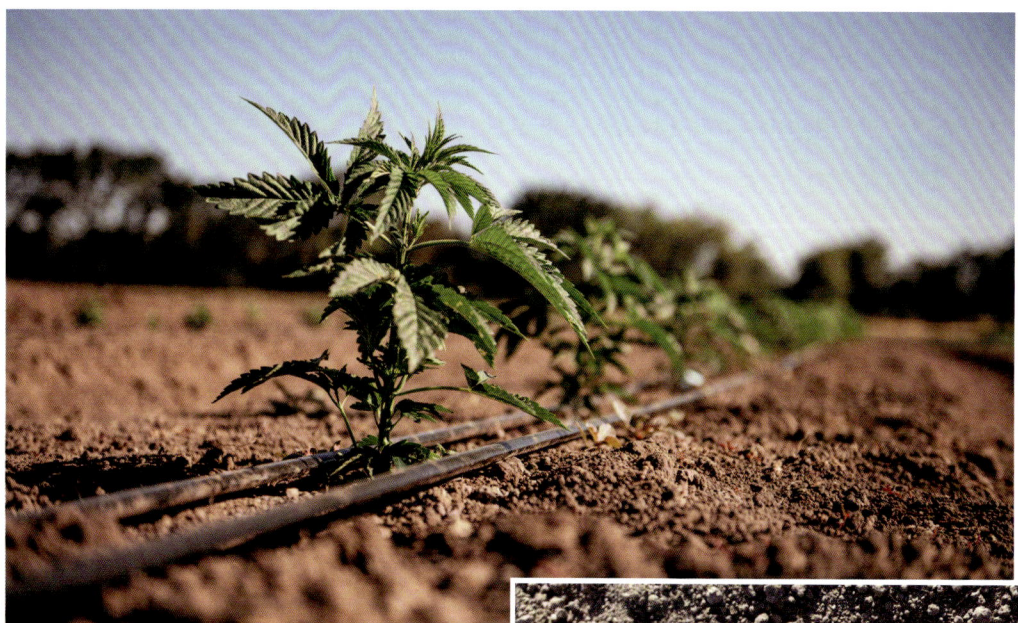

ABOVE: Two lines of drip tape surround recently transplanted clones. It is reasonable to wait to install the second line of drip until after the first cultivation and when the plants are larger and have more irrigation needs.

RIGHT: An autoflower drip line has wiggled off the plants. This can cause a lot of problems. We recommend staking drip lines appropriately.

because the root zones of these taller and broader plants (as compared to autoflowers) are more substantial and thrive when water is delivered to a larger area around the plant.

Depending on plant densities per acre, consider moving these lines of drip tape away from the plants once or twice during the crop cycle to encourage root growth. When deciding where to set your drip lines, keep in mind that clones are very shallow rooted compared to plants grown from seed.

Many farms are beginning to use subsurface drip. Most commonly this technique is used in perennial crops such as alfalfa, where drip tape is buried 12 feet deep and stays in place over three or more seasons. It is much less common with annual crops because they are tillage intensive, and it's a total pain to set the drip and fix leaks during the growing season and an even bigger pain to remove it. However, some farmers are experimenting with drip tape buried 1 to 4 inches deep. Sandy loam with high organic matter is an ideal soil for these buried drip tape systems.

Number of lines per bed / per row

Place drip lines on the inside of the autoflower rows so they cannot fall off the sides of the bed. The second photoperiod drip line need not be placed until the plants are larger, at which time the drip lines can be moved farther apart from each other so irrigation encompasses the entirety of the root structure.

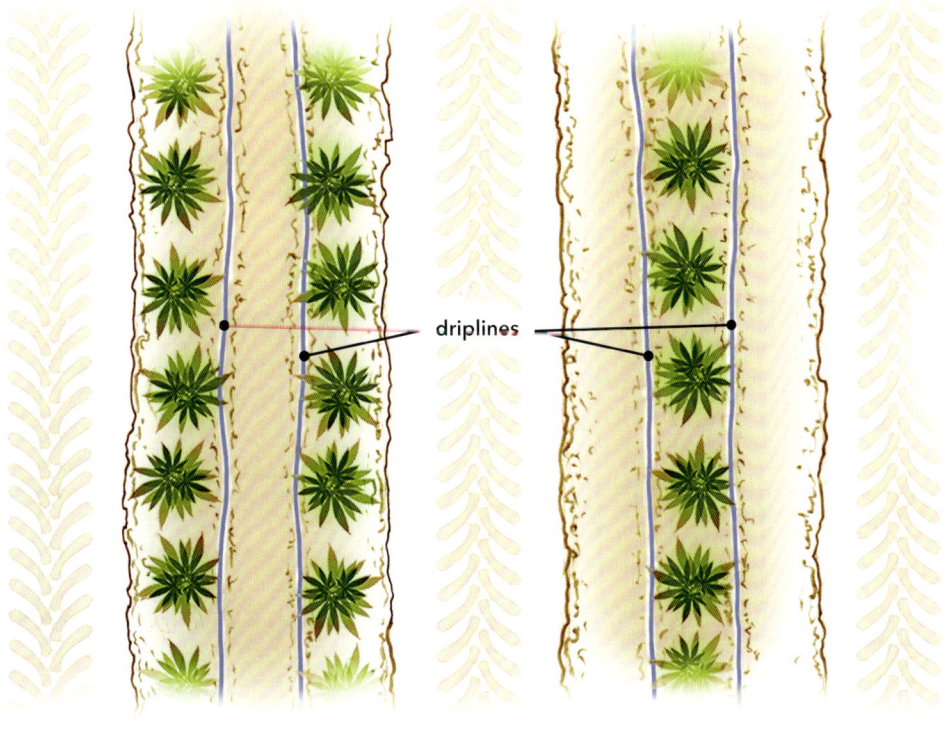

driplines

AUTOS **PHOTOPERIOD**

Cultivating to Kill Weeds

Other than looking bad, a field full of weeds competes with your crop for water, fertility, and sunlight, thereby delaying crop maturation and uniform ripening. Weeds can decrease airflow to your crop and lead to the spread of mold and powdery mildew. Every year we see yellow dock plants with powdery mildew on their leaves reaching into the lower canopy and touching cannabis branches. Weeds also provide habitat and shelter for pests, including birds that can poop on flowers as well as rats, mice, voles, and gophers that can damage your crop. Finally, weed seed can drift into and get caught in flowers as they are maturing.

We ascribe to the ideology of "Weed early, weed often." Weeds are easiest to eradicate when they are small. Our preferred time for weeding is just before they emerge, or in the cotyledon stage. We divide cultivation into two categories: hand and mechanical.

> **We ascribe to the ideology of "Weed early, weed often." Weeds are easiest to eradicate when they are small.**

Hand cultivation is killing weeds either by hand or with hand tools. Mechanical cultivation refers to the use of tractor implements. Deciding between hand cultivation and mechanical cultivation involves several variables. First and foremost is acreage. Farms growing more than 5 acres almost certainly require use of mechanical cultivation, while farms in the 1- to 5-acre range may operate just fine with only hand tools.

The second variable is cost and availability of labor. Cheap and abundant labor naturally encourages growers toward less mechanization, while the opposite is true when labor is expensive and hard to find. On our farm we utilize hula hoes (see below) a day or two *after* we have performed mechanical cultivation to clean up any weeds we have missed. In our climate and soil type, it usually takes a day for the cultivated weeds to fully die. By allowing at least a day between the mechanical cultivation pass and the hula hoe pass, it's abundantly clear to employees what needs to be weeded.

Hand Cultivation

The main tools used at hand scale are the hand hoe, the hula hoe, and the wheel hoe.

The hand hoe is a small hoe with a 6-inch handle. It is used in situations where precision is required, such as weeding within a small circumference directly around the crop. Its use will always be limited, though, because it requires the user to crawl around on their hands and knees, which is both slow and hard on the body.

The hula hoe, also known as a stirrup hoe or shuffle hoe, is a tool that swivels at the point of attachment

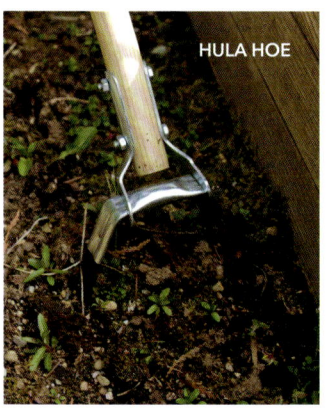
HULA HOE

to the handle, which makes it easy to move it through the soil. These tools come with heads in different sizes, generally 3 to 10 inches wide, and a 4- to 6-foot handle that makes them comfortable to use. A capable user can go through ½ acre or more in a day.

The wheel hoe has a large stirrup head with a wheel in front of it and articulated handles. It is very easy to use—most capable operators could cover multiple acres in a day. The main drawback to wheel hoes is they do not allow for in-row cultivation. You can only move between rows. Thus another weeding pass with a hula is required for thorough weed control.

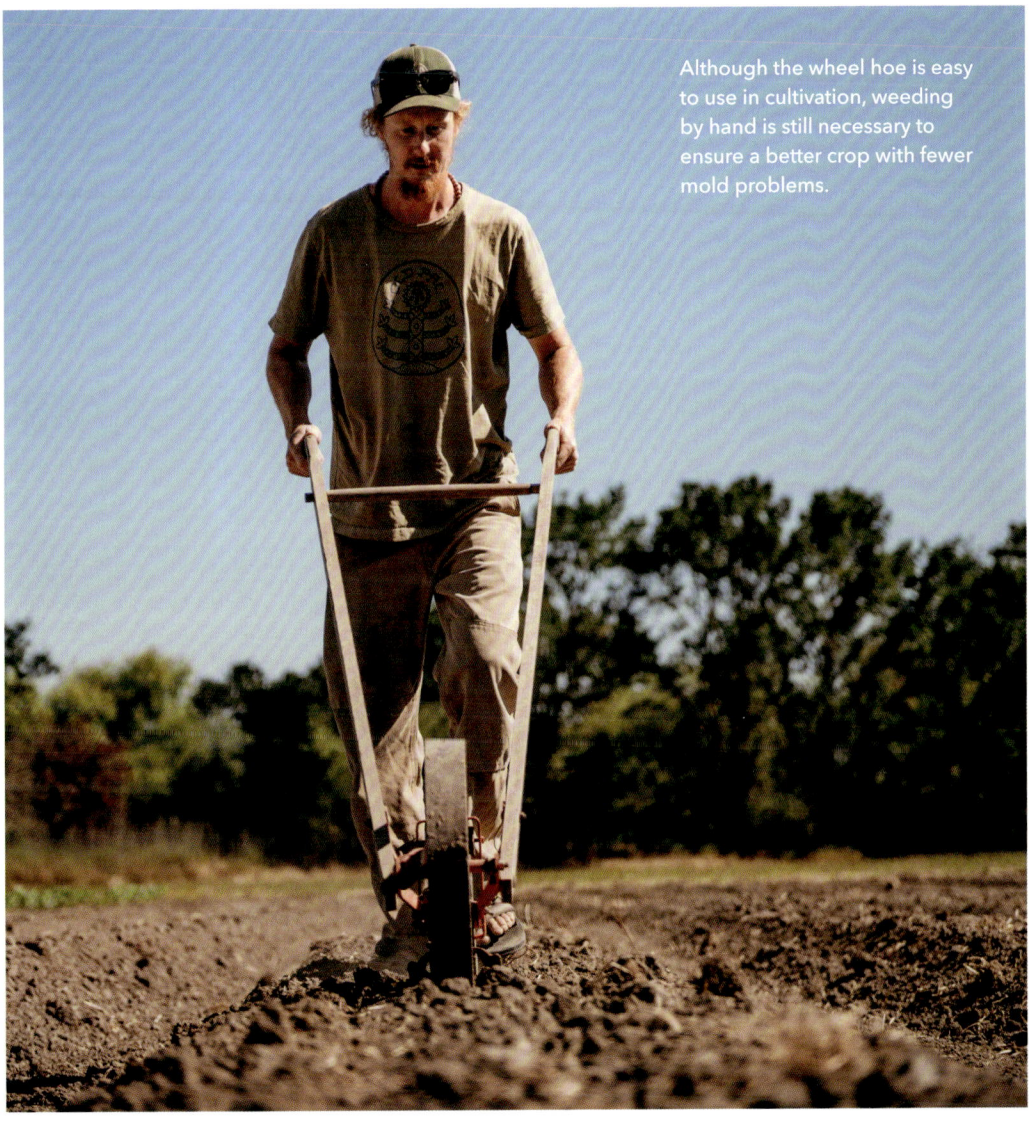

Although the wheel hoe is easy to use in cultivation, weeding by hand is still necessary to ensure a better crop with fewer mold problems.

Mechanical Cultivation

There is a plethora of tools available for mechanical cultivation. When we were still in a more exploratory phase, we researched a Dutch AI-controlled weeder that uses cameras and mirrors to weed with incredible precision. However, the $250,000 price tag certainly requires an economy of scale that we didn't have. After lots of trial and error, we settled on two main approaches to mechanical cultivation.

The first is a rear-mounted, three-point hitch with a toolbar. Depending on the height of the crop and the weed pressure, we can outfit it with a variety of tools, including hilling discs, sweeps, and knives. We recommend utilizing a rear-mount toolbar system because they are inexpensive to set up (less than $1,500), make adjustments and swapping out tools easy, and are simple to use. All you need is a tractor operator who can drive slow and straight. For the largest of operations, many users opt for "sleds," which are essentially multiple three-point toolbar systems mounted together (three at a time is most common, which allows for cultivation of three beds at once).

The other mechanical cultivation tool we use is a finger weeder. We use the K.U.L.T.-Kress finger weeder (around $15,000), though there are other options on the market. The finger weeder employs the use of both sweeps and plastic "fingers" mounted on small spinning discs. These fingers are effective at eliminating in-row weeds in the preemergent, cotyledon, or first-true-leaves stages of growth. Using the tool effectively

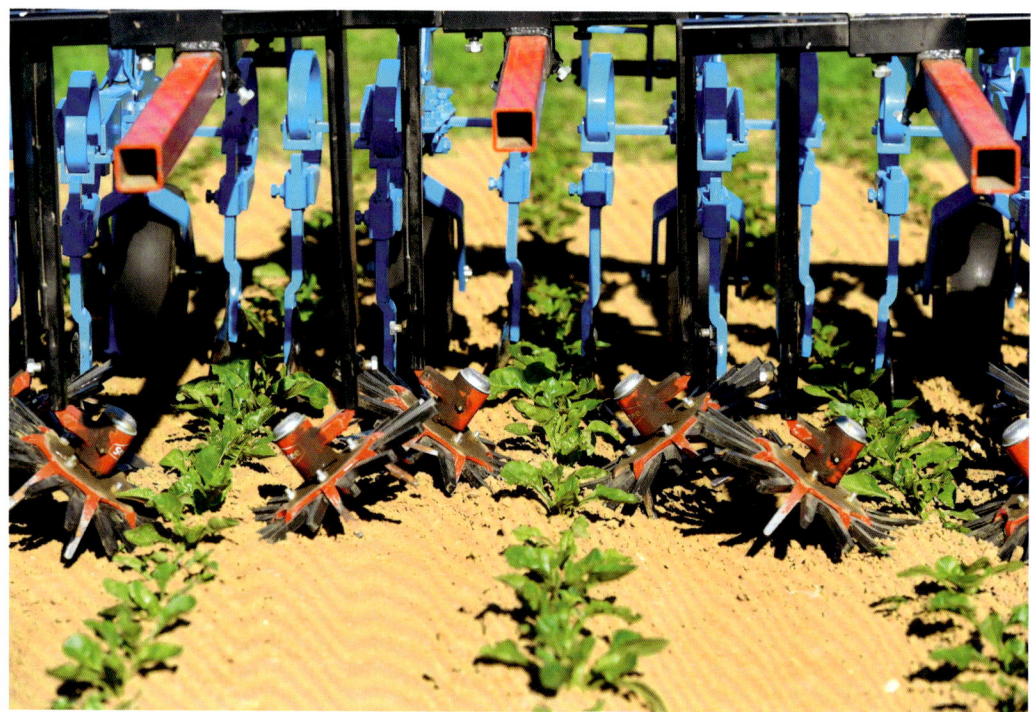

Finger weeders sweep between rows and plants for a very thorough weeding pass.

requires an even more strict adherence to the "Weed early, weed often" mantra, but when properly used it significantly reduces the need for hand cleanup. In some crops, we haven't had to go in by hand at all after thorough and timely use of the finger weeder.

Mechanization begets more mechanization. The efficacy of the tools decreases on uneven terrain. Thus large, mechanized farms go so far as laser leveling their whole fields so all the beds will be perfectly straight and level. Mechanizing a particular task in farming almost always requires that the previous steps also be mechanized or done with precision. For example, performing mechanical cultivation requires straight and level beds with straight planted lines. This means that to shape the beds you need a capable driver who can drive straight, and for the transplanting process you need to employ a mechanical transplanter. You cannot skip steps or do a poor job of field prep and planting and expect to have success in cultivation. Cannabis crops are most often planted on single and double rows per bed, which are easy to cultivate if you have straight lines and well-worked soil.

Depending on the weed seed bank, some growers do everything they can to avoid cultivation at all. This is one of the primary reasons why growers choose plastic mulch. Using plastic mulch eliminates about 90 percent of cultivation requirements. Usually, some weeds will emerge in the same hole as the crop and on the shoulder of the bed. The weeds in these persnickety locations are challenging to remove, and farmers usually elect to remove them by hand or simply leave them.

With either option, if you want a clean field, there will be some element of hand cleanup after mechanical cultivation is complete. We generally weed autoflowers one or two times and full-term and semi-full-term two or three times. There is a point in the crop cycle when most farmers let the weeds go, but good farmers will have already weeded early and often and just have to hope that the weeds don't explode into the canopy at the end of the crop cycle.

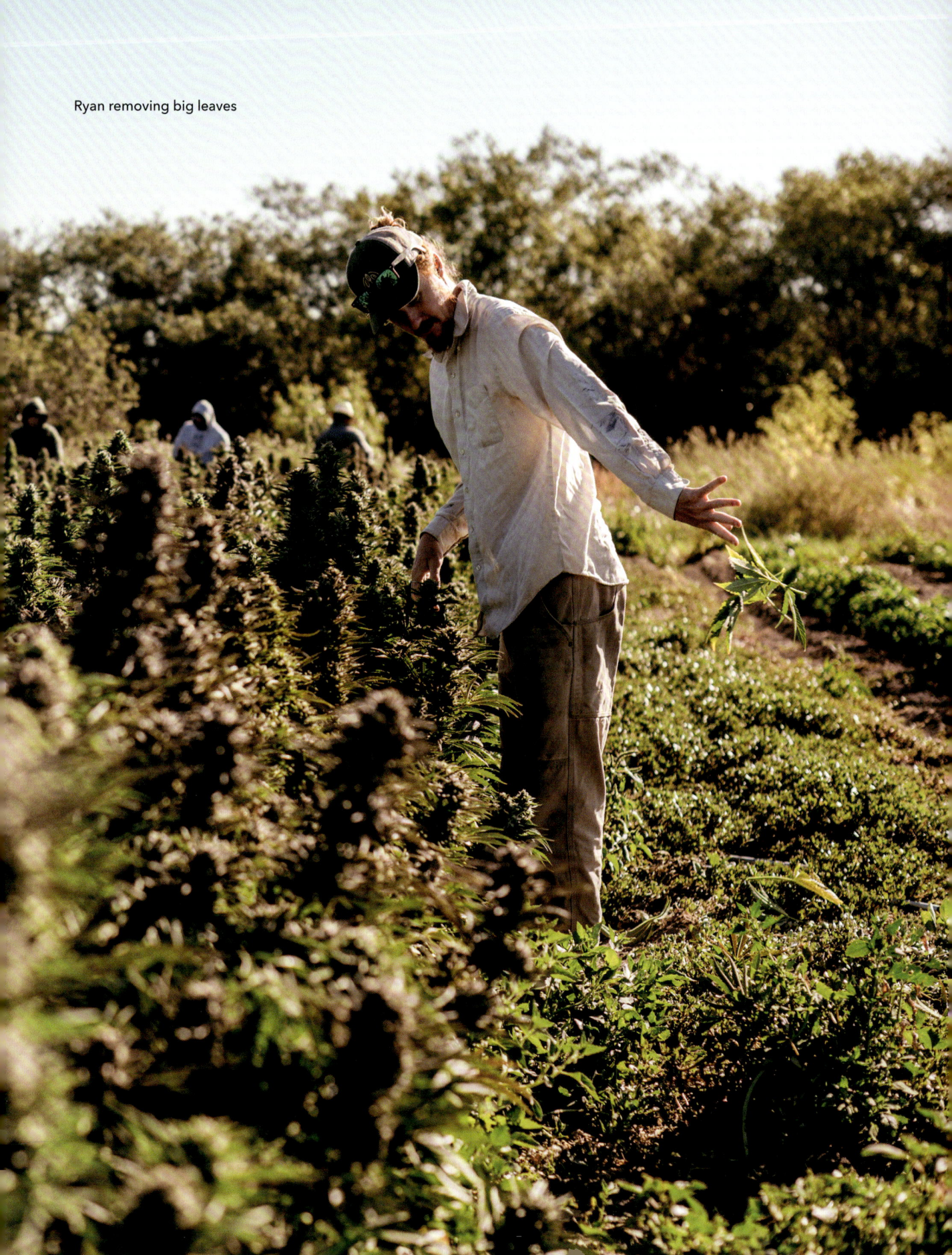

Ryan removing big leaves

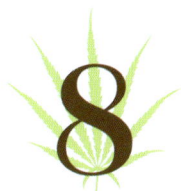

Canopy Management

Cannabis in its native form is an upright, pyramidal plant. This creates severe apical dominance and stratification of flower quality and maturation from top to bottom. Apical dominance is the propensity of a plant to energetically prioritize the tallest shoot, which in turn limits branching and the quality and size of flowers on lower branches. The topmost branches get the most growth hormones and receive full sunlight, shading out lower branches. The lower flowers typically never bulk up and are more prone to mold. In cannabis farming we refer to these as "tops" and "lowers." Tops are the finest quality, heaviest flowers on the plant, so we want to maximize them in our fields.

We have two tools available to us to create an even field of tops—topping and trellising. Topping means pinching off the topmost stem early in the growth cycle, sometimes multiple times, to change the shape of the plant from a single dominant stem to multiple branches. Trellising not only supports the heavy flowers but also trains the plants to grow more horizontally, maximizing their sun exposure.

Topping

Topping takes place during the vegetative stages of growth. It is the practice of cutting the tallest point of growth on the plant or, in some instances, the tallest points of growth. The purpose of topping is to overcome apical dominance and encourage the plant to put energy equally into all the top bud sites. It can be done multiple times or not at all, depending on preference. We decide when to top based on the height of the crop and the time of year, but to simplify labor steps we also do all of our topping at once, ignoring the variabilities among the genetics. We recommend topping plants somewhere between knee and shoulder high, which for us occurs in early to mid-July, but this could vary substantially with earlier planting dates.

How much to cut depends on the vigor of the plant, the time of year, and the desired canopy height. We cut anywhere from ½ inch to 18 inches of plant, though most often in the 4- to 12-inch range.

Topping is not necessary for autoflower crops. Their vegetative cycle is short, and a harvest height of 2 to 4 feet does not warrant the effort. Please note, on large plantings dedicated exclusively for extraction, canopy management is much less important and may not be necessary.

Trellising

We use a trellis system in cannabis for two main reasons. The first is to train the multiple branches gained through topping away from each other and spread them out across a horizontal plane to efficiently utilize all the sunlight hitting a single bed. This increases yields significantly. We want multiple "tops" per plant across the entire field, all spaced perfectly from one another for maximum airflow and light penetration. The second reason for trellising is support: Modern cannabis genetics produce flowers so bulky and heavy that branches will snap off under their weight before harvest, especially in windy conditions. Left alone, plants can lose half of their branches.

We've wondered if we can avoid the need for trellising in the first place. We actively select for thicker stalks in our breeding program in the hopes that one day the genetics will do the work for us. In the meantime we enjoy growing autoflowers because they stay short enough to avoid the requirement of trellising. We have seen other growers plant clones very late in the season so that they never reach more than 3 feet in height and thus never need trellising. And some growers plant very densely so that the plants support each other, and the branches that inevitably break are considered an acceptable loss as part of their crop production system.

Because cannabis is an annual plant, setting up and taking down trellises is an annual chore. Be thoughtful and creative in setting up a trellis system that meets the needs of your crop but is not overly complicated, resource intensive, or labor intensive. To that end there are two main methods of trellising to consider for cannabis: corralling and netting.

Corralling

Corralling is setting up evenly spaced T-posts throughout the bed and running high-tensile wire or trellis rope at several heights along the outside of the plants. This can be accomplished with a single T-post in the center of the bed on narrow bed configurations, or two T-posts flanking the outside edges of the bed in wide setups.

The post spacing depends on the eventual plant height and the prevalence of wind and rain. Larger, taller plants create heavier branching and require more posts and more rope or wire to support them. Plants growing in windy and rainy conditions have similar requirements. You will have to experiment to find what works in your area; however, our advice is to always lean on the side of closer spacing. Corralling is light-years faster than netting to install and take down, but does not include the benefit of training branches and holding them away from each other for maximum airflow. At a scale larger than 5 acres, netting rapidly becomes impractical. Corralling is the best trellis option, if any is chosen at all.

Netting

Netting is the practice of installing plastic mesh stretched horizontally across evenly spaced T-posts that define the outer edge of the bed. Posts are set every 10 to 25 feet, at a height within 1 to 2 feet of the top of the mature canopy. Rolls of netting are attached to the posts at the beginning of the bed and walked out over the canopy and attached to each successive set of posts. The net is then lowered down into the canopy, and branches are trained apart from each other into the mesh to create as much horizontal surface area as possible.

Netting is impractical and annoying, but it does hold the branches upright and protects them from breaking, and in the right conditions it provides the grower with significant value.

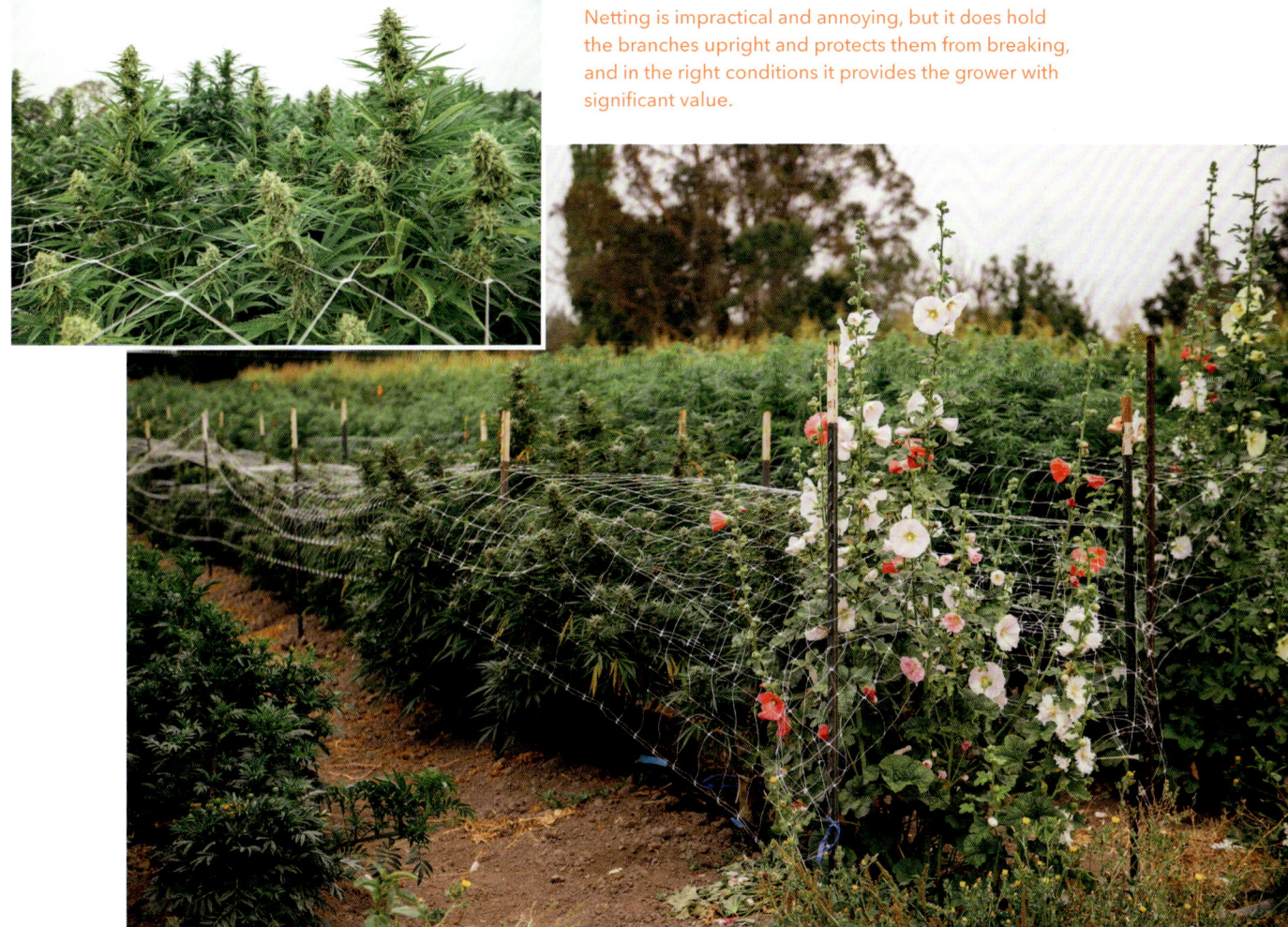

Typically the layers of netting are attached starting at 2 to 3 feet up the T-post and on up at 18-inch intervals. For a plant that reaches 6 feet in height, this means three nets. While netting does the job very well, it is burdensome, labor intensive, and, quite frankly, annoying. In addition to making any canopy activities much more difficult, it is single-use plastic (go ahead, we dare you to try reusing it). Harvests are slow and frustrating even if you cut out most of the trellis prior to harvest. It's surprisingly easy to get your feet stuck in it and trip over it. We often joke that laying netting around the border of the field would make a fine security system.

Pruning

Cannabis is a vigorous grower, and to produce high-quality flowers, some pruning will be necessary once the plants have reached midseason. The first reason to prune is to increase flower size, weight, and quality by removing excess branches. The pruned branches are typically lower in the canopy where they don't receive adequate sunlight anyway. Removing them focuses the plant's energy and nutrition into the high canopy.

The second reason is to promote better light penetration and airflow into the canopy to reduce mold conditions. Flowers that do not see the sun never reach their full size and are more prone to molding.

Pruning is not necessary in autoflower crops because of their short stature and quick maturation. In full-term and semi-full-term crops, pruning is typically done in steps. The first step is usually performed at the start of flower initiation. Removing unwanted growth in the middle and lower canopy is colloquially called "shaving the legs."

The plant on the left has recently "shaved legs." At right is a plant that has not yet been pruned.

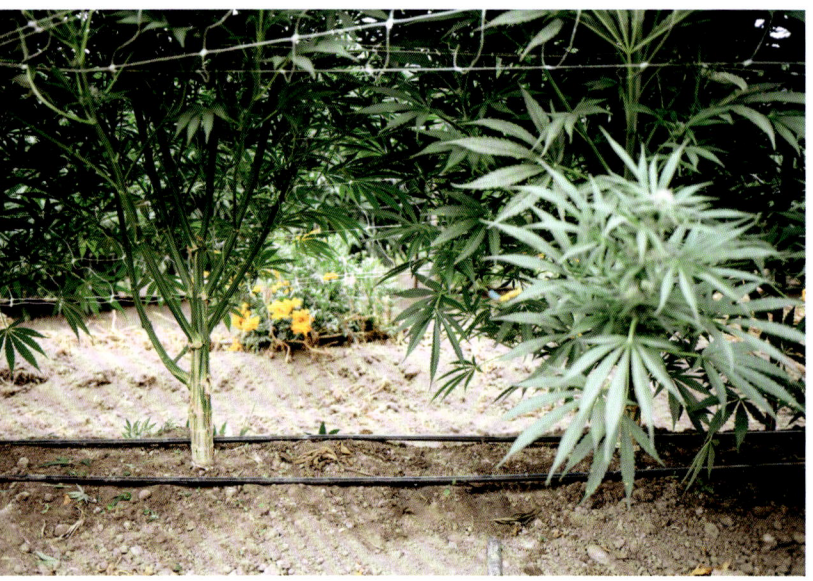

The general idea is to remove weak shoots that will never reach the sun and shoots that are aiming back toward the center of the plant. The goal is to achieve even light penetration on as many colas as you can fit in the upper canopy. Cleanup varies drastically according to genetics. Some varieties will need their legs shaved only once, while others might need it three or four times. This kind of information is not listed in variety descriptions, and the prudent grower will inquire directly to their seed purveyor or nursery regarding how much pruning is necessary.

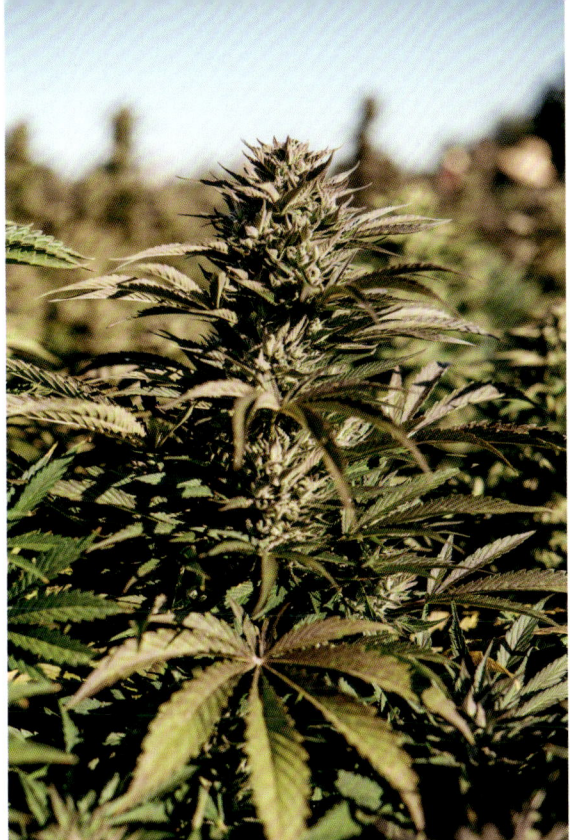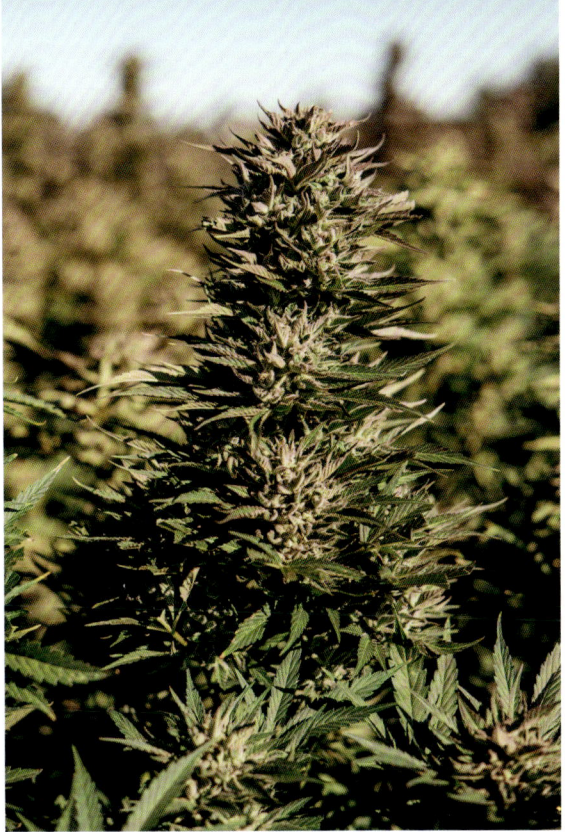

Before (left) and after (right) removing the big leaves prior to harvest

De-leafing

De-leafing is the act of removing fan leaves from plants as they near maturity. Leaves are removed from the upper canopy, specifically on the parts of the plant that will be harvested. Fan leaves are removed for many of the same reasons as pruning: namely, to increase sunlight penetration and airflow in the canopy, to increase the yield and quality of flowers, and to decrease mold, which is most common at the very end of the crop cycle. It is important to note that de-leafing too early or too aggressively can stress the plant and reduce its ability to produce high-quality and high-yielding flowers.

This single act produces greater uniformity of maturation; in some very leafy genetics, it can increase yields by 20 to 30 percent due to light penetration into the canopy. Removal of fan leaves a week or two before harvest also triggers a stress event for the plant, causing it to mature more rapidly. But the main reason the fan leaves are removed prior to harvest is because they have to come off at some point anyway. Nobody smokes the fan leaves, buyers do not want to pay for fan leaves, and in a post-harvest dry/cure system involving mechanical dehumidification (outlined in Section 4), we do not want to use space and energy drying them.

De-leafing is time and labor intensive and costly. There is no effective way to mechanically remove leaves from a live plant in the field, so it must be done by hand.

There is no effective way to mechanically remove leaves from a live plant in the field, so it must be done by hand.

We have found that for an autoflower crop using our planting density, it takes about 200 hours per acre. Note, too, that the plant stature is below a comfortable working height, so de-leafing is a back-breaking job. For full-term crops as we grow them (approximately 3,000 plants per acre 4 to 6 feet in height), it can take 300 to 350 labor hours. We have experimented with every configuration of de-leafing we can imagine. As the price of cannabis flowers decreases, reducing labor hours will become more and more important.

Many farmers are learning to use machine trimmers to perform the de-leafing process on dry material, which allows them to skip field de-leafing entirely. There are notable drawbacks to this approach. Depending on selected genetics (autoflower quality and yield are not as drastically influenced by this step), quality and yield are reduced if fan leaves are left on in the field, because light is required for flowers to maximize potential density and size. Restricting light by skipping or limiting de-leafing may save

LEFT: Genetics with lower leaf mass eliminate a large portion of de-leafing. RIGHT: Genetics with higher leaf mass are much more laborious to manage in cultivation and especially post-harvest.

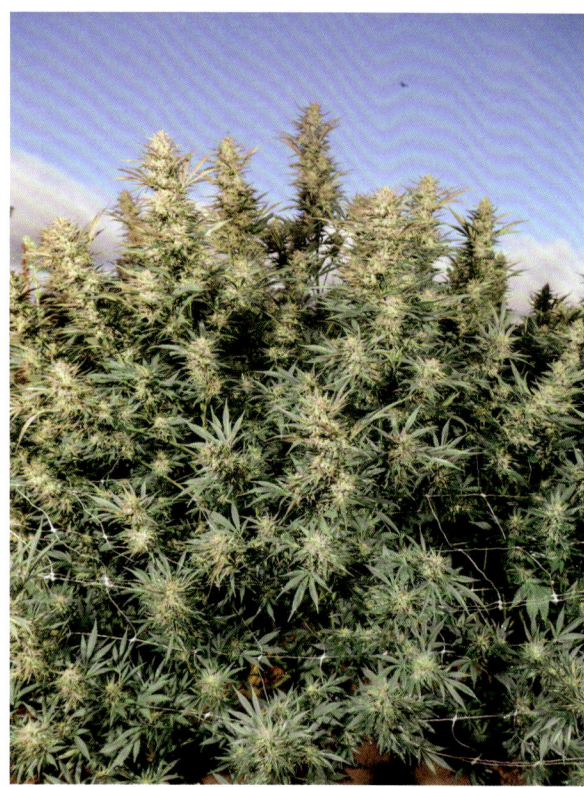
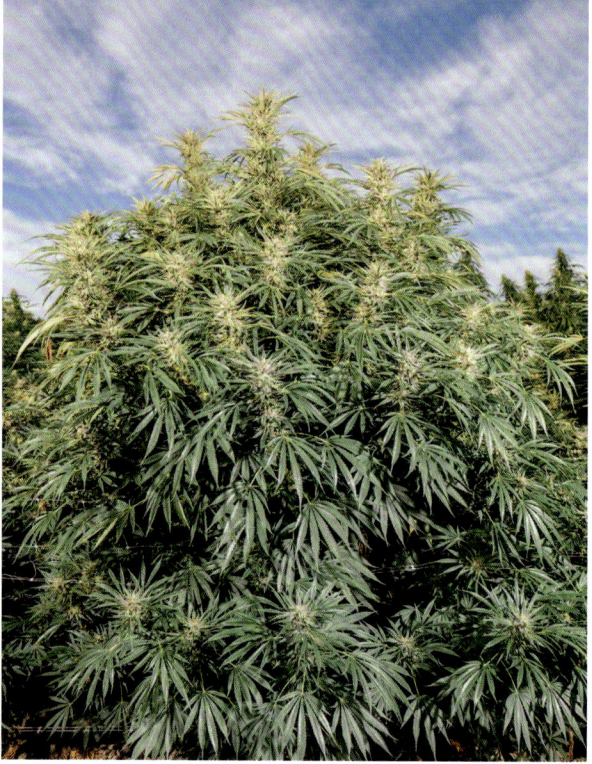

Crop Management

in labor costs but will reduce yields. Additionally, putting unseparated flowers and leaves into a machine trimmer dilutes the cannabinoid content, and thus the value of, your trim, making it less desirable to processors. (Trim is the by-product of bucking; see page 184.)

And finally, putting stalks with fan leaves still attached into your dry room increases the total volume of water that must be removed and decreases airflow onto the buds themselves, which can lead to mold problems in post-harvest. Essentially, using machines to remove all the leaves is a decision to sacrifice value and post-harvest space efficiency but simultaneously decrease labor costs significantly. The cost to produce the finished flower will be reduced, but the overall quality of the crop, ability to sell the trim—which will have a reduced price point due to the presence of leaf matter—will be compromised. When confronted with trade-offs like these, consider the root cause of the dilemma. Over the seasons we have learned to select varieties that have a low leaf mass to begin with. Genetics with this trait will be paramount in the price-compressed future of the industry.

 ## Canopy Management

On a large scale, nonmechanized canopy management is completely impractical. Big operations may choose to selectively harvest tops for a higher-quality product, but pruning and de-leafing would require hundreds of workers at a scale beyond 10 acres. We suspect that these in-crop management practices—including de-leafing, topping, and pruning—will eventually be eliminated, minimized, or mechanized. For example, vineyard pruning equipment could be used to mechanize the topping step.

In terms of genetic selection, it is astounding to experience the difference between a very leafy variety and one with good internodal spacing and low leaf mass. Low leaf mass is one of the traits most highly prized by the seasoned grower with years of harvest and post-harvest experience. Selecting genetics that minimize canopy management is not limited to leafy vs. nonleafy. Plants vary greatly in their branch strength and length and yield per branch (the latter referring specifically to how flowers stack up or grow on a branch.)

Growers at scale will continually look toward genetics and planting schematics that limit canopy management. In Morocco, which is one of the largest hash-making regions in the world, millions of plants are grown without any kind of trellising installation. Growers there limit plant height by planting later in the year, through genetic selection, and by accepting some losses as a trade-off for not having to install annual trellis systems.

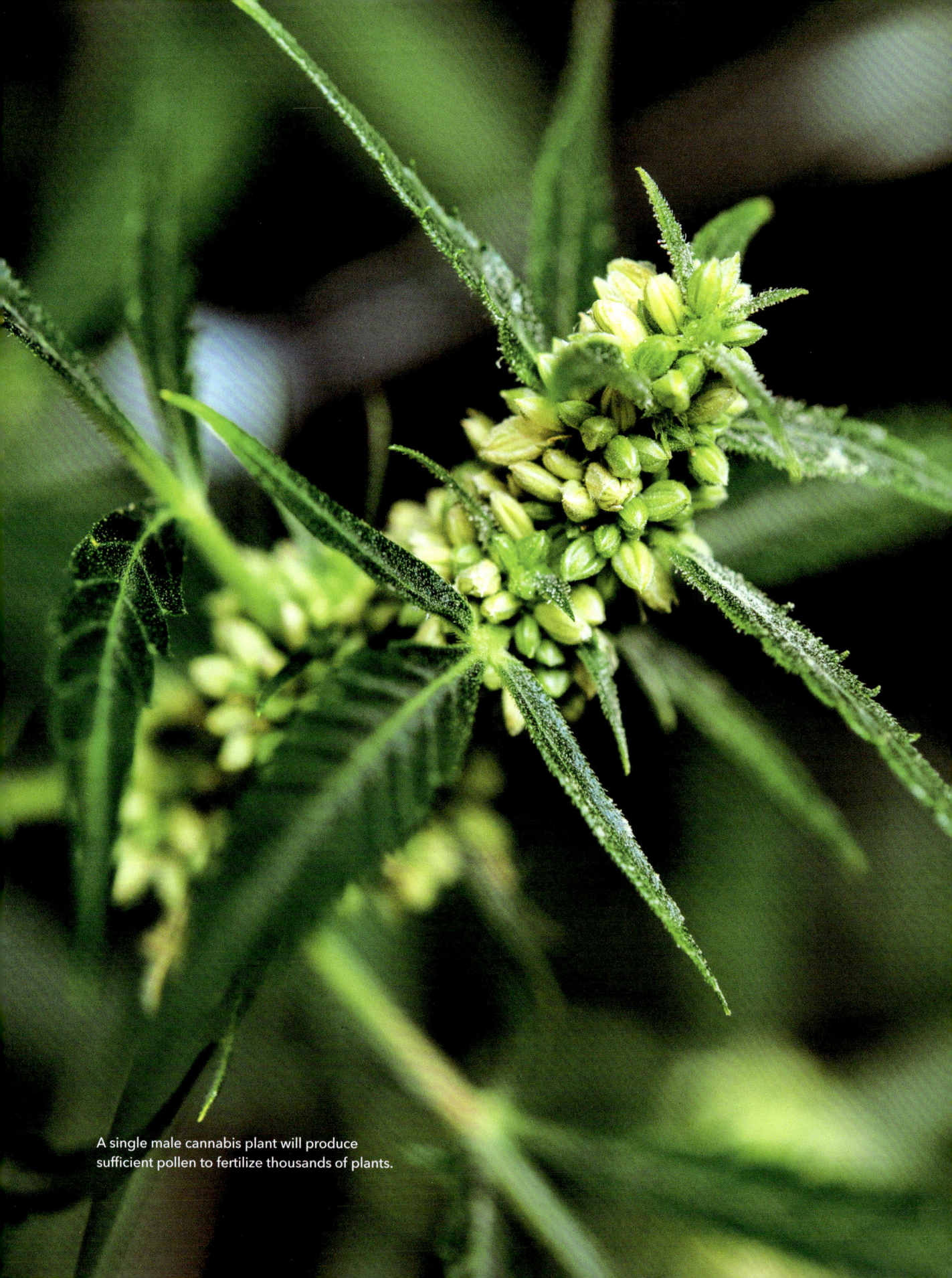

A single male cannabis plant will produce
sufficient pollen to fertilize thousands of plants.

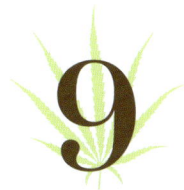

Pollen Management

Pollen and plant sex considerations are factors that set cannabis apart botanically and agriculturally from many other crops. They add a layer of complexity from genetics to in-field management. This complexity is not simply an issue of crop performance but a make-or-break difference. Having a seeded or even slightly seeded crop is a cannabis farmer's worst nightmare. "Seeded" refers to the unintentional introduction of pollen that fertilizes female plants so that they begin growing seed. Seed in the flowers reduces potency and terpenes, changes flower density, changes the color and smell of the extracted material, and creates a reduced-quality product. In such situations, working with buyers becomes tenuous at best, and the most likely outcome is selling the entire yield as trim.

Pollination can occur by means of self-pollination, via male plants in the crop, or from pollen drift from neighboring growers.

Self-Pollination

There are several causes of self-pollination. One occurs with plants that have both male and female parts. Hermaphrodites ("herms" in cannabis speak) can be caused several ways. The first is by poor breeding. A breeder may unintentionally breed from an unstable parent line that displays intersex traits. This parent may pass on these tendencies to their offspring.

The second cause of herms is stress. Since the primary goal of a plant is to reproduce, stress events cause the plant to attempt reproduction in any way possible. For example, imagine a cannabis plant growing in Russia in summer, where in August the nights suddenly turn cold. The drop in temperature triggers a "reproduce at all costs" mechanism in the plant, which can lead to hermaphroditism and the ability to self-pollinate—invaluable traits for passing along genes.

Some breeders exploit this evolutionary response in their programs. The most common method is to create light cycle stress, where a breeder switches the light cycle erratically to force hermaphroditic traits and pollen production. We do not recommend purchasing seed from breeders who use these methods, as using pollen from stress-induced plants can create instability that lends itself to further hermaphroditism.

Plants may also herm from natural stresses such as heat, cold, over- or under-fertilization, wind, over- or under-watering, and the like. Some genetics are hardier than others, though if you stress a plant enough, most cultivars will herm.

Herms may present in different locations on the plant and in different percentages of the population.

Clusters of male flowers at multiple sites on one or more branches. The males do not usually appear until the plants are well into week two or three of flowering, and they can show up right until harvest. Finding them can seem like looking for a needle in a haystack. In our experience, these appear in less than 1 percent of a crop.

Single male flowers at nodes. This form, usually precipitated by a significant or repeated stress event, is the hardest to find, with only a few male flowers per plant. When found in the population, it usually presents in a much higher percentage, 3 to

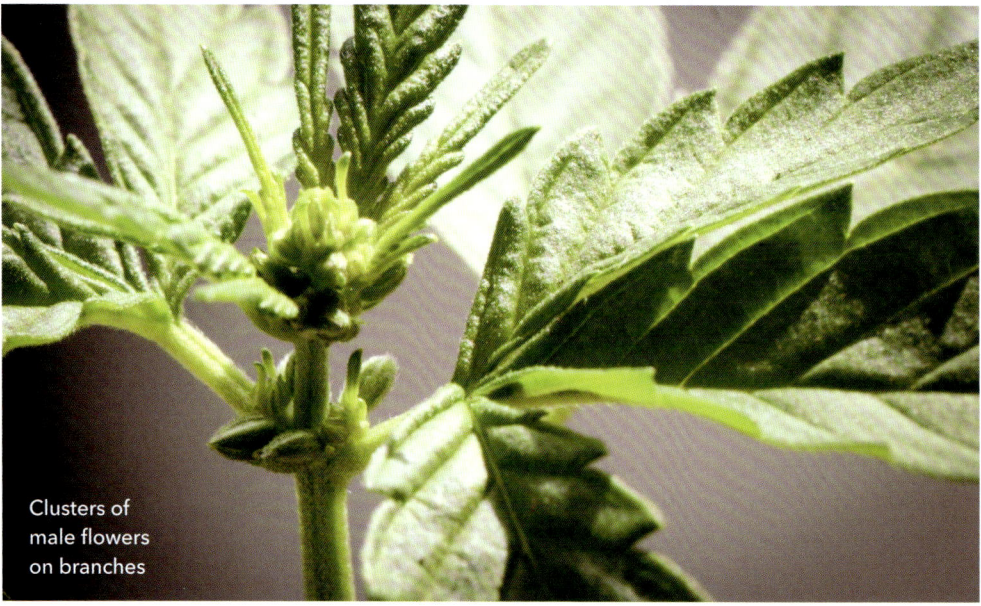

Clusters of male flowers on branches

20 percent. Locating these flowers involves looking closely into the canopy interior. They usually appear from weeks two to four of flowering and can wreak havoc on your crop by setting a substantial amount of seed. But when you use well-bred seed and prevent stress events, this type of hermaphroditism should not be of concern.

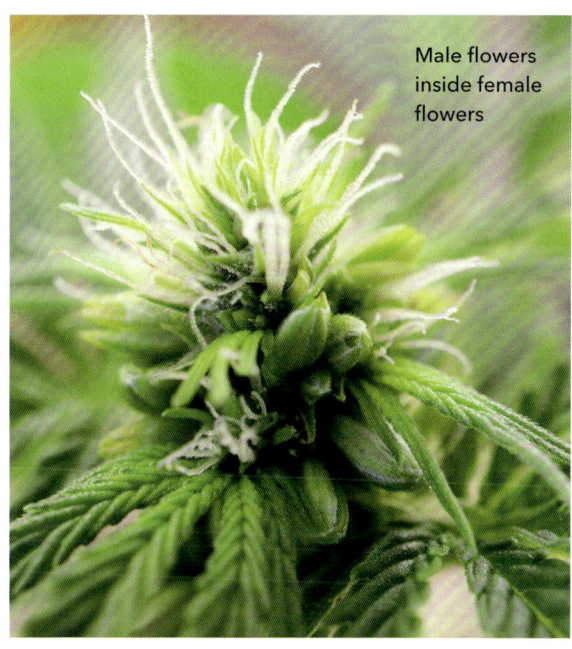

Male flowers inside female flowers

Clusters of male flowers that pop up inside female flowers. These usually appear toward the end of flower maturation and present a lower risk of mature seed set or pollination because very few pistils are available. This form is similar to the single male flowers in that it shows up in the 3 to 20 percent range. With good genetics and no stress events, it shouldn't be an issue.

Male Pollination

The second way plants are pollinated is via males within that population. When planting from seed, farmers *should* use feminized seed; however, even in well-made feminized seed lots there will be roughly 1 male in 1,500 females. Farmers need to take the time to remove these occasional males, a process called roguing. Over the years we have developed a standard operating procedure for roguing plants that has proven very useful (see page 144).

A Hard Lesson Learned

One important rule we have learned is to *never* use regular, nonfeminized seed. Even with rigorous roguing of a crop planted from regular, nonfeminized seed, we always ended up with seeded flowers. One year we planted a crop of regular Blue Dream late and were delighted with our ability to remove all the males. At a certain point we stopped looking because we thought we had removed all of them.

Toward the end of flower maturation, we noticed in the lower canopy a very small male plant just loving life and releasing tons of pollen. Apparently the seed germinated a month or more after all the others, grew very short in the shade of its peers, and went to flower immediately. This single plant no taller than 18 inches seeded the whole crop.

Removing Male Flowers (Roguing)

Plants with male flowers that have already opened should be removed from the field very carefully and treated with the utmost caution so that you avoid spreading pollen onto surrounding plants.

Timing: Every week after the first week of flower

Setup: Two people per bed, walking in tandem, each carrying a large (20- or 30-gallon) trash bag, with a box of extra bags at the edge of the field to resupply as necessary

Scouting: Each person takes one line of plants (assuming two rows on a bed) and looks at every plant. An appropriate walking speed is slightly slower than casual walking speed, about 1 mile per hour. Two people should be able to cover an acre in about an hour.

While scouting for open male flowers, it's critical to take the additional step of looking for "armpit" male flowers in every variety. To do this, choose a subsection of 30 plants and study them even more carefully. Examine the lowest nodes on each plant for more subtle or obvious signs of herm—specifically, male flowers clustered in the armpits of the lower canopy. If a plant looks "funny" or "off" or different in any way, check the lowest branches for early signs of hermaphroditism (especially the areas where the branches meet the main stem, the nodes where flower initiation begins). If you see more than a few signs of male flowers in the lower branch junctions ("armpit nuts") in any subsection, carefully scout the rest of the plants of that variety.

Removal: When you find a plant with open male flowers, put a bag over the entire plant, disturbing it as little as possible. Pull the bag as low as you can, ideally all the way to the ground. Holding the bag closed around the base of the stem, pull out the plant, removing the entire rootball, and immediately tie the bag shut. Do not open the bag again. Plants without open flowers may be combined into one bag. Be very careful when making this assessment, though, as some male flowers open much earlier than others. Throw away the bags; do not leave the plants anywhere near the field. Dead males/herms can open flowers and release pollen days after they have been pulled up.

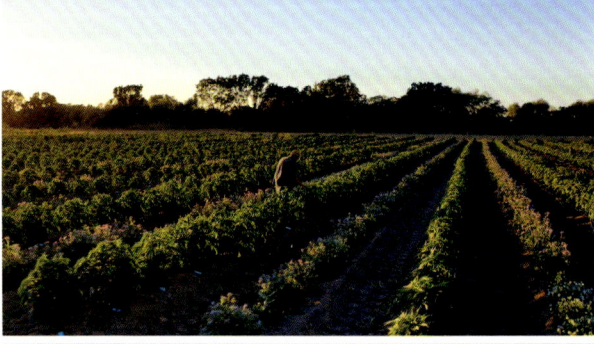

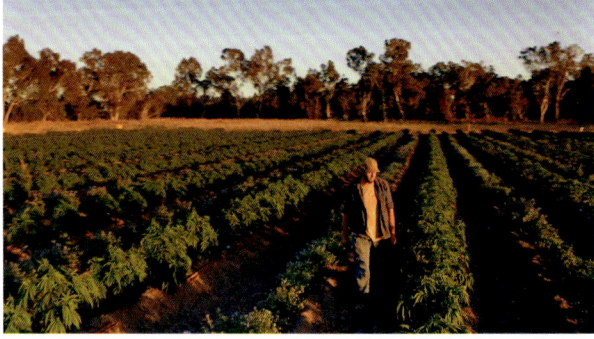

Alex walks a field of autoflowers scouting for males.

Pollen Drift

Cannabis crops can get seeded when pollen drifts in from a surrounding area. We've heard accounts of pollen traveling as far as 40 miles under the right conditions, such as flat topography, low humidity, and prevailing wind. In various parts of the country, especially places where hemp markets crashed, farmers abandoned fields of hemp grown from nonfeminized seed. In subsequent years these hemp fields naturalized and reseeded themselves. In Colorado we've witnessed thousands of male plants releasing pollen into the wind from fallowed fields previously cultivated in hemp. A single male flower can release up to 350,000 grains of pollen, so you do the math. The rogue pollen issue is so dire in some areas, specifically in Colorado and Oregon, that it is likely to limit or impact the way cultivation is done, if it can be done at all.

Some growers have found success using ethephon, a plant growth regulator, to suppress male flower formation or male flower maturation. By spraying ethephon preemptively on crops grown from feminized seed, farmers can eliminate or at least limit potential pollen release and reduce the likelihood of seeding. Ethephon may have detection limits, so please check local regulations before applying. And it is a powerful chemical; we have seen plants with significant reactions, including leaf burning and growth tip death, even at low application rates. We recommend a dilution of 1 to 5 milliliters per gallon, applied out of direct sunlight and not before daytime temps for the next few days will reach 85°F (29°C). If this is not possible, we recommend experimenting with the solution on a few plants and waiting five days to see how they respond.

Breeding for Sterile Plants

Genetics bred to possess three sets of chromosomes (triploid) rather than two (diploid) are essentially sterile and cannot be pollinated. The process involves converting a parent plant to tetraploid (four sets of chromosomes) and crossing it with a normal diploid. All the resulting offspring will be triploid. This process is not uncommon and is used in other crop plant breeding. A chemical process induces tetraploidy, which must be confirmed using a flow cytometer.

A rush to market with triploid genetics includes a caveat: Four sets of chromosomes mean exponentially greater variation in the next generation. Therefore, parent stock used must be very homozygous to begin with, and trialing should be performed before any seed is offered. As an industry we are not there yet.

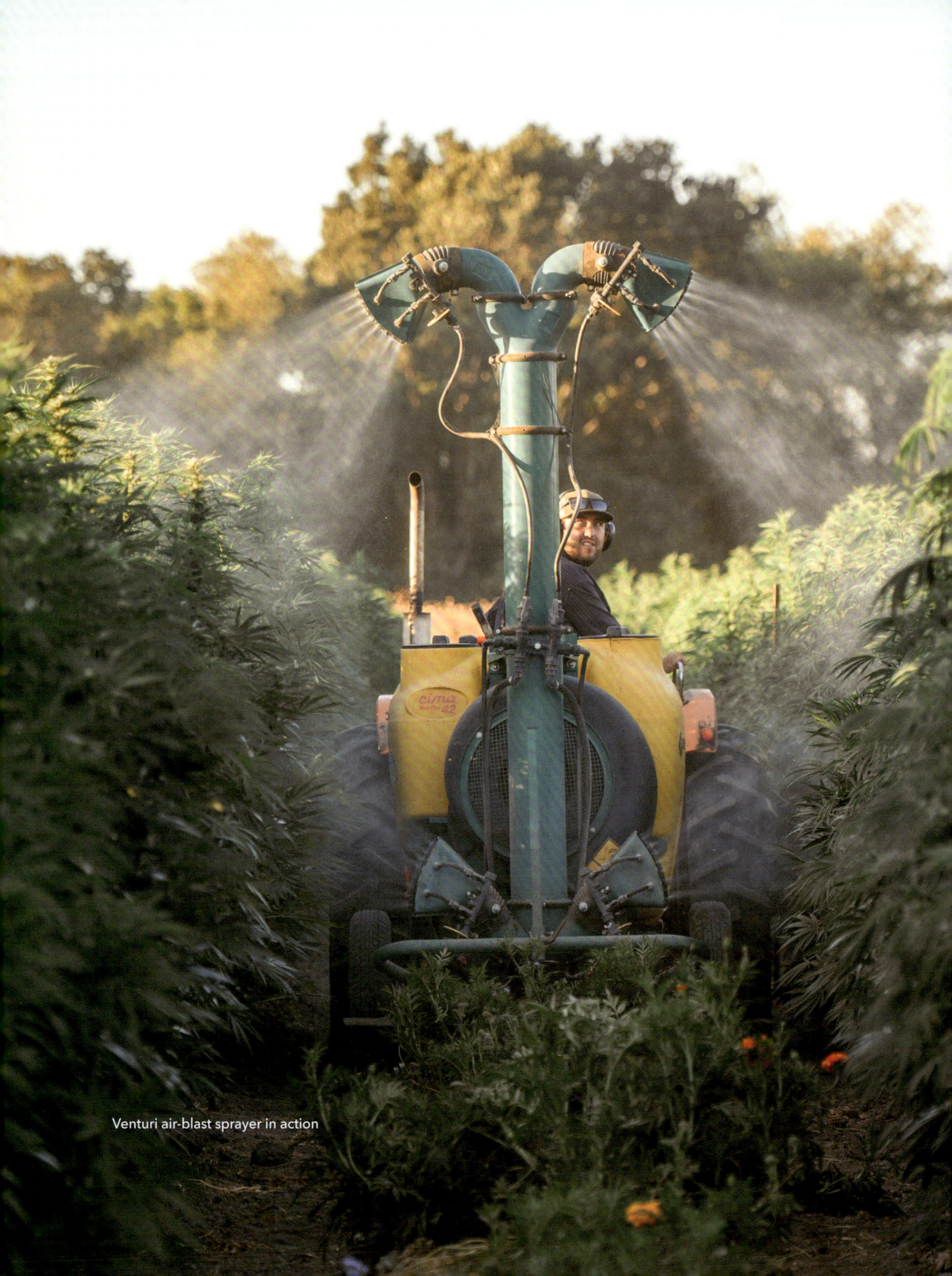

Venturi air-blast sprayer in action

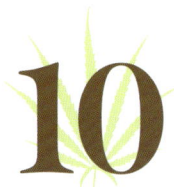

10

Implementing a Spray Program

Many modern varieties of cannabis are exceptionally susceptible to mold and pests. The techniques we've already discussed, including a healthy soils approach and selecting early-finishing genetics, can mitigate some of these challenges, but we still believe that a well-thought-out spray program is an important part of any cannabis farm.

Before discussing the details of a spray program, let's revisit the importance of field layout. For a perennial crop, such as grapes, that requires regular tractor access for sprays during the crop cycle, the rows are laid out only once. As an annual crop, cannabis requires this precision-level field layout to happen every year. The rows must be marked and the trellis installed and taken down annually. Without careful planning, there will be wasted space in the production acreage, or the tractor won't have enough room to pass without driving over dangling branches.

One year after we installed T-posts according to canopy restrictions, we had only 2 feet of clearance on either side of the tractor to fit through the crop for spraying passes. It was nail-biting to make the turns into the beds, and keeping the tractor straight was laughable. Questionable T-post placement further complicated an already dicey situation: We were able to make it through a few of the beds for a few weeks, but for most of them we gave up and didn't even attempt to get the tractor into the field again. As regulations develop, hopefully arbitrary canopy restrictions will fade away, to be replaced by commonsense agricultural metrics.

Sprayer Types

Purchasing the right sprayer for your farm is an important decision. As with any equipment purchase, there are variables to consider when choosing what type and how many sprayers to buy. Key factors include the climate and seasonal conditions of the farm. Does the location have high humidity, reliable summer or fall rain, or particular challenges with pests? Region and conditions also affect the spray frequency, which could vary drastically from three times per week to only a few times per crop cycle. On our farm, we spray our autoflower crop 2 to 5 times, and we spray full-terms 5 to 10 times, beginning a week or two after transplant and ending in roughly week six of flower.

We have tried almost every type of sprayer on the market except airplanes and a very novel motorcycle/scooter that's worth looking up on YouTube for a good laugh. Ultimately we've landed on an efficient and effective combination of sprayers that works well for our farm. When plants are small, we use a traditional boom sprayer that covers three beds at a time. When the plants get too tall for this sprayer to work, we switch to a vineyard-style venturi air-blast sprayer.

Here are brief descriptions of various options.

Backpack sprayers, available in hand-pump or motorized configurations, are labor intensive and cannot achieve uniform spray coverage. Uneven or excessive applications of pesticides can damage your crop. Spraying a large canopy uniformly with handheld equipment is no trivial task in contrast with tractor-mounted sprayers that move through the canopy at a fixed height, in a line, and at a consistent speed. Nevertheless, for a small operator

A boom sprayer gets five beds at a time. Note that it can only spray down and would only work with plants under the height of the boom.

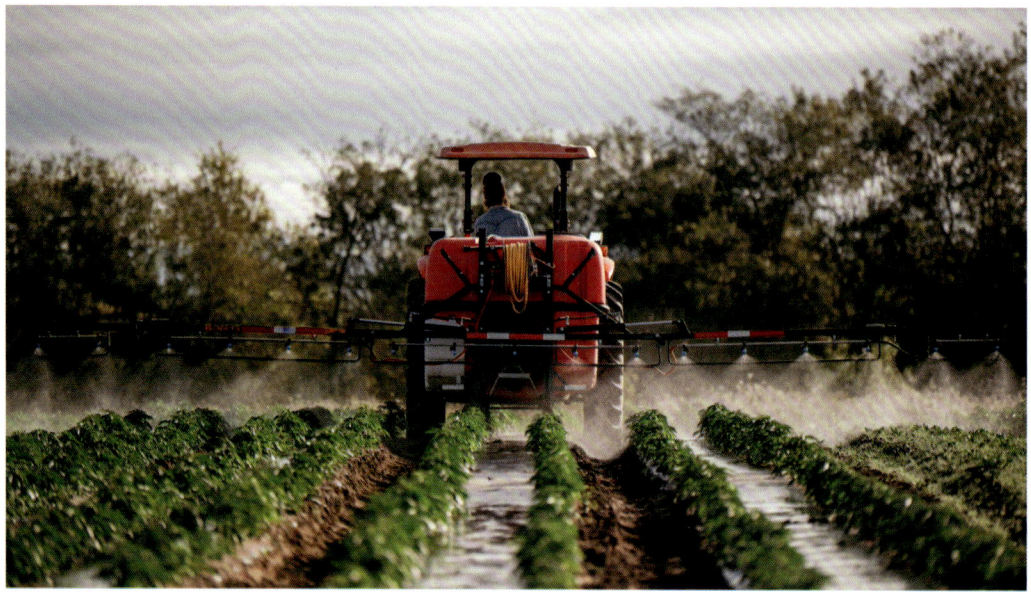

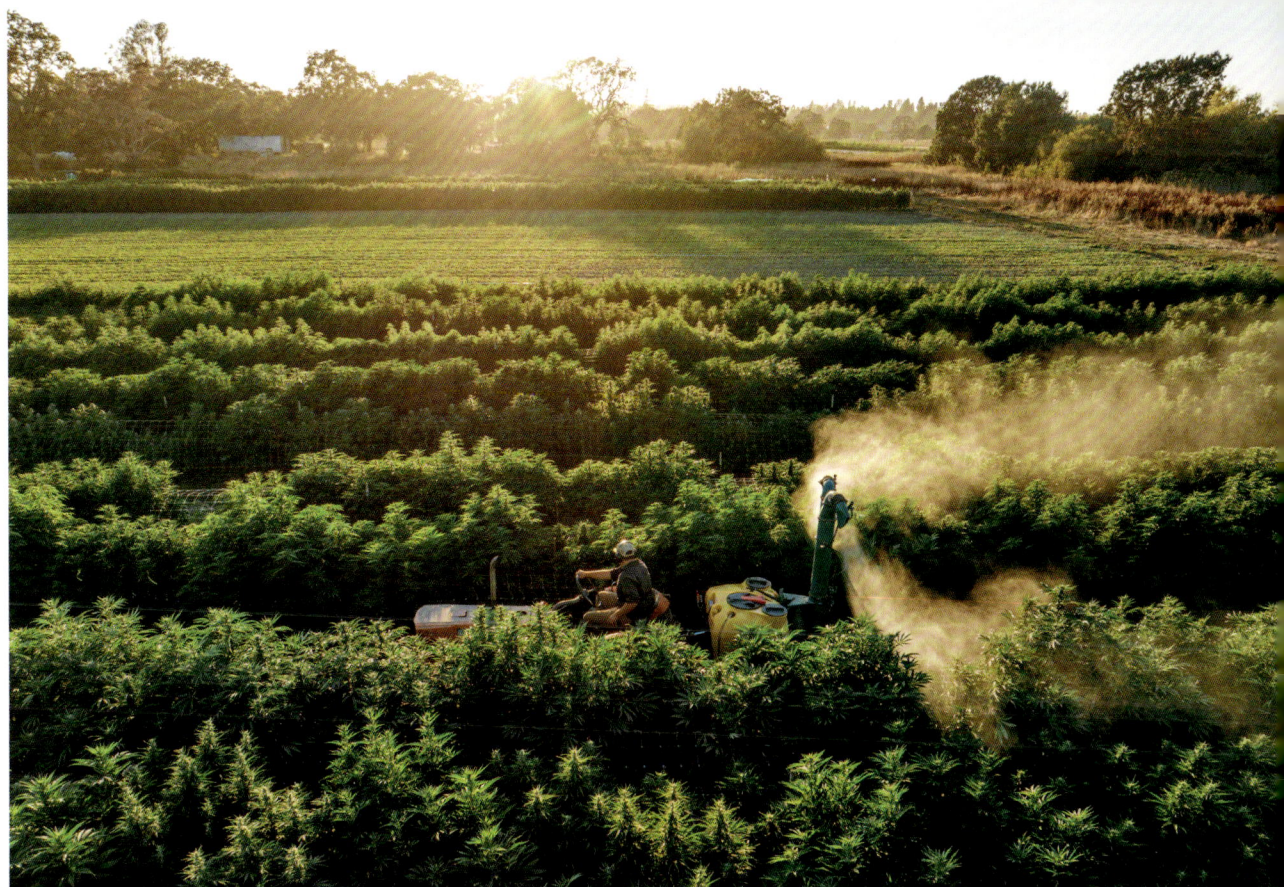

working carefully, sacrificing perfect coverage may be an acceptable alternative to the expense of a tractor-mounted sprayer. For farms at a medium or large scale, backpack sprayers quickly become impractical for the multiple mixings required by the small tank size, which introduces the possibility of error and is very laborious. We do not recommend hand-pump backpack sprayers.

Boom sprayers are available in different boom lengths. Ours is 15 feet, which covers three beds at a time. These sprayers work from the top down and can cover a lot of ground quickly. The main drawback is that they *only* work from the top down, which means that pests on the underside of leaves are less affected—and several of the main cannabis pests (mites and aphids) spend a significant portion of their life cycle on the underside of leaves. Mold also tends to develop in the lower canopy first. The boom sprayer works well for autoflowers because they stay short—generally less than 3 feet—and it can be used throughout the entire crop cycle.

Venturi air-blast sprayers are designed for vineyards and orchards—they reach the plants from the bottom up, the side, and the top down. We like this sprayer for larger plants because it gives great spray coverage and requires low PTO power, which means we can use a small tractor after the canopy has grown in and made access tighter. We believe this will quickly become the dominant sprayer in the industry.

A venturi air-blast sprayer gets excellent coverage by spraying towards the bottom, side, and top of the canopy.

Spray Products

Currently every state has a different set of products allowed for application. Familiarize yourself carefully with these regulations, as we have heard horror stories of accidental misapplication that rendered flowers unsellable. As a foundation for our program, we use a suite of Marrone Bio Innovations products—Grandevo, Regalia, and Venerate—for general prevention and maintenance. These biofungicides and bioinsecticides are derived from living organisms and inorganic materials such as minerals. We add a Bt product for caterpillar management during early flowering.

For most pest outbreaks, we use horticultural oils. Our current favorite is PureSpray Green, though we've used a variety of others in the past with good success. For mites specifically we use sulfur.

It's essential to be proactive with disease and mold management. Once mold or powdery mildew has set in, it's basically impossible to stop growth, and treatment is just about slowing or containing the damage. Products we use for botrytis and powdery mildew include double nickel, potassium bicarbonate, and sulfur. As we discuss in Chapter 3, the best approach is to promote overall agroecosystem health and reduce or eliminate the need to spray altogether.

✳ Sulfur Warning

While sulfur can play a role in pest management, it must be used with caution and careful timing. Many extractors prefer limiting the use of sulfur after transition or early flower because it can give the extractions a sulfur taste. Furthermore, using sulfur and horticultural oils within two weeks of one another can cause extensive plant damage.

Spray Timing

There are various schools of thought about spraying after the crops have transitioned into flower. Some old-school growers believe firmly that nothing should be applied beginning a week or two after initiation. We've taken a modern but still thoughtful and cautious approach to product applications after the crop has entered flower. This is because there is uncertainty about the effects of products on human health, both when spraying the plant and upon later consumption, and also because we want to protect the health of the crop. We've developed some guidelines for sprays after the crop has entered flower.

- Read the labels of the products and follow all the instructions carefully.

- Do not apply products in direct sunlight. We do our applications in the early morning or in the evening after the sun sets.

- Avoid spraying during or right before a heat spell. We use 85°F (29°C) as an acceptable maximum, though in hot climates this may not be possible and upper limits will have to be adjusted based on trial and error.

- Do not apply sulfur after week two. It can affect the smell and taste of the end product.

Foliar Feeding

Plants absorb nutrients/enzymes through their pores. Foliar feeding is the technique of applying fertilizers by sprayer. It is not an alternative to building good and balanced soils. Plants, especially fast-growing annuals, cannot take up enough nitrogen, phosphorus, and potassium via foliar feedings to meet their needs. However, stressed plants or plants undergoing rapid growth can benefit greatly from foliar feedings. It is a fast way to supply micronutrients, such as iron and zinc, that plants do not need in huge quantities and that may exist in limited availability in the soil.

We focus our foliar feeding during the early stages of vegetative growth and not after initiation. We include one or more of the following products in our foliar feedings: homemade compost tea, calcium, nitrogen, and kelp extract.

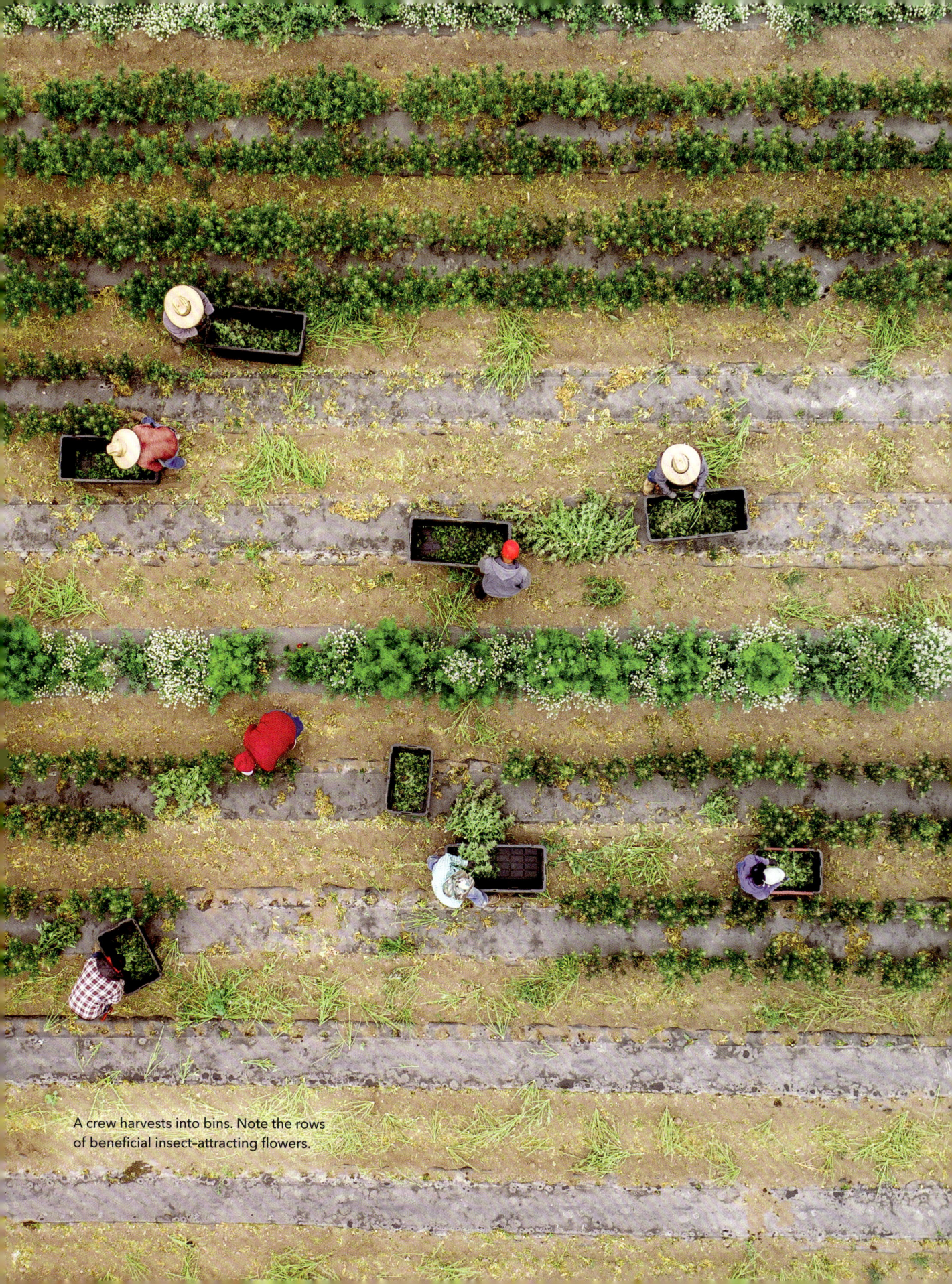

A crew harvests into bins. Note the rows of beneficial insect-attracting flowers.

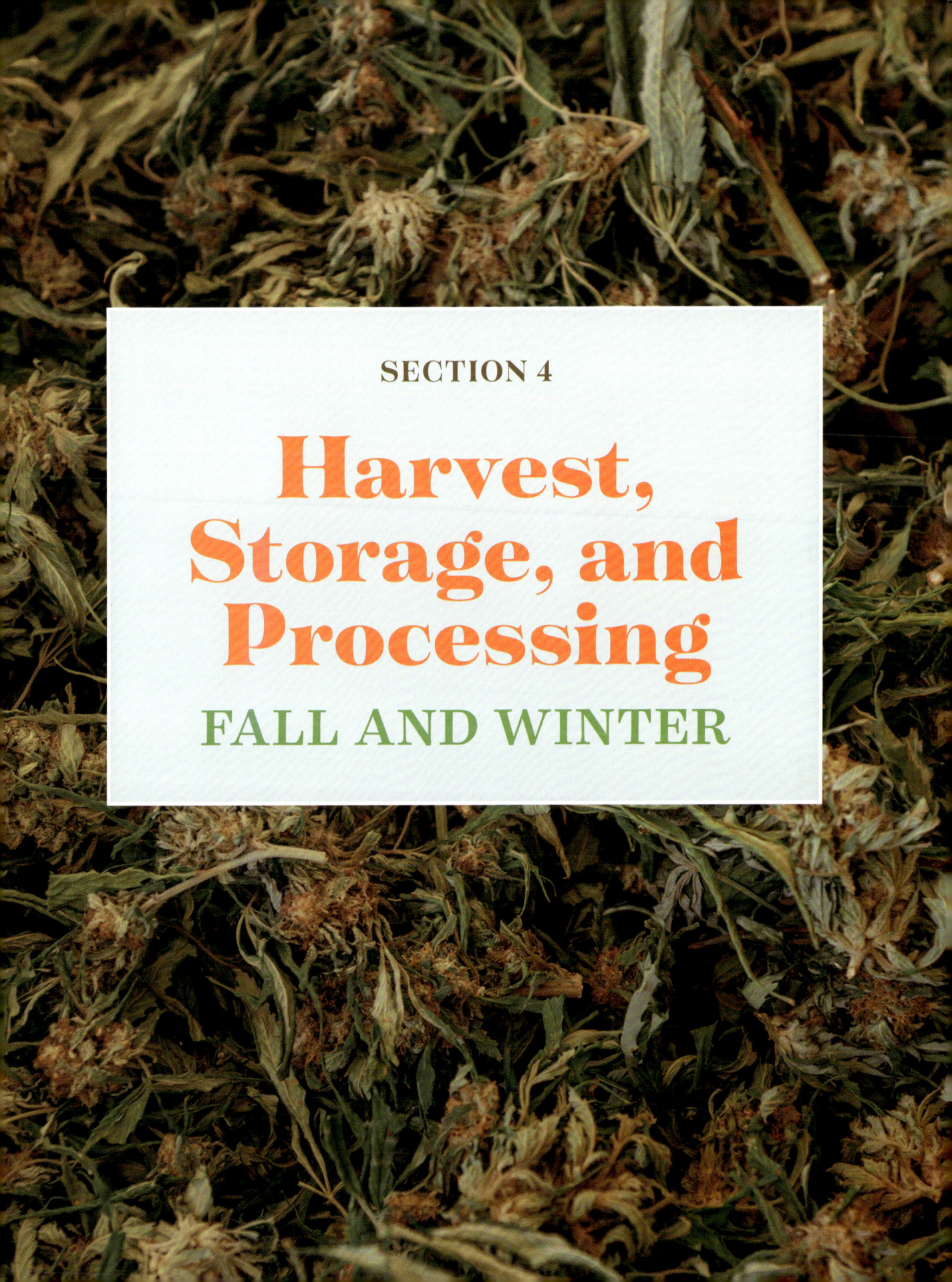

Harvest, Storage, and Processing

FALL AND WINTER

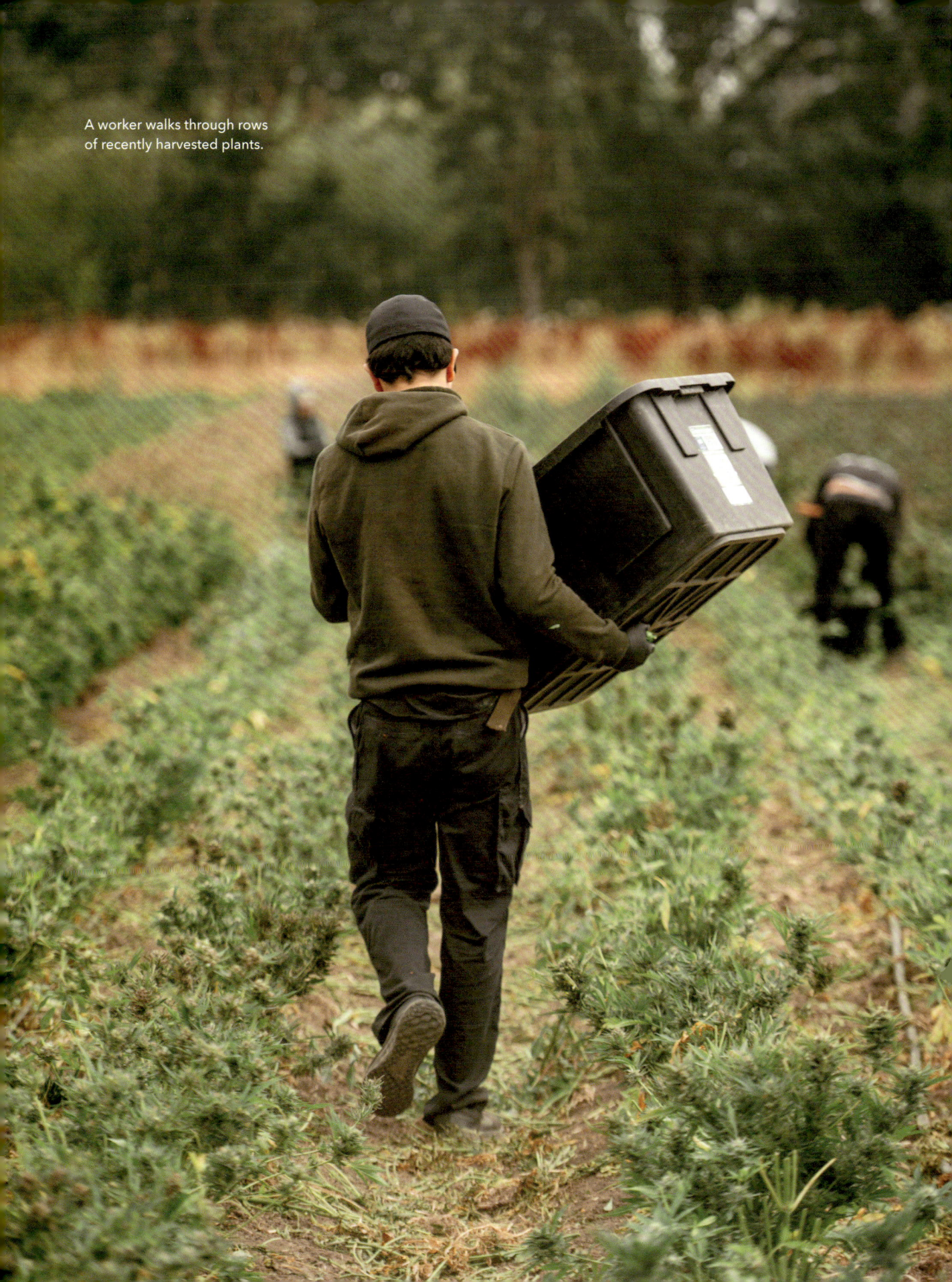

A worker walks through rows of recently harvested plants.

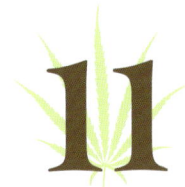

Harvest

All farmers know that after the work of planning, planting, and crop management, harvesttime is the make-or-break season. Crop quality can change in a matter of hours, yields can accidentally be significantly reduced, and extra time is needed to do everything. The harvest time frame is small compared to the entire crop cycle, and yet the stakes are equal to or greater than everything preceding it.

Cannabis farming is capital intensive, with harvest absorbing a significant portion of the year's labor budget. Thus it is exceptionally important to be clear about what you are doing (how you harvest) and why you are doing it (your marketplace). Because the stakes are so high, we recommend you take extra time to review your plan.

Several weeks before our harvest, we dedicate an entire whiteboard to harvest considerations: We map out the expected flow and dates into and out of the dry spaces. We review our labor plan. We make sure we have enough supplies such as gloves, boxes, and scissors. We discuss contingency plans. Harvest begins with clear and conscious decisions, but it's better to start too early than too late.

Recognizing Your Harvest Window

Choosing when to harvest is a complicated and nerve-racking process, with implications that can make or break the success of your crop cycle. For example, waiting for perfect trichome maturity or for additional weight to bulk up your flowers may mean an increased presence of mold and therefore reduced quality and weight. Or there simply may not be enough labor available when you finally decide it's time to begin. There are a lot of variables to help you determine the optimal time to bring in your crop.

Cannabis has a harvest window of roughly 30 days. Flowers harvested in the first 10 days are referred to as "preemies" and are lower in quality in nearly every aspect. Although the flowers are nearly mature, their levels of terpenes and cannabinoids will be lower, with yields reduced by 25 to 75 percent. Additionally, flower aesthetics are compromised, as none of the hairs will have turned color or shrunk, which are clear signs of flower maturity to buyers.

The next 10 days are the ideal harvest window. Flowers have reached their maximum potential terpene levels, cannabinoid content, and yield potential, and the overall flower quality and aesthetics are at their highest. Ideally at this point, you harvest the plants into a dry space large enough to fit the entire crop and supplied with enough power and equipment to dry it efficiently.

Harvest begins with clear and conscious decisions, but it's better to start too early than too late.

The final 10 days of the harvest window are usually characterized by an overmaturation of flowers, which presents in different ways, including an increase or explosion of molds or mildews, flower discoloration (usually darkening), and increased pest pressure. In crops grown for biomass or in situations where yield is more important than quality, farmers may elect to push harvest into this later window.

How do we know when a crop reaches the beginning of its harvest window? We use both the cultivar's days to maturity and our previous experience with it (if any) as benchmarks. Some varieties specify a day range, such as 63 to 66 days, while others provide a number of weeks, such as 8 weeks. Then we turn to the following wide-ranging set of considerations.

Flower Appearance

As harvesttime approaches, we walk the fields daily, looking closely for key changes in flower appearance, such as pistil and trichome color shifts. The flower marketplace has preferences, and flowers that meet those criteria fetch a higher price or are quicker to sell. One thing the marketplace does not prefer is white hair on the flowers, which suggests undermaturity. Thus, we aim to ensure that at least 50 percent of the flower hairs shrivel and turn from white to a darker color (the color varies by strain, generally orange-red, rust, or a variation of brown). The fewer white hairs, the better.

Trichome color is another indicator of flower maturity, so we use a small handheld microscope to study the trichomes. Clear trichomes suggest immaturity, while milky trichomes are considered perfectly ripe. When they begin turning to light brown or darker, they have moved to full maturity and in some cases overmaturation.

Regardless of these somewhat empirical methods, the takeaway is that the flowers themselves look good and "done." After a few harvests, you'll be able to just tell when a crop has reached its peak and will no longer gain weight or quality. Intuition is as important in judging flower appearance as anything else.

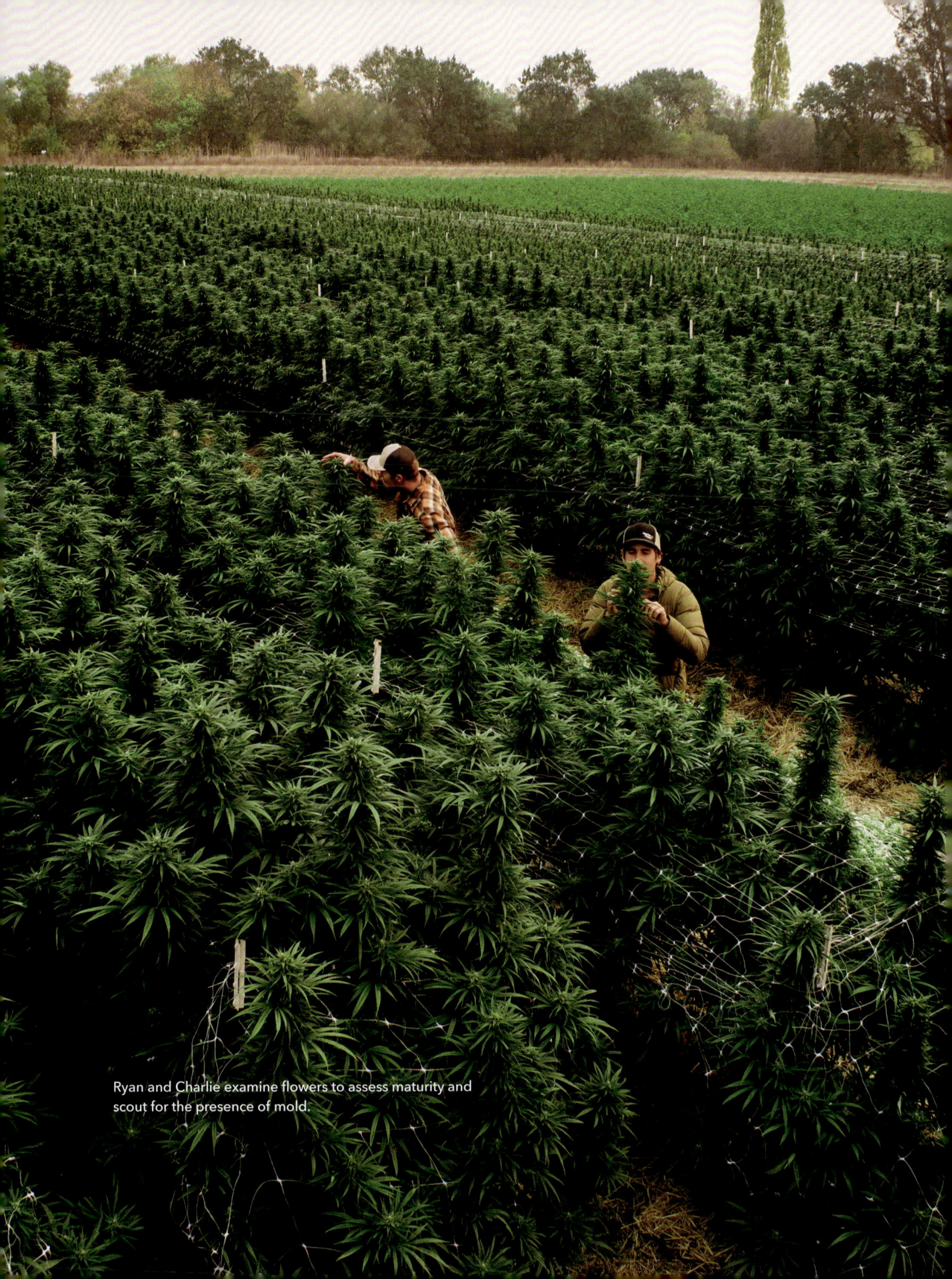

Ryan and Charlie examine flowers to assess maturity and scout for the presence of mold.

Potency

Year after year, cannabis markets have demanded higher cannabinoid content. Buyers demanded flowers with over 15 percent THC, then 18 percent, 20 percent, 22 percent, and so on. While we believe that the infatuation with THC content will wane in favor of unique terpenes or other minor cannabinoids, we do have some control over THC levels by choosing when to harvest. When flowers are maturing and gaining density, there is an ideal intersection between yield and THC concentration. This intersection changes regionally and from season to season and will never be a perfect science. However, we have proven, backed by extensive testing, that potency decreases with overmaturation of flowers. This is due to the overall weight of the flowers increasing while their chemical content plateaus. THC concentration remains the same or decreases while plant matter continues to grow. The ideal intersection can only be understood and judged by experience, but we mention it so you will know to learn about it.

De-leafing

We discuss de-leafing in detail in Chapter 8, but to review: De-leafing too early or too aggressively robs the plant of the ability to produce high-quality and high-yielding flowers. The leaves are like the plant's solar panels or engine. To expand on the car analogy, if the plants have crested the hill, they can roll down to the finish line without the engine.

Understanding that de-leafing takes longer than the actual harvest helps growers to plan harvest schedules accurately. On farms where the crop is all finished in roughly the same 10-day window, the easy and obvious choice is to de-leaf everything all at once, if possible. To help with labor and dry space for a photoperiod crop on our farm, we plant so that crops finish in succession over the course of an entire month (roughly September 15 to October 15). This means we alternate back and forth between de-leafing and harvesting.

Other Harvesting Variables

While the maturity of the flowers is the key factor in determining your harvest dates, there are other considerations.

Weather. Obviously the current and forecasted weather plays a big role in decision making. Starting at the beginning of September, we pay extra attention to the medium- and long-term forecasts. Many times we have begun harvesting before the crop reached ideal maturity simply because the weather was going to turn bad. Wet weather means mold. Conversely, a period of extended fall warmth and sunshine can offer spaciousness in the harvest decision-making matrix, as varieties are given ideal conditions to reach their peak quality before being taken down.

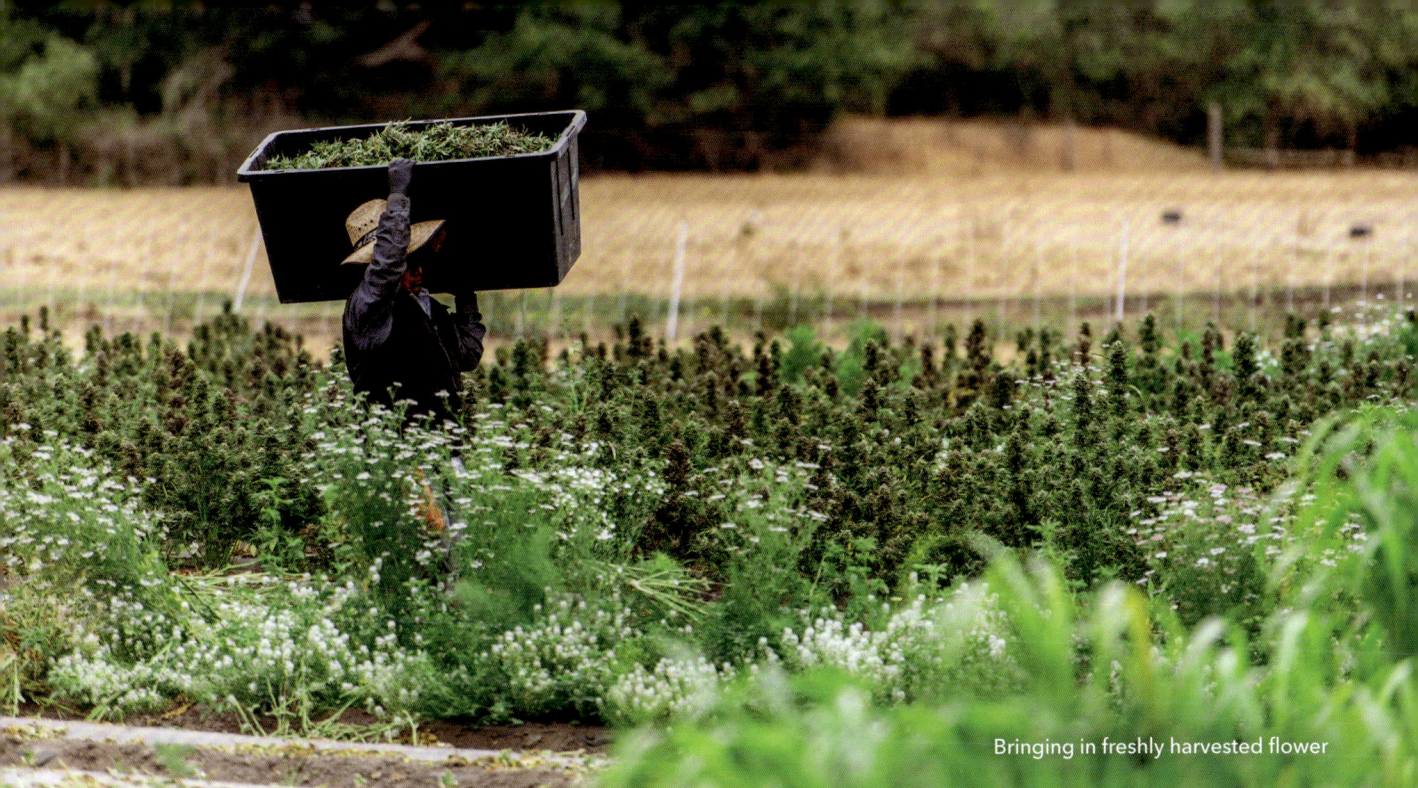

Bringing in freshly harvested flower

Mold pressure. We always consider the current mold pressure and overall health of the plants. A healthier plant has more natural resistance to pathogens and pests. If the plants appear stressed or unhealthy, mold may become an issue quickly. When there is a large outbreak of powdery mildew and we notice botrytis mold, we may elect to harvest early. Specifically with botrytis, in our experience there is always more mold present in the flowers than is visible.

When we observe the onset of botrytis, we take added measures: We pull apart flowers in areas of the field with visible mold, and we cut and break apart random samples of otherwise normal-looking flowers to see if and/or how much botrytis is present where it's not obvious from the outside. Learn to train your eye to recognize an active botrytis infection vs. a dead or dormant botrytis spot. Remember that sprays at this point are essentially useless for mold abatement and potentially dangerous for the consumer. Be aware that, depending on the strain, mold can and will explode overnight.

Availability of labor. Nonmechanized cannabis harvest is exceptionally labor intensive. Every farmer understands the plight of other farmers needing reinforcements to bring their crop in. The size of the crew determines how quickly the crop can get brought in. Many times we've seen beautiful fields of cannabis rot for lack of an effective labor solution. Sometimes harvest must begin early to ensure that the entire field will be harvested before the window closes or the season ends. We recommend checking and double-checking on labor commitments and having a backup plan in place.

Planned number of harvests. Some farmers "cut it once and done," while others make multiple harvest passes on a single plant. This decision may simply be influenced by the availability of labor or dry space. On our farm we have used yield-per-square-foot maximization as a primary consideration in crop management. Thus we frequently opt to do multiple harvests on the crop. We'll take tops, wait four to seven days, then take "mids" after they have bulked up and matured. On that same day we might strip the lower canopy (larf/biomass) and be completely done, or we might wait until a more convenient day or week. Other times we're never able to return at all. Regardless, we cut tops and mids by hand with scissors, and anything left over we strip by hand. When a farmer counts on multiple harvests, starting a little earlier can allow time on the back end to get to the second harvest.

Dry/cure infrastructure. Some farms have more dry space than is needed; some have just the right amount. Most of the farms we encounter either barely have enough or just plain do not have enough dry space. If you have to make harvest decisions with dry space as a limiting factor, we recommend starting your harvest in the early part of the window so that you are harvesting in your ideal 10-day window and not extending further into unfavorable conditions. Map out on a calendar the expected harvest-to-takedown time for each dry space available. Depending on the size of spaces available, the finish times of varieties chosen, and the crew size, some spaces may be utilized four to five times per harvest season. Proper planning is critical to avoid leaving your crop in the field in unfavorable weather or after its ideal harvest window has closed.

Intuition. We encourage farmers to use their intuition, in conjunction with everything mentioned above, to help decide when to harvest. Intuition is a powerful tool and should be heeded when making complicated and high-impact decisions.

✳ Best Time of Day?

Some growers harvest at night or before sunrise to preserve terpenes. It is a logical approach: The field is cool, no sunlight hits the flowers to degrade them, and they do not sit in hot bins for a few hours before going into the dry space. Wine grapes are often night harvested for the same reason—to preserve quality. After an entire season and everything that has gone into a crop, it does make sense to do whatever you can feasibly do to get the best quality possible. While this is not currently standard practice in the industry, we believe that as the industry continues to mature and more research is done, farmers growing for market segments that value terpenes will move toward nighttime or off-hours harvest.

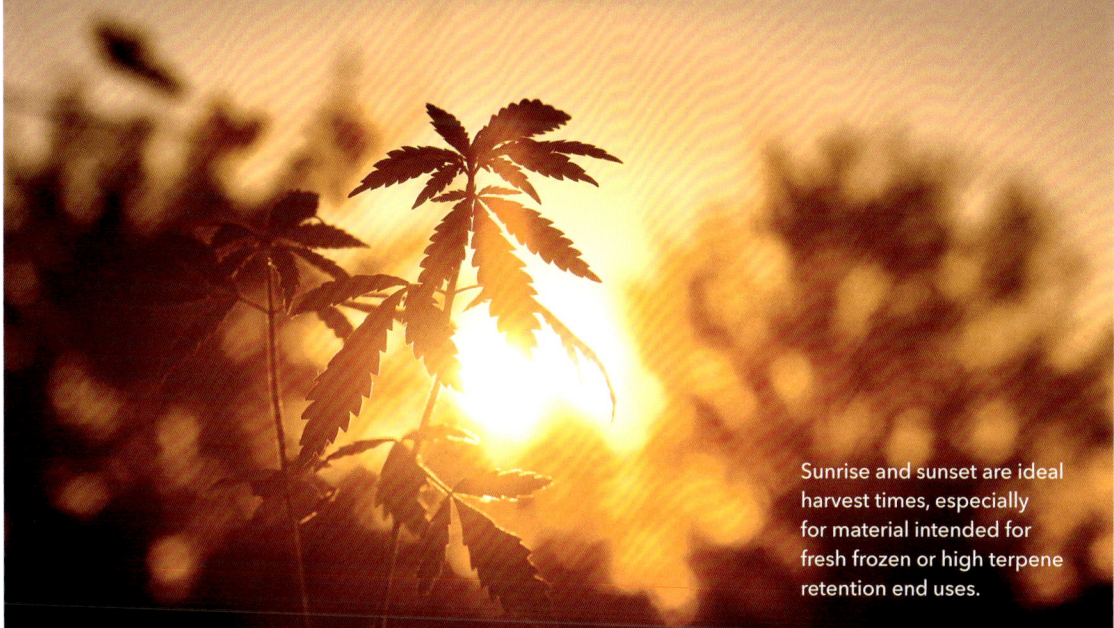

Sunrise and sunset are ideal harvest times, especially for material intended for fresh frozen or high terpene retention end uses.

Preparing for the Harvest

Harvest day approaches. The key steps here are planning and preparation. Before you begin, set up and test everything you need for post-harvest. This may appear obvious, but in the hustle and bustle of harvest season, it's easy to overlook or skip these steps. If you are freezing flowers for fresh frozen, plug in the freezer and make sure it works. Test your backup generator, have enough gas on hand, and confirm that you can easily transfer from the electrical grid to the generator.

If you are going with a traditional drying method, set up your dry space, then turn everything on and make sure the system works the way it's supposed to. Our skipping this step resulted in some stressful (although comical) moments and late evenings, with us scrambling to set up spaces and run tests literally as the rooms were being loaded with racks of flowers. We have seen conclusively that the more thought and time we put into a harvest plan, the smoother and more successful the harvest is.

Once you've got a plan in place, what does the actual harvest look like? How will you get the flowers off the plants? How you harvest should be determined primarily by the market for the crop. Each product requires a different method.

Product: Extraction

If a crop is going exclusively to extraction and therefore fetching the lowest price, limiting labor should be priority number one. In this case, the flower's presentation and structure are unimportant. Harvesting by hand—wearing thick gloves and pull-stripping the buds and leaves off each stem—works but is physically taxing. This product begs mechanization. There are several viable approaches to a mechanized harvest, and we are confident that more will emerge in the coming years.

One option is a modified stripper header, which is a combine attachment traditionally used in grain crops. These machines strip the flowers off the stalks while the plants are still rooted in the ground. Another approach is to put the plants through a wood chipper, then dry the crop and use a sorter to separate out stems and leaves, which have different densities and weights than crumbled flowers. Yet another approach is to cut whole plants, field dry them in rows on a tarp or directly on the ground, then feed the plants by hand into a thresher.

Whichever method you use, in this high-growth industry we will continue to see rapid innovation in harvest techniques, which currently constitute the largest portion of the labor budget and, really, of the crop production overall.

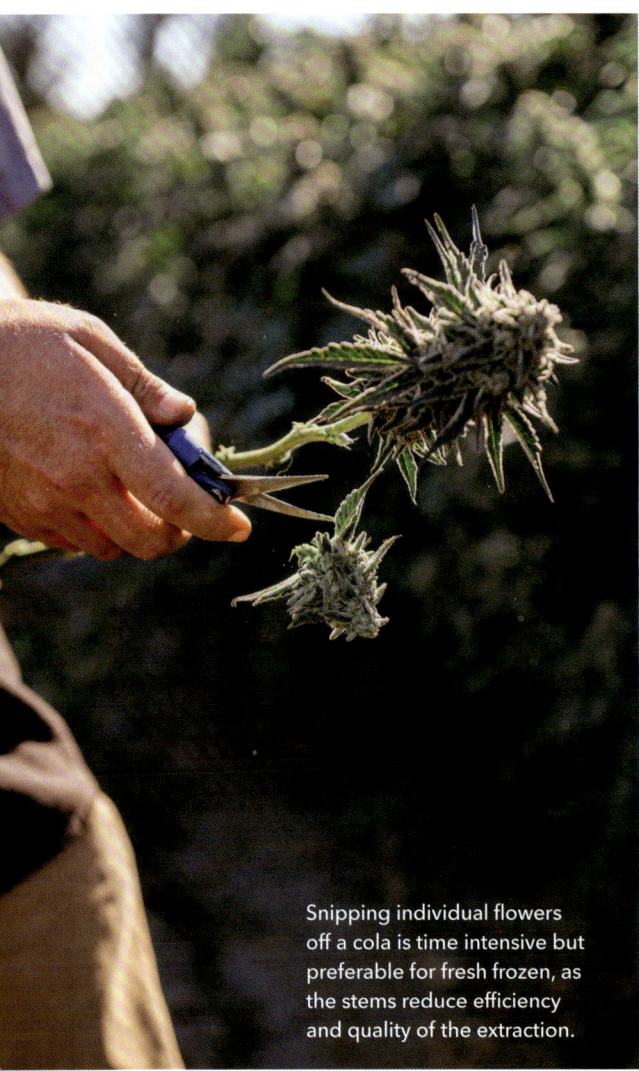

Snipping individual flowers off a cola is time intensive but preferable for fresh frozen, as the stems reduce efficiency and quality of the extraction.

Product: Fresh Frozen

Fresh-frozen flowers are used to make high-quality extracts such as live rosin or "diamonds," which have a special niche in the marketplace. They are often harvested under contract, especially when done at larger scales, because the market is specialized and the large freezers required are capital intensive to buy or rent. Harvesting involves wet bucking the flowers directly into bags and freezing them immediately. *Bucking* means separating flowers from stems, using scissors for hand-trimmed flowers as described here. Wet bucking is done with fresh flowers. For fresh-frozen product, bucking must be done wet so only flowers are frozen. It can be done mechanically or by hand.

There are myriad ways to go about harvesting flowers to freeze, though buyers can be picky about the specifics of the harvest process. It is important to remove as many of the leaves as possible before freezing because leaves can change the color, smell, and potency of the extract. Best practices involve getting the flowers into the freezer within an hour, or less, of harvest. We want the flowers to freeze as fast as possible to ensure they stay turgid and desiccate as little as possible when frozen.

Flowers are packed into bags ranging from 1 to 25 pounds. To limit condensation, remove as much air from the bag as possible without crushing the flowers. This can be done by hand by gently pressing the bag until the air is removed and then sealing it with a twist-tie. Bags are typically racked, so that bottom layers are not flattened, in a freezer truck or insulated shipping container. The material remains frozen until use and is extracted frozen as well. This product has its challenges: We have heard many horror stories of entire shipping containers full of frozen material losing power and thawing.

Product: Smokable Flower or Dry Extraction

With packaged flowers, where the presentation and structure of the flower matter, harvesting by hand is more appropriate. Specifically this means using scissors or clippers to cut plants into pieces to go into the drying room. We stress again that the ideal situation is to harvest an entire crop during the perfect maturity window into a dry space large enough to hold it all and equipped to dry it efficiently. All bucking would take place after drying and curing.

In this perfect setup, horizontal racking wins out over hanging for space and labor efficiency, both in terms of loading trays and unloading them after drying is complete. If this is not possible, one of the following methods should be employed. As you will see, horizontal racking vs. vertical hanging aside, the total time required to harvest and buck a crop of cannabis is roughly the same in every method. What varies is *when* each step is performed. Different approaches must be utilized in a time pinch or when dry/cure space is limited.

Cutting the Whole Plant

With ample available dry space and time flexibility, hanging whole or half plants is probably the most common method and will take roughly 300 labor hours per acre. To cut whole plants, you need good hand pruners or loppers; in some instances a small chain saw might be most appropriate. Cut the plants at the trunk of the main stem. Standard 27-gallon totes may not be big enough, so consider using a pallet-size macro bin, such as those used for grape harvests. Large plants can be unruly to transport, so in these instances making a few additional cuts may make it easy to move them around and get them into the dry space.

The time saved at harvest relative to other methods is spent breaking down whole plants and dry bucking after dry/cure is complete. A benefit is that this breakdown step can be performed indoors or in the shade with less of a time crunch. Because the plants must be removed from hanging before being bucked and stored, total labor is slightly higher in the end, roughly 1,050 to 1,100 hours per acre.

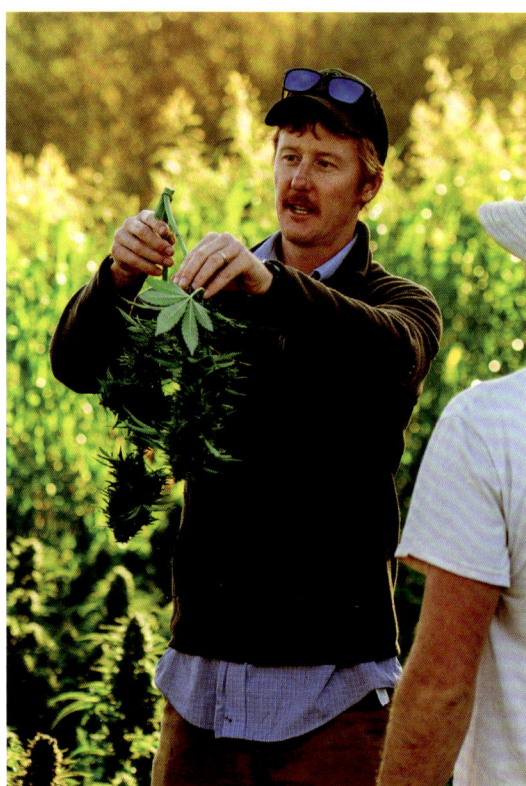
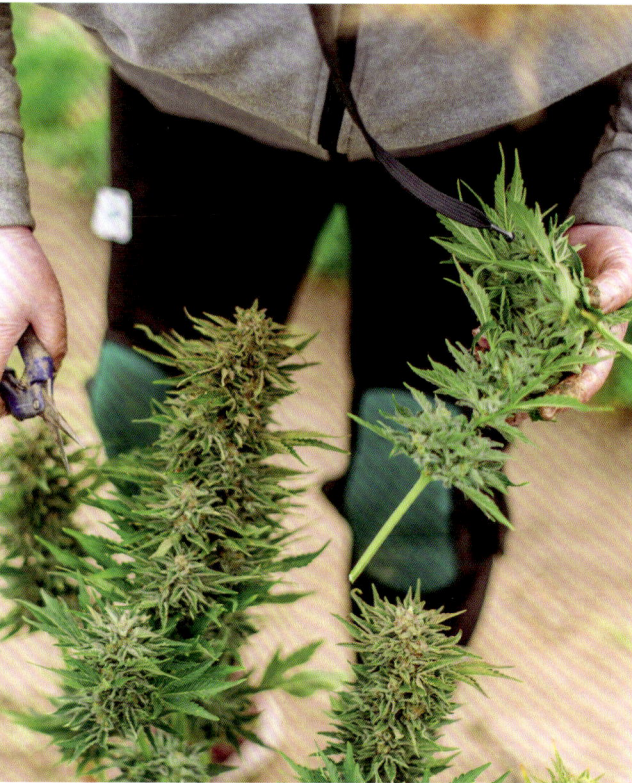

LEFT: Leaving a hanging hook while cutting stems   RIGHT: Partial bucking

Cutting Stems with Hooks

Instead of cutting the whole plant, the stem is cut into sections measuring 12 to 24 inches. Branches are trimmed with pruners or trimming scissors at nodes, leaving a 1- to 4-inch hook for hanging the stems on a vertical trellis system to dry. Sometimes the plant needs to be hung from a flower site, which is not ideal because the stems that lead to flowers are less robust and regularly break, and the branches fall onto the floor.

This method takes around 600 labor hours per acre. Bucking must still take place after the material is dry. Removing the stems from the hanging trellis is very time consuming.

Partial Buck

Rather than removing the flowers from the stems, partial bucking is the process of breaking the plant into 6- to 12-inch sections of stem with flowers still attached. Because a lot of extra stem is removed, this system is more space efficient in that flowers can be packed tightly into a crate or vertically hung, but it does require more handling simply because there are more pieces. Total labor hours for this method comes

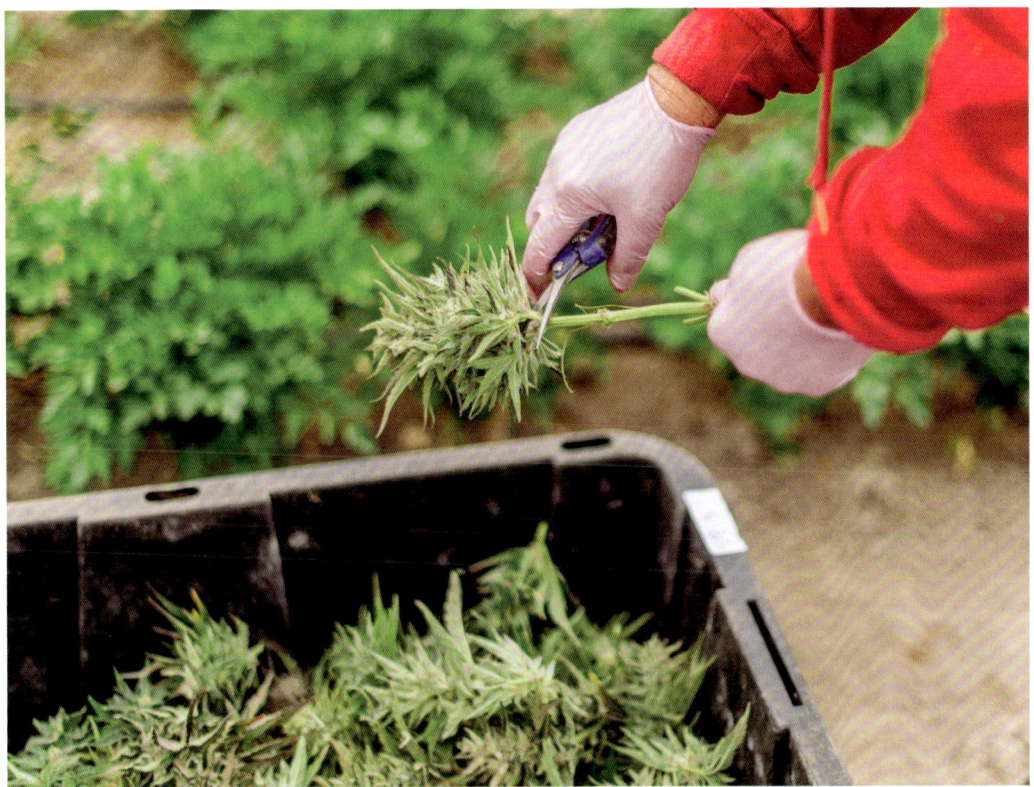
Wet bucking into a harvest bin. This makes the dry/cure more space and time efficient.

to between 500 and 600. Racking, as we describe in Chapter 12, is much more efficient than hanging, specifically when it comes to removing material from the dry space after dry/cure is complete.

Wet Buck

Wet bucking means removing flowers from stems at the time of harvest. Typically branches are cut in the field, brought into the shade, and then big-leafed and bucked as they are loaded onto dry racks. We've calculated, not including any de-leafing beforehand, that it takes about 1,000 labor hours to harvest and wet buck an acre of cannabis when breaking down the plants into approximately 4-inch pieces to be placed on drying racks. This is the method we currently employ because it front-loads labor input requirements at the beginning of post-harvest while vastly increasing dry space efficiency. The limiting factor in our context is dry space, and since we will eventually need to remove excess stem and leaf, we do it at a point in the process that will allow us to optimize dry space efficiency by a staggering margin.

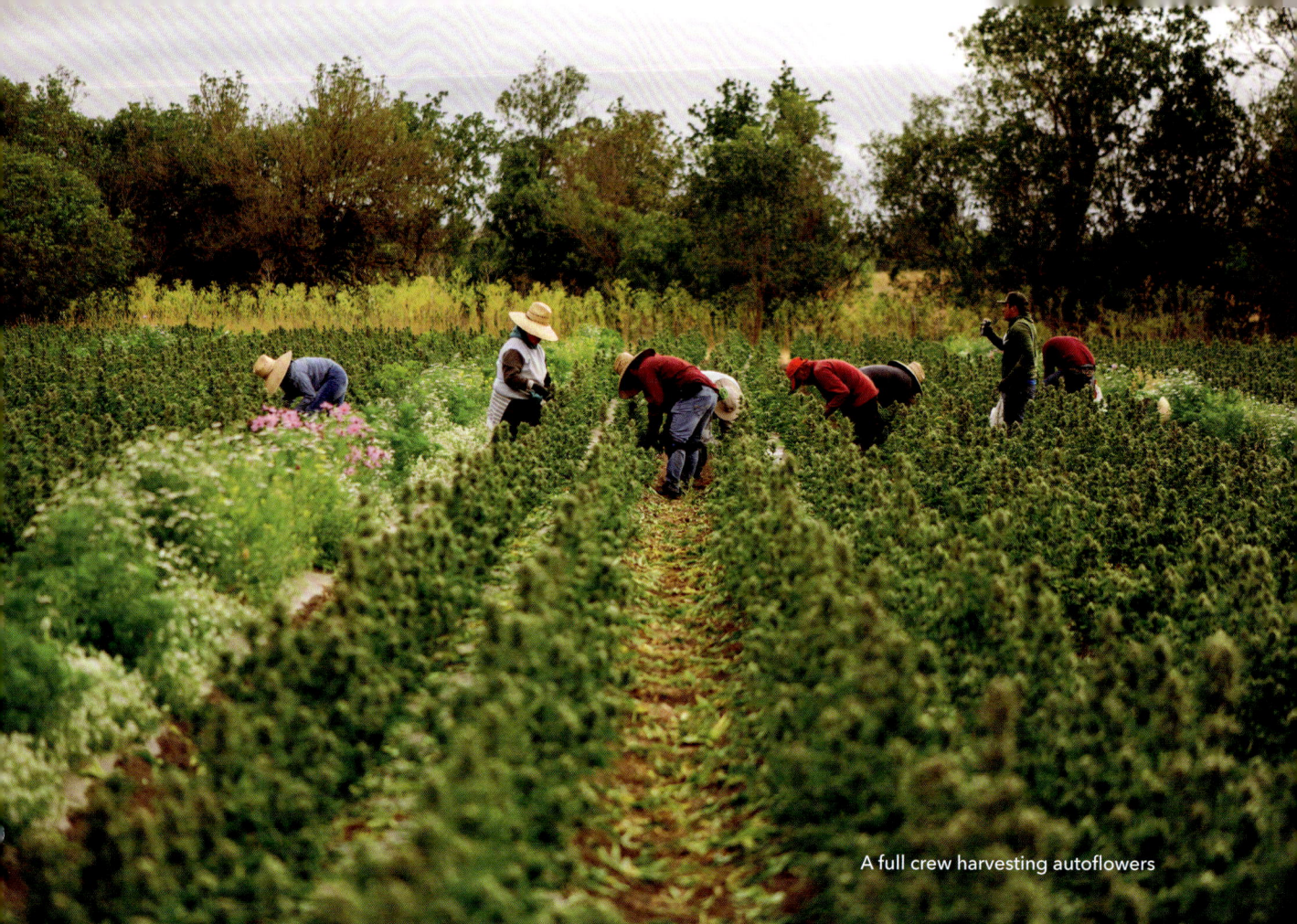

A full crew harvesting autoflowers

Getting the Crop In

In the field each employee has their own harvest tote. Currently we use 27-gallon plastic totes, but anything stackable that works within your system will suffice. Select harvest totes that are easy for workers to handle but are not so deep that material at the bottom is squished. We tried to imagine a system where our thin drying racks could double as a harvest tote to eliminate a handling step, but it was not practical from an ergonomic or workflow perspective.

Full totes are brought to the edge of the field and stacked in the back of a shaded box truck. Depending on field layout, some farmers may drive a tractor or truck into the field to limit the amount of time employees carry totes into and out of the field. Some farmers use a refrigerated box truck for short-term storage (2 to 12 hours) before product is transported to dry space.

After a few hours some crew members begin to put material into the dry space while most of the crew continues to harvest.

Estimating Harvest Costs

Because harvest is one of the biggest line items in the budget, it's critical to estimate the cost. There are many variables in harvesting an acre, including how much canopy is occupied (autoflowers vs. small photoperiod vs. large photoperiod) or how your dry space is set up, or if you plan to wet buck. With these variables in mind, we offer these per-acre estimates.

- Whole- or half-plant harvest: 100 to 300 labor hours

- Breaking plants down into 10- to 24-inch "hangable pieces": 400 to 600 labor hours

- Wet bucking or breaking plants down into 4- to 10-inch pieces: 800 to 1,500 labor hours

As you can see from our projections, harvesting by hand is time and capital intensive. Furthermore, just as with wine grapes, it needs to happen when it needs to happen. Waiting a few days extra could result in massive decreases in yield or quality. This is why we believe so strongly that medium-to-large acreages and/or acreages grown for extraction will move quickly toward mechanized harvest.

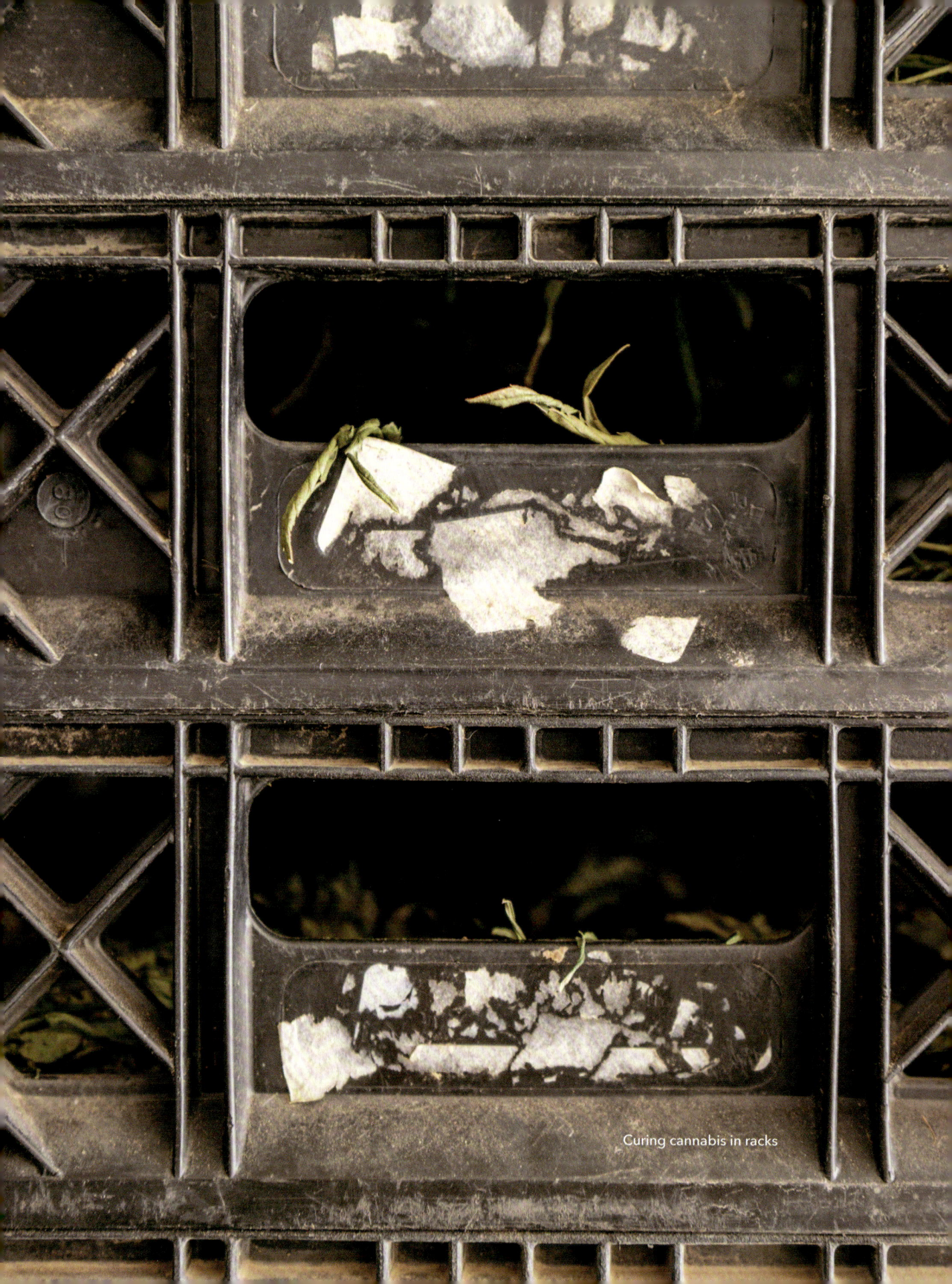

Curing cannabis in racks

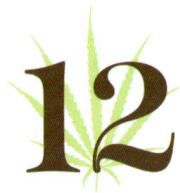

Post-Harvest

Have you ever rolled a joint only to find it keeps going out and you have to relight it? Or inhaled some smoke from fresh-looking cannabis flowers only to find that the flavor was off? Both situations are a result of poor post-harvest practices, namely drying and curing. Although cannabis is a plant like any other, in practice it's far closer to chocolate, mezcal, and wine than to tomatoes, potatoes, and celery. Cannabis has an elaborate and long-standing culture as an artisanal good, and post-harvest is where the artisans are separated from the bulk commodity producers.

Before we get into the specifics of drying and curing, let's define the goals for the process. And note that they are not necessarily the same for all markets.

For smokable flower, or flower sold in its dried form (buds, ground pre-rolls, etc.), the purpose of the dry/cure process is to preserve the terpene profile, cannabinoid content, flower structure, and color and then to store it with the proper moisture content. All these yardsticks help ensure that the consumer has safe, aesthetically appealing flowers that are rich in flavor, easy to burn, and offer a consistently enjoyable smoking experience.

For flowers going into markets for hash and extraction, the criteria vary drastically depending on the type of extract to be made: Live rosins require strong terpenes and color preservation for a quality extract, so flowers are frozen fresh. On the other hand, flowers slated for ethanol extraction do not need to be dried and cured in a way that maximizes terpene retention because the process strips the terpenes out of the flowers completely. Drying and curing is expensive, complicated, and time consuming, and the quality, infrastructure, and effort should match the product marketplace. Growing cannabis is easy compared to getting the crop picked and dried. We always tell people, "I'll grow you 50 acres of cannabis no problem, I just do not know how to harvest and dry more than 10 acres of it."

☀ How's It Hanging?

The history of drying and curing on our farm reads like a good novel. It meanders around with funny interludes and the requisite drama but ends "happily ever after" with a working solution. We started out drying on lines of baling twine hung between the rafters in a 600-square-foot garage. We would cut the plant into sections that could be easily hung by leaving one branch whole and cutting the other at node to create a stub that acted as a hook. We ran a few residential dehumidifiers in the garage and fit in box fans wherever we could to circulate air. This provided good airflow but was not space efficient.

As we planted larger crops, we created a hanging "wall of weed" where we hung trellis netting vertically instead of horizontally. These walls were up to 8 feet high and hung 6 inches above the floor for ample airspace. We could pack in 10 times more product than previously, but it still was not enough space.

Next we rented 20-foot shipping containers, installing frames in each container so we could use the same hanging system. There were a couple of clear drawbacks. First, the containers were not insulated, so the heat produced from the dehumidifiers coupled with the sunlight directly on the containers made them too hot during the day. And even with fans in the corners, the herb in the middle of the container would dry much slower.

The next problem, which took a while to solve, was access. With the trellis netting running from wall to wall on the inside of the container, we couldn't easily reach any material other than that which was directly against the door. We did leave 18 inches of space at the bottom of the netting, allowing us to army-crawl into the container. Every time we ventured forth to test dryness or check the conditions in the middle (a daily task), we would emerge out of breath and covered with cannabis dust.

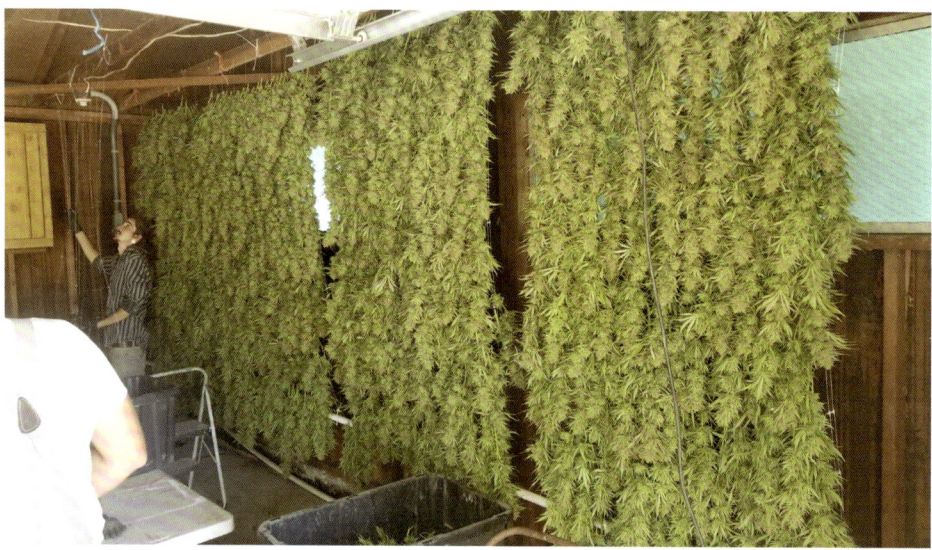

The wall of weed looks amazing but is not the most efficient way of doing things.

Renting uninsulated containers and framing them out, only to have to remove the framing when we returned them, encouraged us to purchase our own containers. When we found two 40-foot insulated high-cube containers, we were off and running. Instead of the trellis net system, which constantly snagged and tangled, we used metal hog panels as drying racks. This system was clean, fairly easy to use and reuse, and provided the correct amount of airflow. We put air conditioners in the containers so we could dry at cooler temperatures. We ran perforated 4-inch PVC below the hanging weed and hung it from the ceiling, with small Can-Fans blowing from both ends distributing air evenly throughout the container. The only problem was that the galvanized hog panels had a heavy metal on them that was on a banned substances list. This was somehow getting on the flowers and causing failed tests in the parts per billion requirements for extracted material. So back to the trellis netting we went.

We quickly outgrew those containers, so we rented six 53-foot reefer trucks with diesel air conditioners. Using our "walls of weed" system once again, our main issue was that we had an even longer distance to army-crawl through and had to use more perforated PVC that was cumbersome to install and remove. At this point we were filling multiple shipping containers and 53-foot reefer trucks twice per season. It also became clear how painfully slow the process of hanging and then removing all of the branches was. It is cumbersome to remove the branches once they are dried because they constantly snag or break, leaving the floor littered with flowers. Material near the dehumidifiers or fans always finished days before the rest. We couldn't achieve uniform results.

For our next iteration we partnered with a professional industrial designer with the hopes of inventing a drying system, for rent or purchase, that would build upon the concepts we had developed and the lessons we had learned. After a six-month process of design and refinement, we concluded it was too capital intensive and we did not want to take on debt to start a new business. Instead we found someone who had started a comparable business and bought their unit. This company started out in the wood-drying and -curing business on the East Coast and transitioned to the hemp and then the cannabis market. The system used a vacuum pump to pull water from the herb quickly. We would be able to achieve a proper dry/cure in less than a week! We bought one, had it shipped across the country and set up, and gave it a try. And it just plain didn't work. So back it went, thankfully covered by the "satisfaction guaranteed" contract.

Back to the drawing board. We had heard of farms using horizontal racking systems and went to investigate for ourselves. Our biggest concern was "pancaking" the flowers: When the heavy, wet flowers are laid onto a horizontal surface, sometimes the bottom side flattens against the rack, throwing off the aesthetic quality of the finished product. But we found that after being trimmed, mechanically or by hand, the pancaked side is indistinguishable. The way we make this system work within our existing spaces is outlined under Racking System (page 174). While this is not the end of the story, we haven't made many meaningful changes to our system since the adaptation of drying in racks.

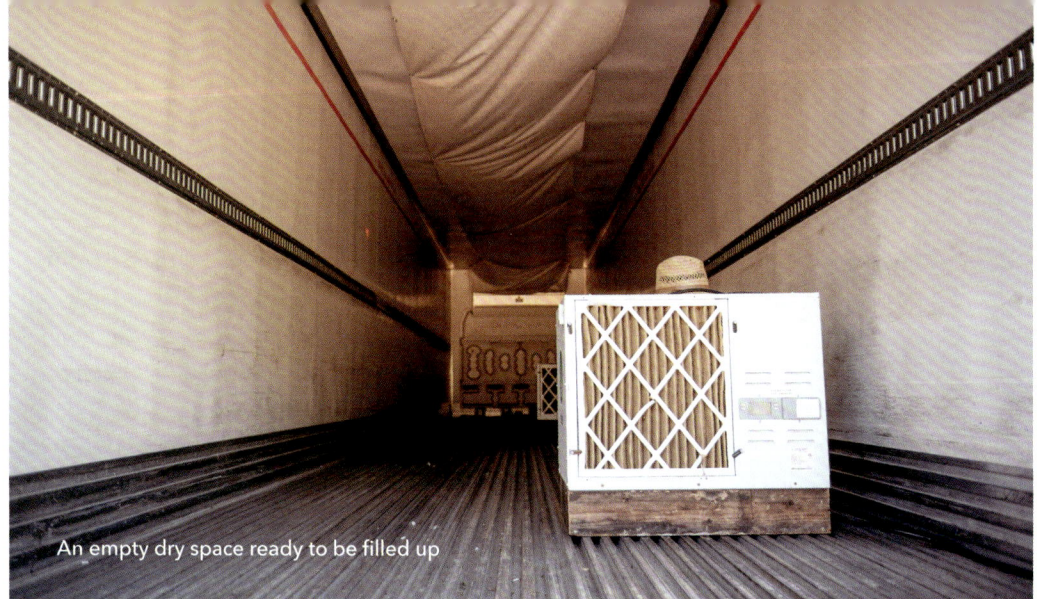
An empty dry space ready to be filled up

The Ideal Dry Space

Creating the ideal dry space is like buying a mattress. If you buy one that's too small, you'll be forever wishing you bought a bigger one, or you'll soon find yourself upgrading, but you'll never regret buying one that's too big for your current needs. An ideal dry space needs to check a lot of boxes. A building with the following characteristics is the best option.

Ample space and accessibility. Build a structure that is large enough to dry the whole crop for the year. Ideally it will have enough room for easy future expansion. Provide room for walkways and sufficient workspace to accommodate hanging, racking, or whatever system you employ. You want plenty of open airspace to allow for air circulation but not so much that it increases heating, cooling, or dehumidification costs. Specifically, the ceiling shouldn't be excessively high, which can cause large temperature gradients. A flat ceiling minimizes air pocketing and temperature gradients, so go that route if it's economically feasible.

Include large doors or a loading dock that allows easy access for a tractor or large truck.

Temperature and humidity control. The space needs to be insulated, with proper levels of dehumidification, heating, and cooling. Consult with HVAC professionals to make sure you are getting the appropriate equipment. For cannabis a good metric to use is dehumidification capacity of 200 pints/day or more per 2,000 pounds of wet material.

Airflow. A dehumidifier is only as good as the fans supporting it. Excellent air exchange is necessary for a quick and uniform dry down. In some cases powerful floor fans suffice. The best we have seen are V-flow fans, designed to hang above confined animals in inhumane feedlots. Mounted from the ceiling, these high-amperage, extremely powerful fans move huge volumes of air and don't need to be removed between cycles. Other options include vent socks (large tubes, usually made of plastic, that transport air), traditional HVAC venting setups (very expensive), or wall-mounted oscillating fans.

Ease of cleaning. As material dries, dust, leaf matter, and buds fall to the ground. After every cycle, a thorough cleaning is necessary. The floor should be a smooth, easily cleaned surface. Poured concrete is the standard in warehousing; it allows for heavy equipment ingress and egress. Cleaning practices will vary based on state regulation and operators' preference, though we recommend regular organic matter and dust removal after every dry/cure cycle and occasional bleaching or deep cleaning.

Low lighting. Drying and curing cannabis flowers should never receive direct sunlight.

Once your dry space is in place, you need to implement a hanging system. Use our story, How's It Hanging? on page 170, as background to your own planning. Depending on the scale of your operation, there are various options for hanging whole plants, chunks of plants, or branches.

Vertical Hanging System

Vertical hanging systems use trellis net, mesh fencing, or any material formed of squares or rectangles roughly 8 inches square (size can vary depending on availability and preference) to provide efficient use of space to dry crops. Cut branches into similar lengths so that the layers are as uniform as possible. Pack these squares so that branches are nestled against but not layered on top of one another. A completed wall should allow minimal light and air penetrability. As drying begins and the flowers and leaves shrink, air will flow better.

Loading the panels is time and labor intensive, but the main drawback to vertical systems is the unloading of the material after the crop is dry. Branches and flowers catch easily, and a significant portion of the crop, in the form of broken flowers and trichomes, ends up on the floor. Trellis netting tangles quickly, so it's important to develop a system for storing it when it's not in use.

The best hanging systems utilize pulleys, eliminating the need for ladders, which are both dangerous and hilarious in dry rooms. While we've done plenty of cringeworthy things ourselves, it always makes us shudder to witness people repeatedly walk up a 12-foot ladder carrying a 30-pound bin of fresh flowers. Then they pause and balance their bin at the ladder top, reaching over precariously to place branches in the wall of weed. A pulley system allows workers to hang stems on an entire net safely from the ground and then hoist it mechanically.

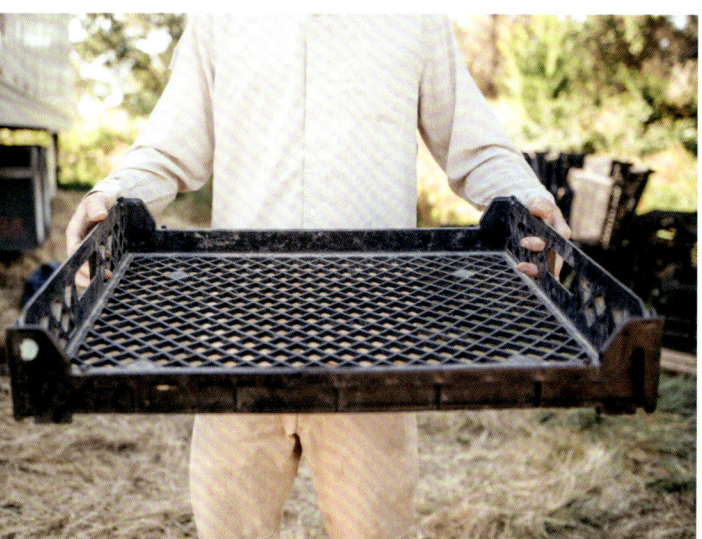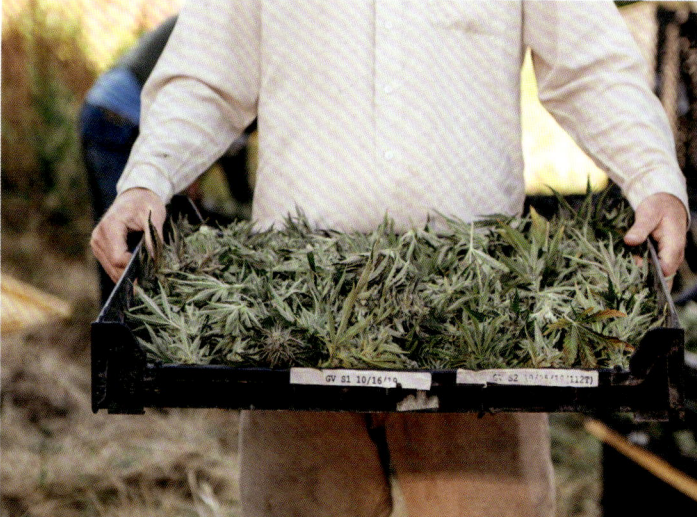

An empty rack is filled. Note the flowers are packed in but do not extend over the top rails.

Racking System

We highly recommend using a horizontal racking system instead of a vertical one. At a conservative guess, working with racks requires about half the amount of labor as a vertical hanging system. Select bulb or bakery racks or other inexpensive and easily available stacking racks with slots or holes for maximum airflow. One of the main advantages of racks is the simplicity of unloading them. Since they are small and lightweight, workers simply dump them gently into larger storage containers one at a time.

We've adapted the racking system for use in 53-foot reefer trucks. Renting the trucks and running large diesel generators is expensive, but the combination allows us to circumvent both building compliance and cannabis compliance requirements (they're on wheels!) and control the temperature. Since our dry space is so valuable, we make sure there is ample airflow and dehumidification power so we can pack the racks and fully load the space. We use racks that measure 16 × 24 inches, typically loading two or three pounds of wet-bucked flowers onto each one. When putting unbucked flowers onto racks, we fill the racks with a similar volume of flowers, though the weight is greater because stems are much heavier than flowers.

We make two lines of racks, stacked to within a foot of the ceiling, and leave an ample walkway down the center. To ensure good airflow, we use six 24-inch hurricane fans on the floors spaced equidistantly in the reefer and two dehumidifiers placed roughly 18 and 36 feet into the container. When the reefer kicks on for cooling purposes, it blasts a massive stream of cold air into the container, providing additional airflow, albeit inconsistently. The reefers also provide drying power, as they blow dry, cold air.

In terms of cost to set up dry spaces, we recognize that the industry is moving quickly, and we have done our best to minimize expenditures into hard assets. We chose to invest tens of thousands of dollars in dehumidifiers, fans, and electrical supplies, but it was an easy decision to rent the reefer trucks from roughly June through October instead of purchasing them. Even buying used ones would be a major expenditure compared to the cost of rentals. The main drawback to renting is that we have to set up the electrical boxes and service to each container every year.

Our racking and drying system works exceptionally well, though if we lived in an area with different building regulations, we would absolutely do it differently. Having an onsite warehouse with concrete floors and built-in dehumidifiers would simplify our process considerably. When considering where and how to dry your crop, review the totality of your situation—including existing structures, building and permitting costs, access to power, field access, climate, and so on. In very arid areas, dehumidifiers are unnecessary, and only airflow is needed. Ultimately the main goal for drying and curing is the ability to control conditions, which, regardless of anything else, means a well-insulated space with ample power.

LEFT: Racks are loaded into the dry space. RIGHT: Racks are stacked along the length of a reefer truck.

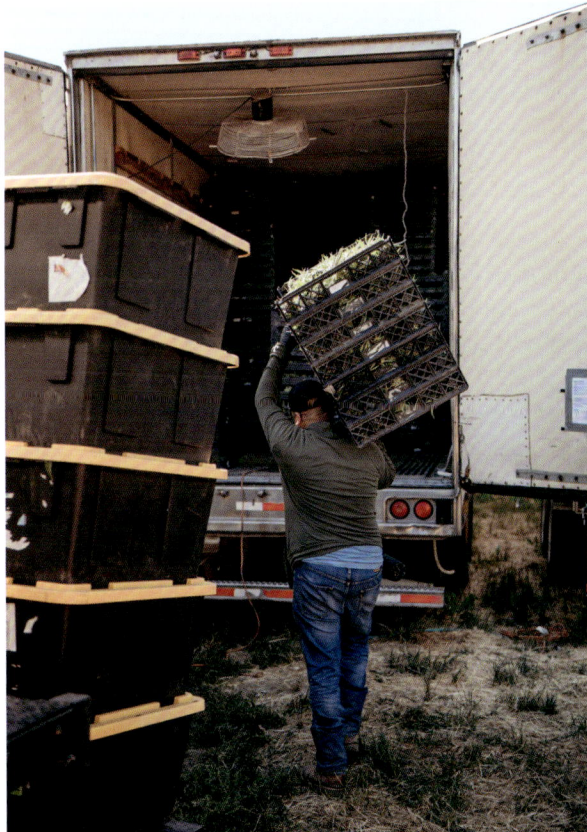 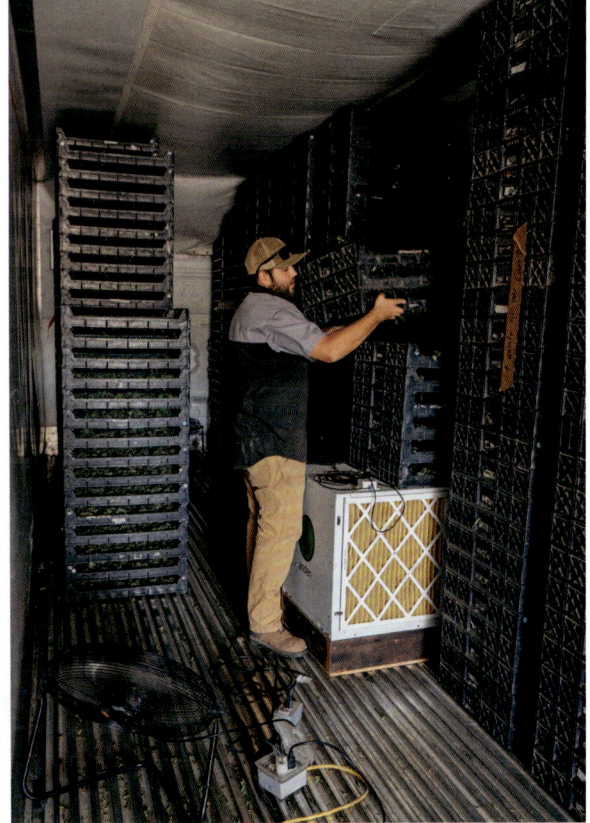

Overhead view of a dry space setup

Our dry spaces are in 53-foot reefer trailers and look like this from overhead. The ideal dry space would have better access, with the dehumidifiers and fans placed out of the walkways, either hanging from the ceiling or ducted in from outside the space entirely.

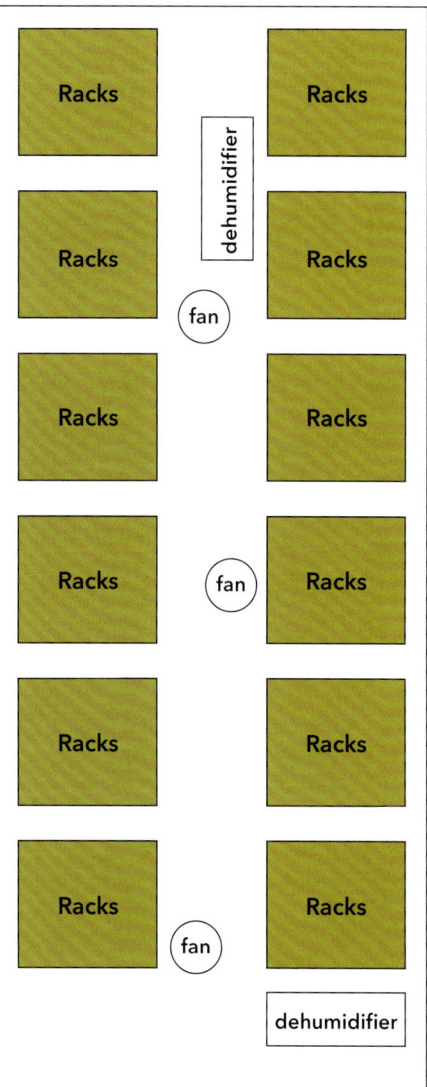

Drying Cycle

There are two distinct phases of drying. The first is what we call the initial sweat. This is the period where you're removing free water—that is, water not chemically bound. In the second, or equalization, phase, which occurs at the end of drying and into curing, the bound water, which has markedly less volume, evaporates more slowly. A key factor in the initial sweat is the exponential relationship between dehumidification and temperature—that is, drying happens *much* faster at higher temperatures. The caveat for cannabis, outlined in more detail below, is that higher temperatures can spoil the crop, volatilize terpenes, or severely reduce quality. It is a careful balance of drying fast enough to prevent mold from developing and making efficient use of space while keeping temperatures low enough to maintain high quality.

For smaller lots of premium-grade cannabis, the rule "slow and low" (a slow dry/cure at low temperatures) is the best method. The slow and low standard we learned from Mendocino growers is the 60/60 rule—that is, 60°F (16°C) and 60 percent humidity. In small-scale, craft scenarios, this is a great metric to aim for to produce the best possible product. In larger systems with higher throughput producing a lower quality, a modification of this rule might be something like "medium and balmy," meaning that you're aiming to get as close as possible to the 60/60 rule within the parameters of your context but that you may have to compromise a bit, specifically on the temperature.

When we've been backed into a corner with our available dry space and the need to get product out of the field and pushed through our post-harvest infrastructure, the best place to make a modification to 60/60 has been in the initial sweat phase. The modification we've made is keeping temperatures around 80 to 85°F (27 to 30°C) during the first few days of the initial sweat, since dehumidifiers are much more effective at pulling water out in warmer temperatures. In theory, concerns about volatilizing terpenes are assuaged by the presence of the free water in the plant tissues, which buffers somewhat against degradation of the material.

After the initial sweat is complete, we enter the second phase of drying. We call it the equalization phase because while the flowers may be perfectly dry, the stems and interior of the flowers still contain water and will continue to remoisten the flowers. During this phase the goal is to aim for 60 to 68°F (16 to 20°C) and 53 to 60 percent relative humidity across the entire space. This phase lasts until the water content is the same among the different-size stems and flowers. It can last between 4 and 10 additional days, again depending on the amount of material, presence of stems, thickness of material, and ambient humidity.

Technical Specifications for a Dry Room Setup

Expert operations manager Jake Brookes of Ladybug Farms in Watsonville, California, shared the following notes for his dry room specs, with the note that this setup provides oversize dehumidification power to get the relative humidity (RH) down to 60 percent within 12 to 18 hours to reduce water activity and microbial growth, and to finish the entire process in 10 days at 60°F (16°C) and 58 percent RH.

- ❏ Max capacity: 10,000 plants at max, 10,000 pounds wet
- ❏ Two 506 PPD dehumidifiers (1,012 pints per day max dehumidification)
- ❏ Five vertical-flow fans, 15,500 CFM
- ❏ Three-ton condenser

How to Tell When Your Crop Is Dry

"It's snapping and perfectly crispy."
"My stems are still bendy, and this one is even peeling."
"Dude, it's done."
"Dude, no, it's not."

After having way too many variations on this conversation, we purchased a water activity (a_w) meter. This device, commonly used in the prepared-foods industry, measures the chemically bound water in the stems and flowers. Anything above 0.65 a_w can and will mold; anything below is shelf stable. Using a meter has been extremely helpful in standardizing our system and taking the guesswork out of it. However, the machine is not perfect, and it requires users to take uniform samples to get accurate readings. We generally do not even begin taking water activity readings until day five of drying, at which point we see readings anywhere from 0.65 to 0.85 a_w. Based on our readings, we can adjust the settings in the dry spaces to meet our desired timeline for emptying out the space. We consider the drying phase finished when representative samples taken across the entire space (at least five samples taken from lower racks, higher racks, and in different areas of the container) reach 0.6 a_w.

At this point we assess the quality of the flower—it is crucial to double-check the measurement against physical reality. While the benefits of a meter are clearly demonstrable, growers should not ignore or discount their experience in making post-harvest decisions just because they bought a fancy new piece of equipment. We have bagged up flower that was supposedly dry according to the water activity meter that then rehydrated in the bags and spoiled. This is usually due to moisture left in the stems. The first qualitative indication to look for is a clean snap of the stems. If the stems still bend or peel apart, they need more time. Second, we test the flower itself. How squishy is it? It should be crispy on the outside but still have a spongy core.

Overdrying

Keep a close eye on the outside humidity and humidity forecasts during the drying period. It's easy to be caught off guard when the ambient humidity outside suddenly gets very low, or the temperature in the dry space spikes for the night, speeding up the dry-down process and increasing the risk of overdrying.

Adding humidity to the dry spaces with a swamp cooler or humidifier is an option, though not ideal. A powerful humidifier with a humidistat controller may be necessary to maintain the proper RH in the dry space. Overdrying permanently reduces the quality of your product. Though overdried material can be remoistened to proper levels, unfortunately it will never regain its former quality.

Arid Climate Caveat

In some areas the ambient humidity is low enough that dehumidification is entirely unnecessary. This saves a lot on equipment and electricity. In these places the concern is not material staying wet for too long but rather the material becoming too dry. Here the focus is on proper airflow and air circulation so that material dries uniformly, and then taking it down into storage at the right time. The other option is humidifying the space with industrial humidification units so that the material can dry more slowly and then properly cure.

Curing

We distinguish between the drying phases and the curing phase. To summarize what we have discussed about drying, the goal for the drying phase is to remove all free water from the plant as quickly as possible and at the lowest possible temperature. After drying is complete, we enter the curing phase. The plant material is properly dry but is still going through an enzymatic process of chlorophyll breakdown and is therefore not ready to be sealed for storage.

During this phase we leave the flowers in the drying racks until or beyond day 14. If dry space is needed for a successive harvest, the material can be moved into secondary conditions such as cardboard boxes with airflow (provided by a few fans to make sure there is some gentle air circulation) or stored in a container that utilizes two-way polymers that can regulate interior RH below 62 percent. Flowers cannot go into plastic until curing (chlorophyll breakdown) is finished, or the terpene profile will be diminished or ruined—a situation known as "haying," meaning flowers that once smelled beautifully suddenly smell like freshly cut grass. This is extremely undesirable in cannabis because it indicates the unique and distinct terpene profiles have been ruined, rendering a crop with less than 50 percent of its original value.

We commonly hear the question, "How do you know when the flowers are cured?" Flowers are properly cured if they can be sealed into plastic without rapid flower degradation, which includes color, smell, flower structure, and general appearance. We continue to use the water activity meter in this phase, though mostly just as a final check before we decide to move the flower into sealed plastic. We have found that a minimum of 10 days beyond the initial sweat, or removal of the free water, provides an acceptable cure. Therefore we allow for a minimum of 14 days to do our drying and curing. When we have more time, because of sales flow, storage space, time of year, and so on, we allow for a longer curing period, up to an additional 14 days.

 ## Remote Monitoring

Monitoring dry space conditions is extremely important. We used to check each space in person multiple times daily, which worked fine until it didn't. During our July 2021 autoflower harvest, everything was going smoothly until one evening, after our last check, an air-conditioning unit on the rented reefer truck started blowing warm air instead of cold. When we did our morning checks, the trailer was reading 130°F (54°C), and all the flowers were brown because they overheated. We had to sell 750 pounds of flower as biomass instead of machine-trimmed flower, and we lost at least $30,000 overnight due to a preventable error. Ever since, we've used a remote monitoring service for all our dry and storage spaces, with temperature alerts sent to our phones.

Post-Harvest Flow Chart

Bucking can be performed before or after drying and curing, depending on available time, climate conditions, or available dry/cure space.

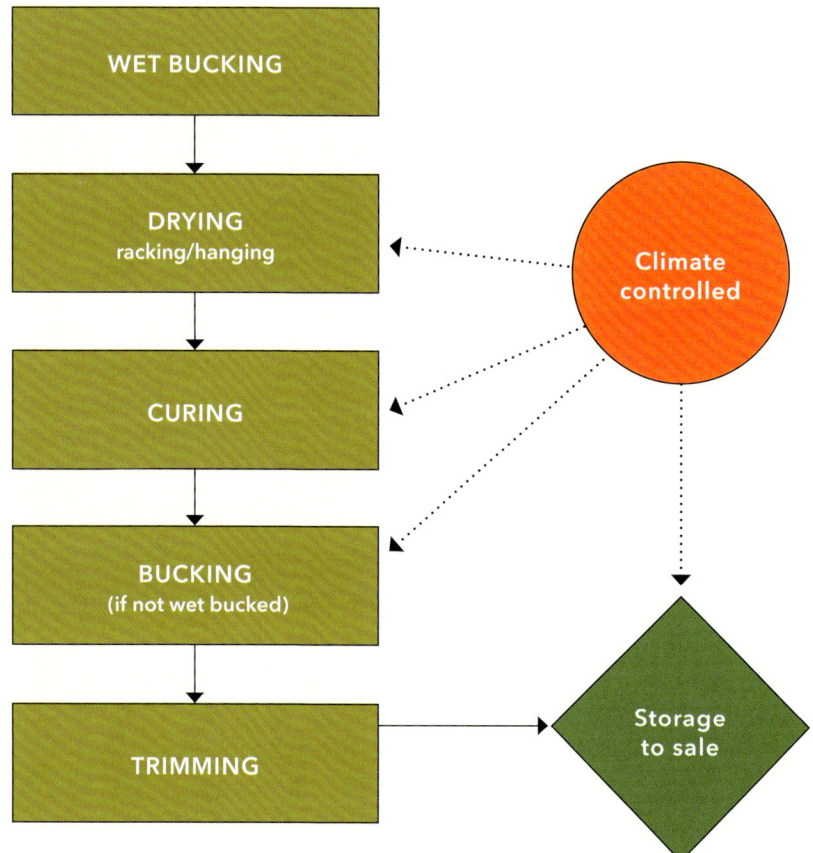

Storage

As the dry room is emptied, boxes of flowers are stacked into one group and kept in the storage container until sale. They need to be checked and burped every few days for the first seven days after they are put into plastic, and once they are clearly stable, they can be checked every two weeks to ensure product quality. Burping—opening the bags and reclosing them—is the process of allowing CO_2 and moisture to leave your sealed flowers and allowing fresh air in. The frequency of burping depends on how long the product has been cured for. We aim to burp as little as possible, no more than once, by not sealing flowers in plastic until they are thoroughly cured.

Proper storage is key for flower preservation. We have seen many bags of beautiful flowers ruined by improper storage. For smokable flowers going into jars or bags, proper preservation is even more important. Without proper storage, flowers lose their color, usually trending toward an off-putting shade of brown, and terpene profiles fade, degrade, or sour.

After extensive research, we settled on an inexpensive, low-tech solution for storage that keeps flowers exceptionally preserved for a year or longer. We use the following parameters for long-term storage, which we consider anything greater than two months. For less than two months, we simply focus on temperature and humidity.

Store at 55°F (13°C) and 57 percent relative humidity. A few degrees in either direction shouldn't make too much difference, but we've found those conditions are ideal.

Leave flowers on the stem. Storing entire branches is not space efficient and makes handling difficult. We have found 6 inches or more of stem is acceptable. Long-term storage of flowers on the stem does not align with a system set up for wet bucking, so it requires extra communication and planning to make sure it's done correctly.

Trim or process the flowers right before sale/packaging/shipment. Even if you follow all the other steps recommended here, flowers will not preserve nearly as well if they have been trimmed.

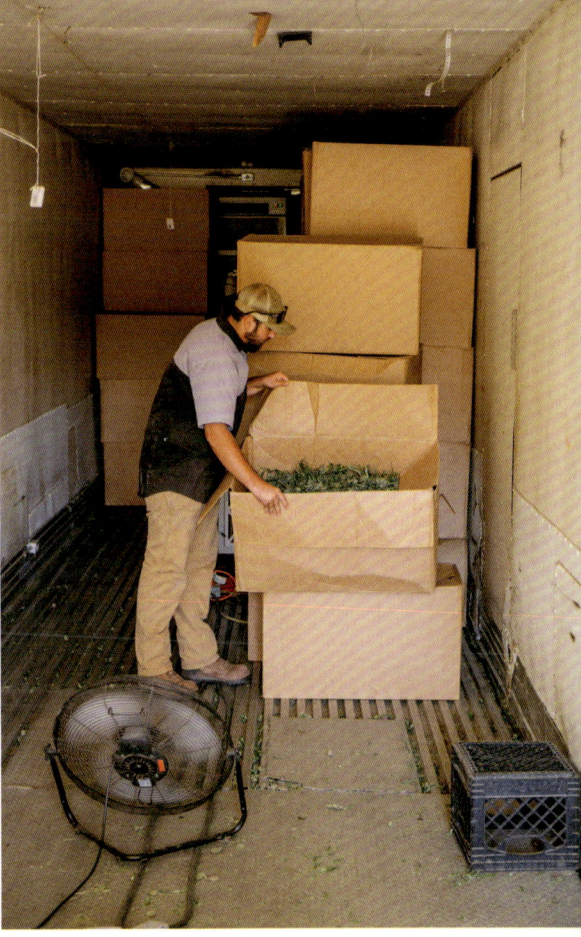

Checking stored flowers to ensure proper conditions is an important part of storage. Sometimes, mold may be present or flowers may be too dry.

Store in sealed plastic bags or airtight containers. The purpose here is to expose the flowers to as little oxygen as possible. We've looked into fancy systems that suck the air out of a room or a container, but we ended up pushing the air out of the bag with our hands (the concept is the same as pushing the air out of an air mattress) and sealing it with a zip tie. We normally store 10 to 15 pounds in a bag nested into a cardboard box.

Always maintain stable conditions. Use remote monitoring (see page 179).

Post-harvest is where most of the money is spent and the biggest mistakes can happen. Frying an entire dry space, haying the crop by bagging it too soon, or overdrying can spoil the efforts of an entire season. Absolute attention to detail and proper planning are necessary, even after years of experience, to make it through unscathed and have a high-quality, salable product in the end.

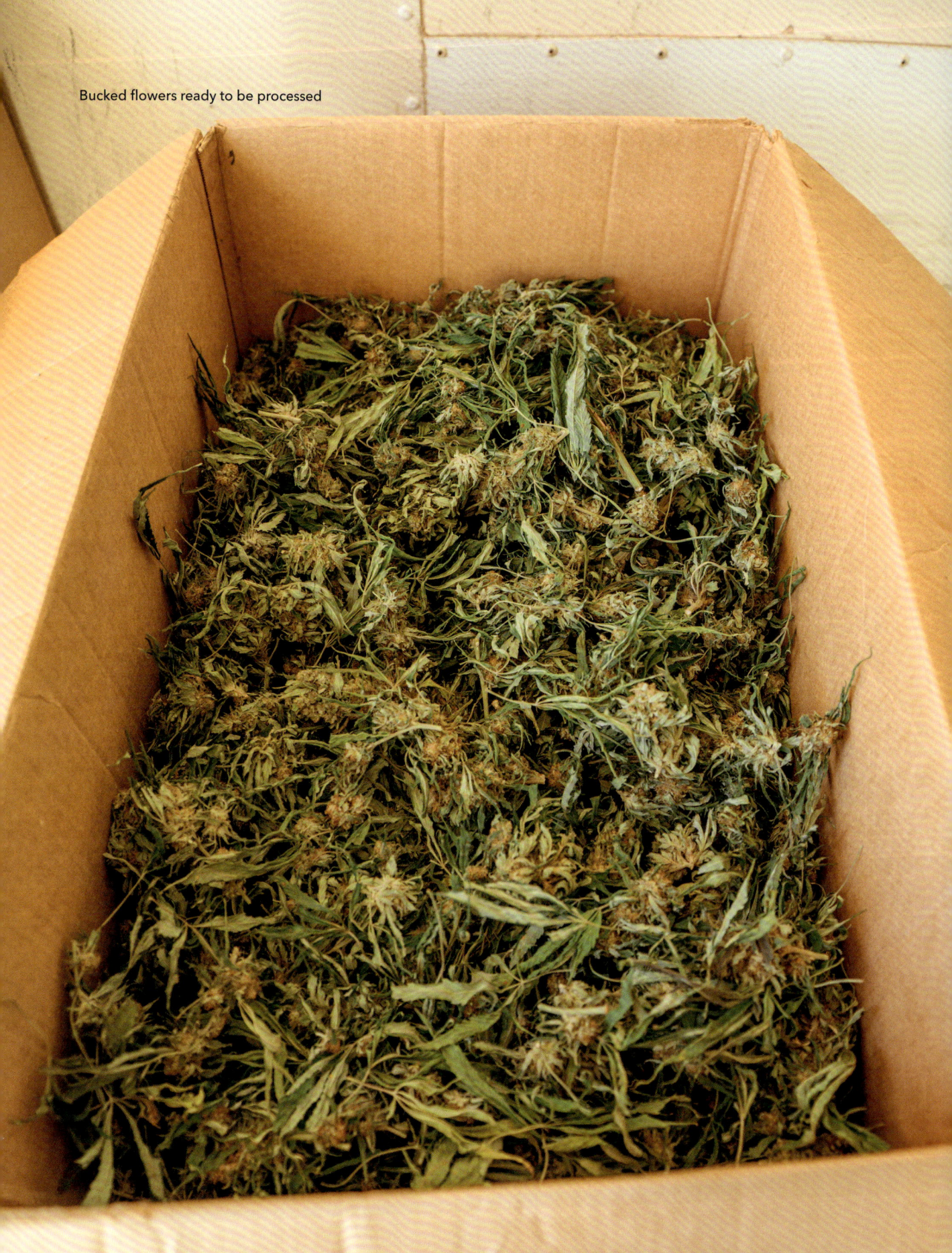

Bucked flowers ready to be processed

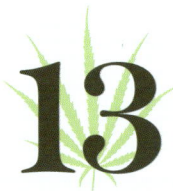

Processing the Product

Processing is the step in the crop cycle that really brings the quality of your material to light. Most cannabis is eventually smoked or vaporized, and yet its size, smell, and appearance matter. Just as wine enthusiasts enjoy looking at the color of the wine while they drink it, cannabis connoisseurs and buyers love to look at, smell, and enjoy the flower before eventually burning it up!

After the extensive (and expensive) process of dry/cure comes the physical preparation of material for sale. For smokable flowers this means bucking and trimming. In western United States wholesale markets in the 1990s through the early days of legalizing recreational use around 2019, cannabis flowers were carefully hand-trimmed and sold in one-pound bags. Workers known as trimmigrants would come from all over the world, flocking by the thousands to growing regions for a blitz of fast-paced, high-paying work that lasted a few months. Due to the risky nature of working on illicit or semi-illicit farms whose privacy and security were paramount, trimmers made good money ($150 to $300 per pound trimmed) for their willingness to show up and for their discretion. Trim scenes, as they were known, could sometimes include up to 100 people sitting at tables working 10- to 14-hour days.

Today processing sun-grown cannabis is a regular, seasonal job. Growers can outsource this task to the distributor—indeed, some buyers prefer to handle processing in-house and will buy material bucked but untrimmed. This fetches a lower price, as the process of trimming on average removes 50 percent of the weight before the flower is considered finished and ready for sale! This laborious trimming process is becoming increasingly mechanized. It begins with bucking.

Bucking Dry Material

When material has been dried on the stem, it must be removed from the stem, or bucked, before it can be trimmed. As mentioned in Chapter 11, bucking is laborious and time consuming, and machines do not necessarily improve the process. Most are modified cotton gins where you insert the stems, then pull them back to strip off the flowers. They are no quicker or better than bucking by hand. They also break apart the flowers, producing too many "smalls," which reduces the overall value of the crop.

Newer designs that allow operators to feed material much faster, essentially serving as threshing machines, save a lot of time compared to hand scale but again break the buds into many small pieces. To produce high-grade smokable flowers, the material still must be bucked by hand to preserve the size and shape.

Trimming

The final step in the crop cycle is trimming the green leafy plant matter, leaving only trichome-covered flowers—the good stuff. Trimming creates two products—the finished flower and the trim or "shake." The process was traditionally performed by workers using small scissors and wearing rubber gloves to keep the resin off their hands. This method is still widely used to achieve the highest-quality product, either directly after bucking or sometimes after an initial pass through a trim machine that removes most of the leaf matter so the trimmer can work more efficiently.

Trimming removes a lot of weight, and the process used can significantly affect the overall yield of salable flower. We once hired a mixed-mechanized trim crew to process our entire harvest. We agreed on a price per pound, and they brought in their custom machine and a supplemental crew to perform the finish work. They utilized the machine as much as possible to expedite the process, because the sooner they finished, the more money they made per hour. After a few days we noticed quite a few bags of shake next to the bags of finished flower (which also appeared on average too small)—the ratio didn't seem right.

A review of the system found that the process of trimming had netted under 45 percent salable flower from the bucked weight. We had lost significant weight that, even at modest prices, meant thousands of dollars. This experience gave us a laser focus on the trim process. It is a complicated intersection between efficiency, quality, available labor, standing orders, and time.

Trim Machines

Trim machines are almost all variations on a drum tumbler that rolls the material around. Blades or very small wires on the inside of the drum remove leaf matter, and the actual contact of flower on flower rolling around likewise removes leaves.

There are many options, with the least expensive starting at several thousand dollars. The more expensive models have options to set up an assembly-line flow with conveyors and sorters as add-ons. We have purchased and used several of the cheaper options, which worked acceptably for our needs. We have also seen and used some of the very expensive models and were impressed. The size and cost of the unit should correspond to your scale.

Spreading Labor Out

Trimming is a good task if you want to keep your crew busy through the winter months—sometimes it's the only task available! As described before, material that is to be stored for longer periods of time should be dried and stored still "on the stick," to preserve the flowers' quality. Having a large harvest on hand throughout the offseason can help alleviate the seasonal aspect of work that makes keeping good employees around so difficult for small farms.

Trim, a.k.a. Shake

The by-product of trimming, called trim or shake, is the leaf matter and small pieces of flower that still contain THC. It can be used in extraction, or in cases of exceptional quality, in pre-rolls or ready-to-roll products. We noted in Chapter 8 some of the decisions that affect the quality of trim and will review them here.

The quality and sale price of trim are determined by the ratio of flower to leaf matter. The more leaf, the lower the THC and terpenes will be. "Sugar trim" is a high-quality product containing little or no fan leaf. "Shake" is lower quality, as it typically contains a higher volume of leaf matter and even some stems.

When fan leaves are left on during harvest and are not removed prior to trimming, the quality of the trim will be very low. When fan leaves are removed and just the smaller leaves (sugar leaf, which is often coated in trichomes) remain, then the quality of the trim is higher. Processing by hand is necessary to achieve the highest-quality trim, although an initial quick pass through a trim machine to remove most of the leaves, discarding the trim, and then running material a second time will yield an acceptable product. Storage parameters are identical to flower.

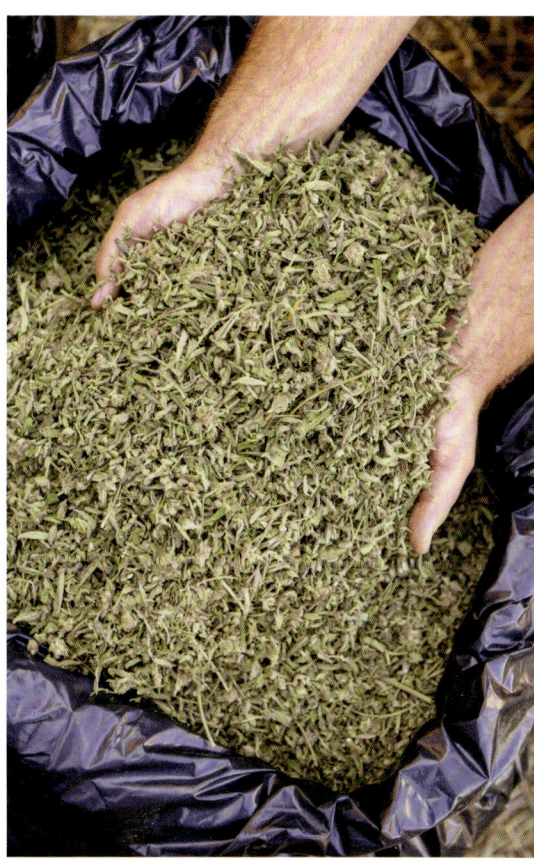

Shake, with leaves and flowers present

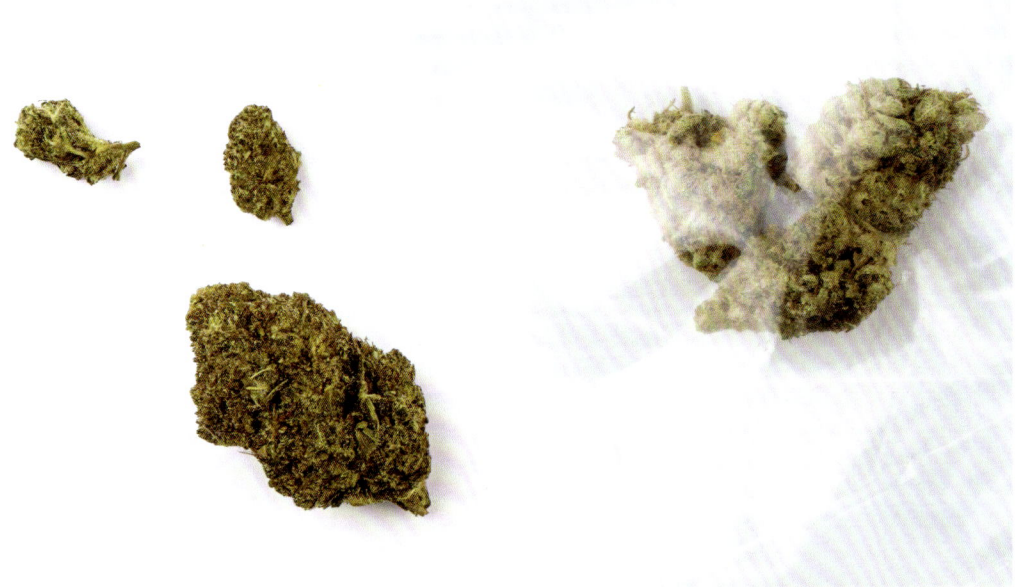

Smalls, mids, and tops should be separated prior to sale.

Grading

After trimming, material is graded in preparation for sale. There are three grades of cannabis flowers—smalls, mids, and tops.

Smalls are flowers smaller than a dime. These are usually from the lower portion of the plant but also can be formed when larger flowers break apart in processing. Smalls can fetch a fine price, as there are relatively fewer of them produced, and their quality is still high.

Mids is more of a quality statement, referring to the middle of the spectrum. They are also known as mid-grade. These may be discolored, overdried, irregularly sized, or odorless and/or hay-smelling. This can either be due to a mistake in cultivation, an early or late harvest, or post-harvest handling. Flowers that looked amazing in the field but were dried too quickly or at too-high temperatures can easily become mids.

Tops refer to the top of the plant and the flowers that received the most sunlight and growth. These are the finest quality and often the largest size, although there is a limit. Flowers must be broken down into individual buds and not left on the stem. As noted above, beautiful-looking tops can become mids with improper dry/cure.

Combining sizes or qualities all together makes sales more difficult. Buyers are looking specifically for smalls, mids or mid-grade, tops, or AAA tops (best of the best). Grading the crop appropriately is important to maximize value and sell the crop efficiently.

Packaging and Final Storage

Until you sell your finished flowers, keep them under the storage conditions outlined in the previous chapter. Finished flowers going out to a client have traditionally been put into turkey basting bags in one-pound portions. This is still common practice, though more frequently we see flowers go directly from the trim line into branded packaging, with the most common size being one-eighth ounce. Our system is to process and package according to order or keep a minimum of inventory. Once processed, cannabis degrades much faster.

Trimming to order, or at least with sales flow in mind, reduces the risk of product degradation. Some cultivators put finished material in plastic bags within cardboard or plastic sealed drums or bins to exclude light and add an additional layer of protection. Humidity-regulating packets can be used within storage containers to maintain perfect conditions if controlling the ambient temperature or humidity is not possible.

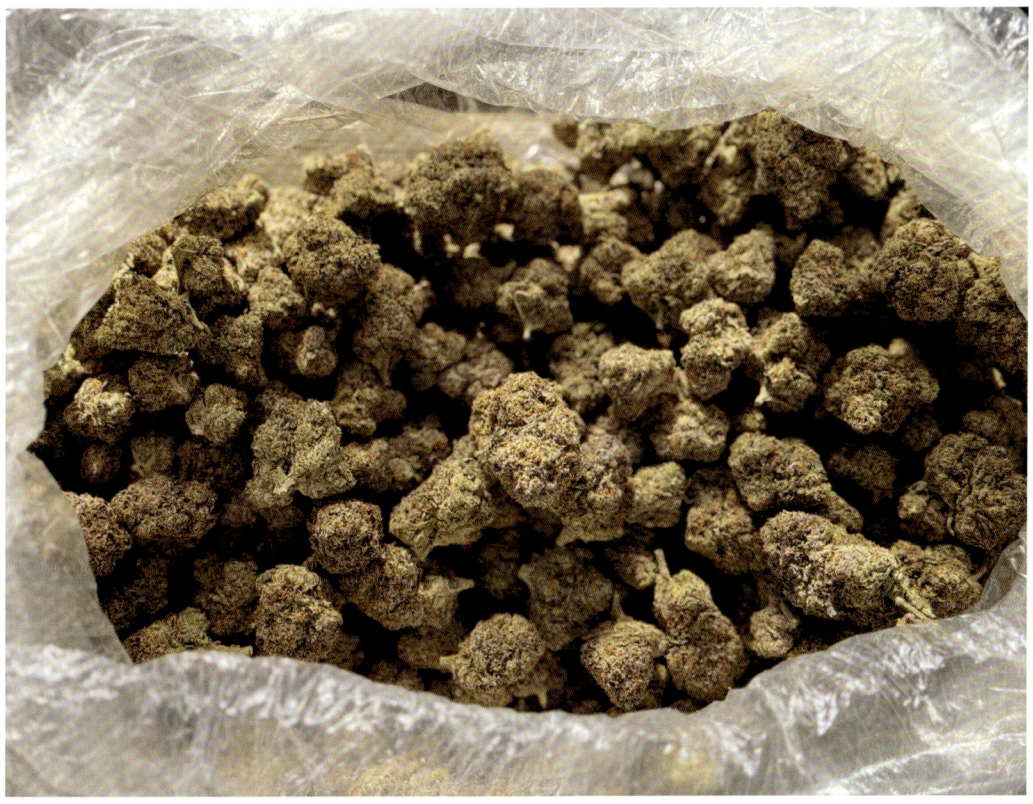

Well-manicured flowers in a turkey bag—this is the traditional way of packaging pounds.

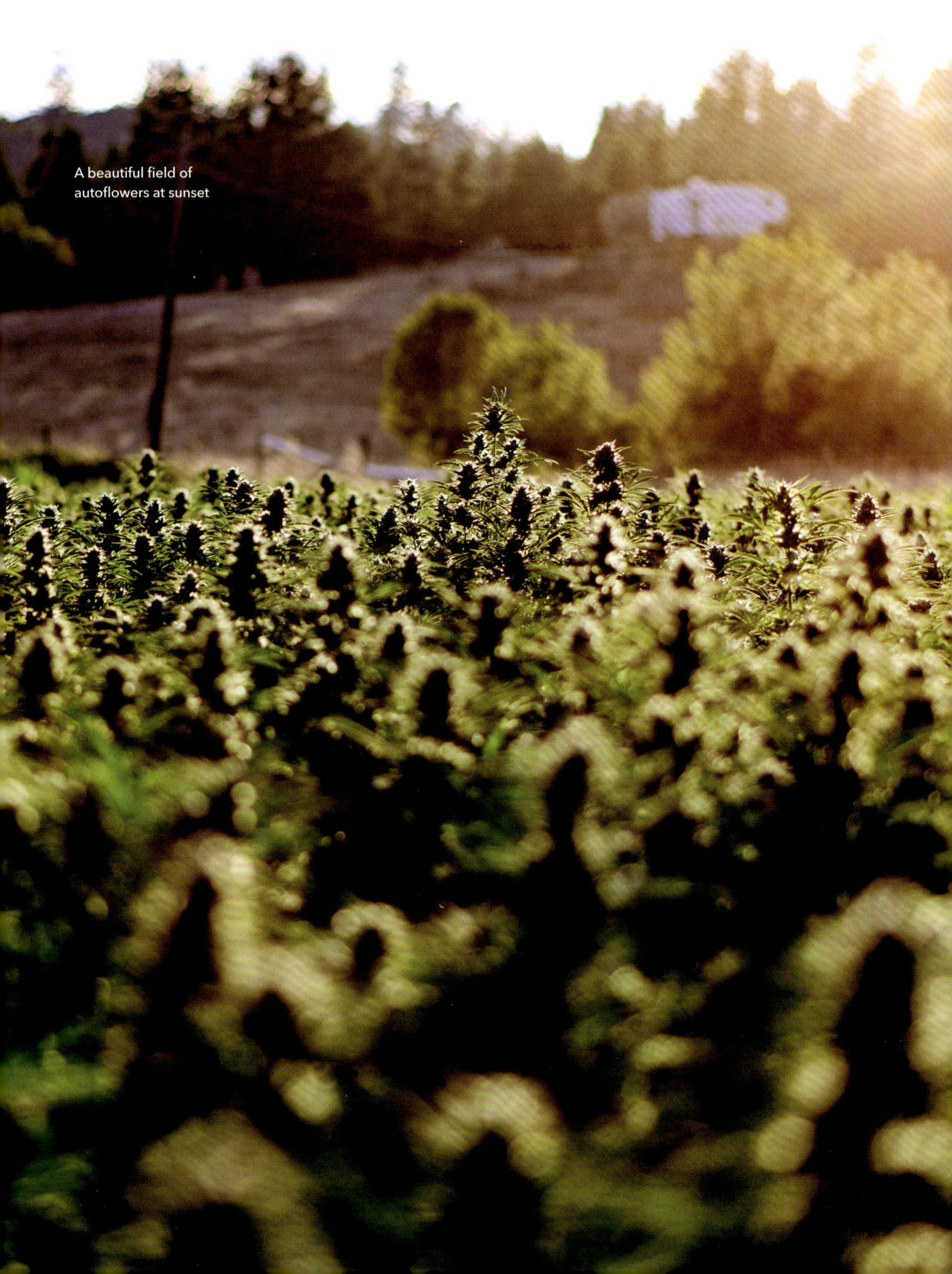

A beautiful field of
autoflowers at sunset

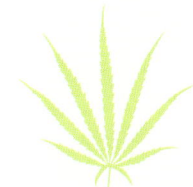

Epilogue

Looking to the future, we believe that the major growth in outdoor cannabis will be in larger crops grown specifically for extraction to be used in manufactured products: edibles, sodas, vape pens, and so on. Farmers will produce mixed products ranging from pure biomass for extraction to flower for pre-rolls and value-brand flowers. There will always be consumers who want to smoke actual flowers, but these segments will see much slower growth and occupy increasingly smaller sections of the marketplace. Within this subset of smokable flower cultivation, we will see mostly bulk commodity flower. Think budget beer vs. a fine wine.

Cultivation systems will evolve to meet the demands of the marketplace and will increasingly deliver quality, potent flowers at lower and lower price points. New equipment will be designed to eliminate the most labor-intensive steps in production: harvest and post-harvest. Ideal growing locations with low taxes and regulatory oversight will determine where cultivation hubs establish.

The Future of Cannabis Products

This does not mean all small-scale producers are doomed. Cannabis is a luxury plant like the wine grape and will therefore see a more stratified market ranging from boutique, regionally specific flowers to bulk distillate vapor pens. Wines range from $2 bottles produced in vast, mechanically managed vineyards of California's Central Valley to single bottles of rare vintage fetching thousands of dollars. Cannabis will most likely follow suit. The wine grape yields different aromas, tastes, and alcohol concentration depending on climate, location, genetics, and many other factors. The cannabis plant produces a complex array of cannabinoids, many of which we are only beginning to

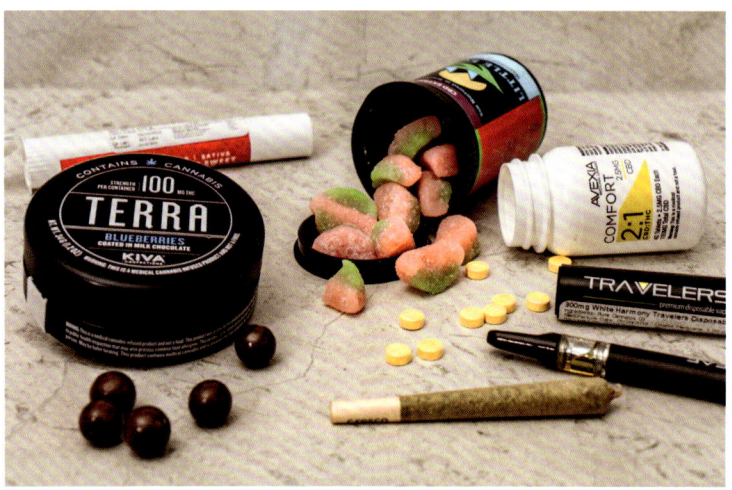

The majority of cannabis product categories are value-added items such as gummies or pre-rolled joints. These are derived from bulk-produced flower.

understand. Some of these have profound medical value.

Cannabis also produces a huge diversity of terpenes and potency, which gives it a natural variation. The sensation from smoking a heavy, *indica*-dominant flower with diesel-fuel terpenes is very different from an almost fake candy fruity–smelling *sativa*. Artisanal cannabis breeding and cultivation will highlight these qualities to be enjoyed by connoisseurs. Within this category will be more diversity still, from the organic/biodynamic outdoor producers in the hills of select regions to the light-assisted greenhouse growers producing immaculately fresh flowers throughout the year.

On the other hand, large-scale agriculture sees cannabis cultivation as essentially growing the active chemicals. Indeed, growers are already paid by the percentage concentration of THC for trim and flower grown for extraction. Pre-rolls and cheap bags of weed will likely be the most abundant items in the market and are easily produced at scale growing autoflowers. The resulting by-products are the raw inputs for edibles, sodas, and other manufactured products, which likewise command a large portion of the market.

Evolving Cultivation Systems and Mechanization

The salient theme of industrial agriculture is mechanization. The bottleneck of scaling up cannabis production is harvest and post-harvest. This problem has already been solved to some degree in the CBD sector in industrial hemp. Stripper header combines can pull the leaves and flower from the stalks in the field, and large, temperature-controlled dry facilities can efficiently process thousands of pounds. However, these processes eliminate what in hemp is known as "smokable flower." In large-scale cannabis systems, we expect to see selective harvest of the top colas to be used for smokable flower products and then mechanical harvest of the rest of the plant.

Eventually the stripper header is likely to predominate and eliminate even a selective harvest step, but the process of removing leaves to produce smokable flower remains unsolved. Assembly lines on conveyor belts, fan-driven wind systems, and novel alterations on trimming machines are all potential solutions in the short term.

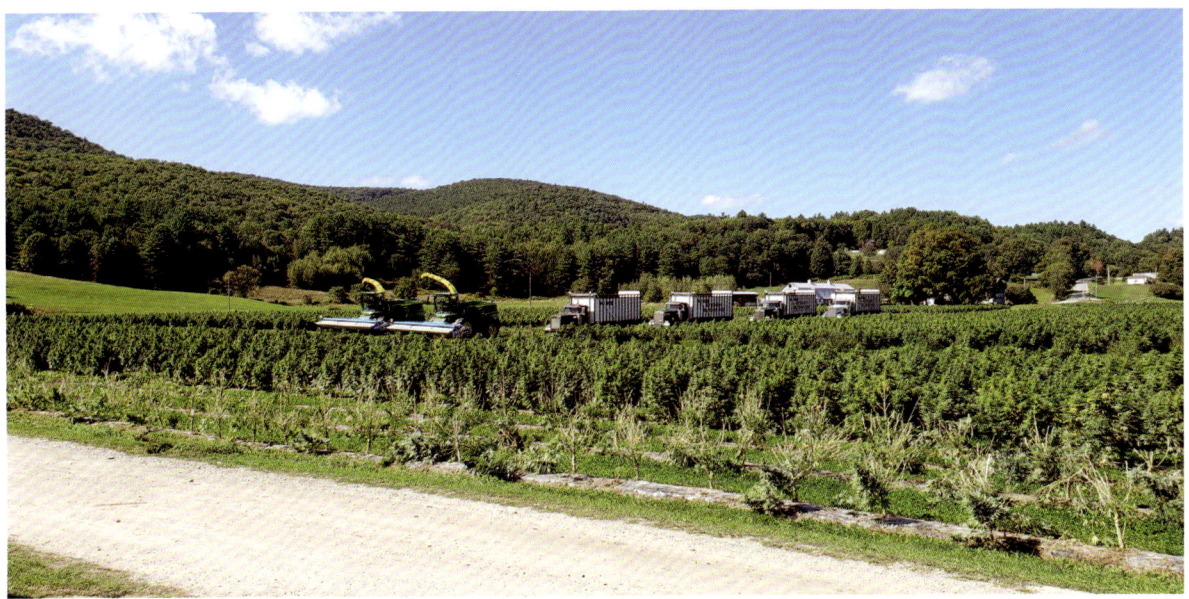

Certain chemical sprays may be developed that cause the leaves to fall from the plant in the field. Additionally, genetics with low leaf mass and other agronomic traits will become increasingly essential.

The stripper header at work in England. This implement will rapidly become the standard in large-scale cannabis agriculture.

The Future of Genetics

Sinsemilla (seedless) cannabis has been developed under prohibition for a generation. As the industry expands and larger acreage is planted, genetics developed specifically for this application will be paramount. Field-ready traits are currently not favored by the industry, but we expect to see the development of some interesting new varieties that will look very different from what we see today. The exaggerated focus on the dense, sparkly, and terpene-rich flower that may look prettiest to consumers has not necessarily led to the best adaptation for efficient field production. This trait of having dense, beautiful buds is often accompanied by relatively high leaf mass, and is therefore more susceptible to mold issues and takes longer to dry and cure.

In an industry where mold is the primary pest and dry space is the bottleneck of scaled production, plants with low leaf mass and elongated, airy flower structure will mature more evenly and dry much faster. The increased air circulation between the flowers will decrease mold pressure, and the low leaf mass will make post-harvest more efficient. The elongated and airy flower structure means the product is already half ground up and will require little to no grinding for its end use. When the product is bound solely for extraction or pre-rolls, how pretty the flowers look is unimportant. What matters is overall yield, potency, and terpenes, combined with a plant suited specifically for this crop system. This is one example among many, including novel concepts we have yet to discover.

Ploidy breeding is commonly used in the vegetable seed industry in crops such as seedless watermelons. Polyploidy is the condition in which a normally diploid (two sets of chromosomes) cell or organism has acquired one or more additional sets of chromosomes. In cannabis specifically, the condition is induced chemically and plants that are tetraploid (with four sets of chromosomes) are identified. These plants are inbred and eventually crossed with inbred diploid stock to create triploid (three sets of chromosomes) seed. This seed will produce plants that are virtually sterile. This means they cannot get pollinated and produce seed. This is particularly useful in cannabis because even if you rogue out any males in your fields, neighboring growers can release pollen that will travel many miles on the wind. Additionally, seed producers are able to protect their work because triploids cannot be used for breeding or seed production.

Stable, uniform F_1 hybrids like we see in all other annual crops are currently in development for cannabis and will become the industry norm. As of yet, most cannabis seed stock is highly heterozygous, which is why the industry still leans heavily on cloning. Traits such as vigor, cold hardiness, potency, and consistency will one day accompany desirable flower qualities. Creating stabilized lines takes years and requires massive research and development investment. As the market is decriminalized, we expect to see multinational seed genetics companies with huge budgets enter the space and quickly monopolize genetics through plant patents, genomic intellectual property patents, and the ensuing litigation that accompanies them. Privatizing the genome is an unfortunate consequence of the political economy we live within today, and the complete commodification of cannabis will be the result.

A Plant Unlike Any Other

While cannabis is just a plant with its own peculiarities, its cultural, medical, and spiritual significance is completely unique. From the hashish growers of Morocco to the Rastafarians of the Caribbean, the plant is embedded in cultural and religious traditions the world over. Scientifically it is fascinating that this plant produces cannabinoids and that the human body produces endocannabinoids and thus has receptors for them. The overlapping miracle of life never ceases to amaze. The use of cannabis is mind opening. Bob Marley once said, "When you smoke the herb, it reveals you to yourself." It alters the way you perceive the things around you; likewise, it alters the way you perceive yourself. It's almost like changing the filter or the lens with which you see the world. Things, patterns, or behaviors you have seen a thousand times can suddenly become visible in a new light. You can find yourself looking at something you normally take for granted and observe fascinating details you'd never noticed before. It provides perspective for personal and cultural introspection.

This spiritual and emotional dimension of cannabis use is sacred to many, and its inevitable commodification is therefore somewhat sad. Fortunately we will always be able to grow our own, and the traditions of reverence will not die out with the clandestine cultivation culture of the twentieth century. It is our hope that respect will always be given where it is due, and that the continued privatization of the commons will soon fall into the pit it has been digging for the past 500 years. Cannabis has helped us remember what is truly important in life, and we hope it will do that for people in coming generations. No matter how you grow cannabis, remember that it is a medicine plant.

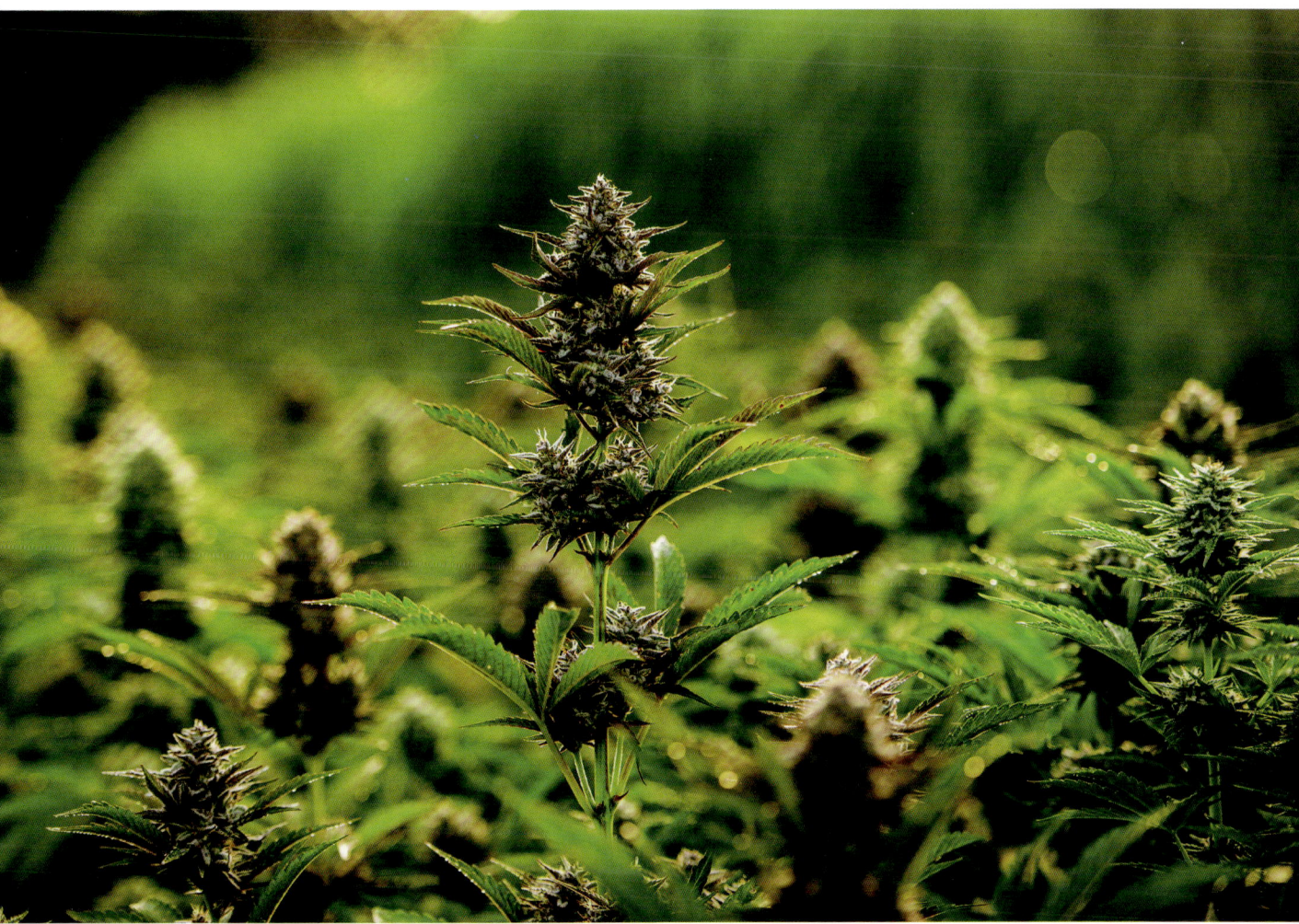

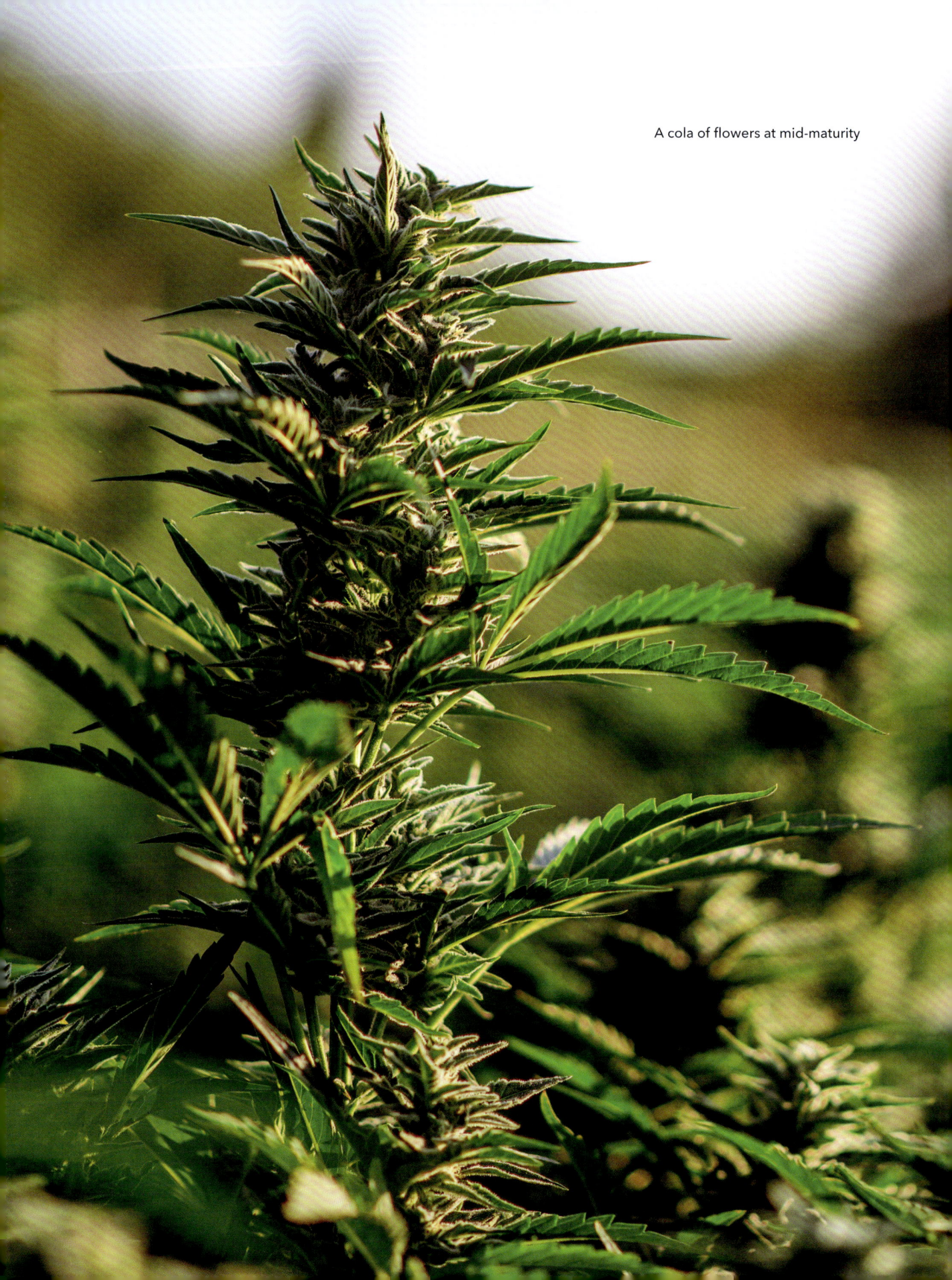

A cola of flowers at mid-maturity

The Effect of Regulation on Cultivation Culture

Cannabis has been an illegal, Schedule I drug according to federal law. Modern cannabis horticulture has evolved in a very particular way within this regulatory context. Until recent years, it was one of the last remaining cottage industries. People originally grew it indoors to keep it secret. It is still grown indoors in part due to this legacy and in part due to the unique and enhanced flower qualities growers can obtain in meticulously controlled indoor environments. That said, there is no economical reason to grow plants indoors under electric lights other than this. It is true that indoor cannabis quality is very high (though the criteria are mostly subjective), but the costs of production are also drastically higher than outdoor. During its prohibition (and to this day) outdoor cultivation was found in rural, remote places such as the mountainous Emerald Triangle of Northern California—Mendocino, Humboldt, and Trinity counties. These hills often have poor, rocky soil. Plants had to be grown in big pots or grow bags with imported potting soil. Sheriffs and federal agents would fly helicopters through these areas and pick off operations based on mysterious criteria. Growers kept operations small to avoid detection from above.

As states made medical cannabis legal, other production models surfaced, though again conformed to the regulatory environment. In California and in other states, cultivators were limited to 99 plants, or in some counties fewer. Therefore, people grew the biggest plants they possibly could to obtain the highest yields. Growers would often achieve impressive results—10-plus pounds of flower per plant—using 400-plus-gallon grow bags filled with expensive, imported potting soil. Some plants would reach 20 feet in height and width. To manage such monstrous plants is a laborious process: Inputs are greater (imagine the fertilizer and water demands!); potting soil is expensive and increases water usage significantly; and trellising and pruning must be done with ladders. Big plants are fun to look at but are challenging to manage. From an agricultural perspective, they make little sense.

Greenhouses came next. To limit discoverability and to manipulate the light cycle to force plants into flowering during the early season, growers began erecting greenhouses. Informal arrangements between law enforcement and growers arose, regarding cultivation under plastic and its identification from above. Who's to say that's not tomatoes growing in there? Don't ask, don't tell. By covering the greenhouses with silage tarps to place the plants in total darkness for select portions of the long summer day—a process called light deprivation—growers could obtain harvest in midsummer and get a high price (colloquially termed "ticket") before replanting for the standard fall harvest. Remnants of clear plastic, silage tarps, and irrigation tubing can still be found scattered throughout gullies and hillsides all over Northern California.

Genetics were likewise developed under these regulatory conditions, specifically bred for indoor production where all conditions are meticulously controlled, and so often lacked vigor, mold resistance, and other agronomic traits in favor of a pure focus on the quality of the flower.

 ## Backcountry Cannabis

This is a true story from one of our longtime friends, a traditional cannabis farmer from the early days.

"After two hours of driving up a dirt driveway, you arrived at a little cabin. No electricity, just a Honda generator and gravity-fed water. From there, we would take ATVs down rutted mountain goat trails that wove along the edge of a 300-foot drop down to the valley floor. Eventually we would arrive at our destination, a grow spot we called the ridge. On the top of 14-foot orchard ladders, precariously perched on the rocky ridgeline, we would big-leaf for days on end. The plants were huge, 15 feet tall and at least as wide, in 300-gallon grow bags. All the soil we brought in bag by bag on the back of the trusty ATV.

"Whenever we heard the *thump-thump-thump* of an approaching helicopter, we would scramble down our ladders and hide in the surrounding trees, praying that the helicopter hadn't seen us and wasn't headed our way. A few times it did, hovering just a few hundred feet above our garden. You could feel the wind generated by the helicopter rotors, blowing the plants about like those crazy clown guys you see at car washes. You could taste the fear and sweat as you waited out those minutes, asking yourself, *Why the hell am I doing this?* Then would come the inevitable debate that would last the rest of the night of whether to chop down early to avoid any potential prosecution. That was how it felt on the hill."

Modern Regulations—Canopy Taxes, Acreage Limits, and How These Change Cultivation

In every state but Oklahoma, the process of obtaining a legal license to cultivate cannabis is difficult and expensive, requiring interacting with multiple government agencies. There is the county or city application, the state application, and, when it's all said and done, a specific tax accountant to prepare taxes under a tax code from the days of Al Capone—280E. These factors create an entry barrier that is extremely hard to pass through, limiting growing access to groups with substantial capital and perpetuating unfair social systems.

Current rules and regulations are often arbitrary at best and influence the cultivation of cannabis just like prohibition and medical rules once did.

Canopy tax. Agricultural businesses pay taxes, like most businesses, based on profit. Cannabis cultivators aren't so lucky. In some states and/or counties, in addition to being taxed on profit (and only able to deduct costs of goods), farmers are also charged a pay-to-play tax (or a fee in some jurisdictions) based on the number of square feet being cultivated.

Setbacks, field placement, and security. We are allowed to grow vegetables all the way to our property line, but cannabis must be 100 feet from the fence line (even though we own the neighboring parcel). Most state regulatory systems additionally require that farm parcels take on prison-level security with fencing and cameras. This creates more waste, up-front capital investment, and additional resources to monitor and maintain.

Acreage limits. These rules, which compel farmers to maximize yield per acre, vary from municipality to municipality. These limits are often not based on any practical consideration.

Track and trace. Perhaps the most frustrating regulation is the requirement that growers place plastic tags on every single plant that identifies it with a barcode and serial number. Every single act involving each plant, including de-leafing, is supposed to be reported, and a final harvest logged. This harvest then travels through the supply chain and ultimately to the end consumer. A private company called Metrc has won the bids for most if not all states to perform this compliance tracking oversight. State regulators have access to Metrc files and can use them when inspecting. Why legislators believed this would benefit taxpayers or consumers in any way is beyond us. How they believed it would eliminate the possibility of backdooring product into legacy markets is also laughable. It is a waste of time and money. Thousands of pounds of useless

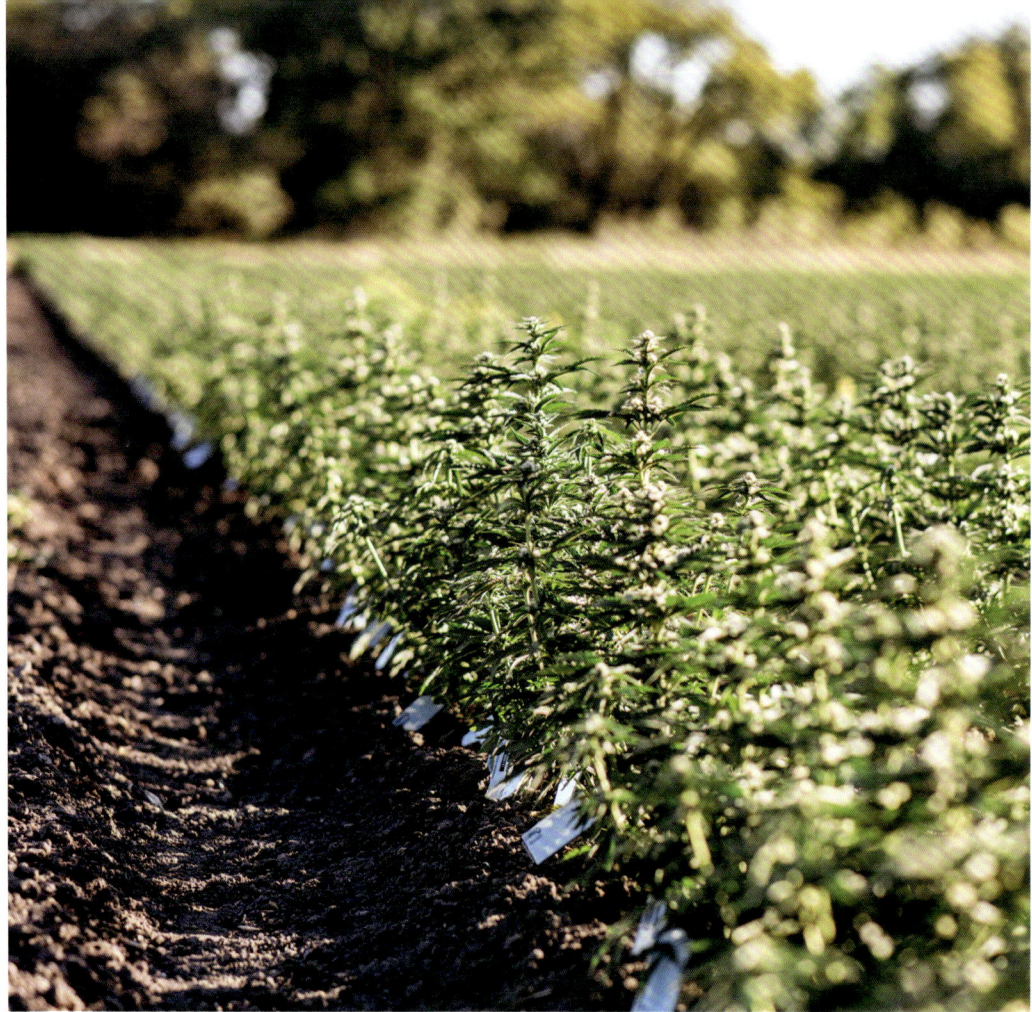

Autoflowers bear plant tags that are on the plants for roughly 30 days and then disposed of.

plastic are thrown away yearly for the impossible (and needless) bureaucratic task of knowing everything.

Pay-per-plant tags. In some states, cultivators are charged *per plant* for their track-and-trace tags, directly influencing genetic selection and crop systems. Many growers will pay more for tags than they will for seed (not even including the labor to apply the tags).

Taken together these taxes and regulations are as limiting as the old 99-plants rules. They force farmers to use cultivation methods that may not be appropriate for their soil type, climatic region, marketplace, equipment, labor pool, preferences, and so on. They stifle innovation and efficiency and supplant them with administrative hurdles and hoops of fire. When farmers are hyper-focused on maximizing yields per square foot because of poorly written regulations, they are forced to abandon some basic tools in their toolbelt. Further, farmers are forced to conform with regulations that may lead to higher cost of production, higher ecological impacts, or just plain poor farming practices. These include the following.

Crop rotation. Most farmers employ some sort of rotation. Larger farmers employ a classic corn/wheat/soy cycle, while smaller farmers simply make it a point not to plant the same crop in the same spot two years in a row. Our cannabis licenses have made it impossible to do any sort of crop rotation.

Genetic selection. Requiring farmers to pay per tag for every plant they grow creates a disincentive for developing diverse crop plans in favor of higher-yielding, lower-plant-count-per-acre plans, similar to the ethnobotanical constraints under the old 99 rule.

Tagging plants is a pointless activity that epitomizes bureaucratic overreach—not to mention it is expensive. In 2021 we spent close to $10,000 putting tags on plants, while a neighboring farm spent over $25,000. When farmers are forced to pay out extra, superfluous labor costs, they may have to cut corners on or completely abandon more fundamental labor costs.

General field layout. Farmers have lots of natural variables to contend with when deciding how to lay out a field. These include slope, drainage, soil uniformity, available sunlight and shade, and access for equipment.

These natural variables sit in second place to additional bureaucratic requirements (such as setbacks), which just increase the cost and difficulty of simply growing a plant and sometimes eliminate the obvious ecological or practical options entirely. As a side note that exemplifies the mysterious and oxymoronic cannabis regulatory environment, it is highly ironic that hemp (which is literally the same species as THC-producing cannabis) is not subject to any of these asinine rules and regulations, although it does have its own (albeit single) impossible requirement—less than 0.3 percent THC. This leads to all kinds of regulation dodging—harvesting samples early, selective sampling, etc. The rule itself is not consistent with botanical reality.

While some states or counties do not have canopy taxes or acreage limits, others issue few permits at all. Furthermore, the way these permits are issued, and who they are issued to, is dubious at best. Cannabis is a highly regulated, confusing, and complicated industry with regulations that box out too many blue-collar working farmers and narrow industry evolution. In many ways, it was easier to grow weed *before* it was legal. But the fact of the matter is, the state of cannabis is where it is today because a certain set of cowboys, curanderas, trailblazers, and innovators with a high tolerance for risk have continued to push forward despite massive systemic resistances.

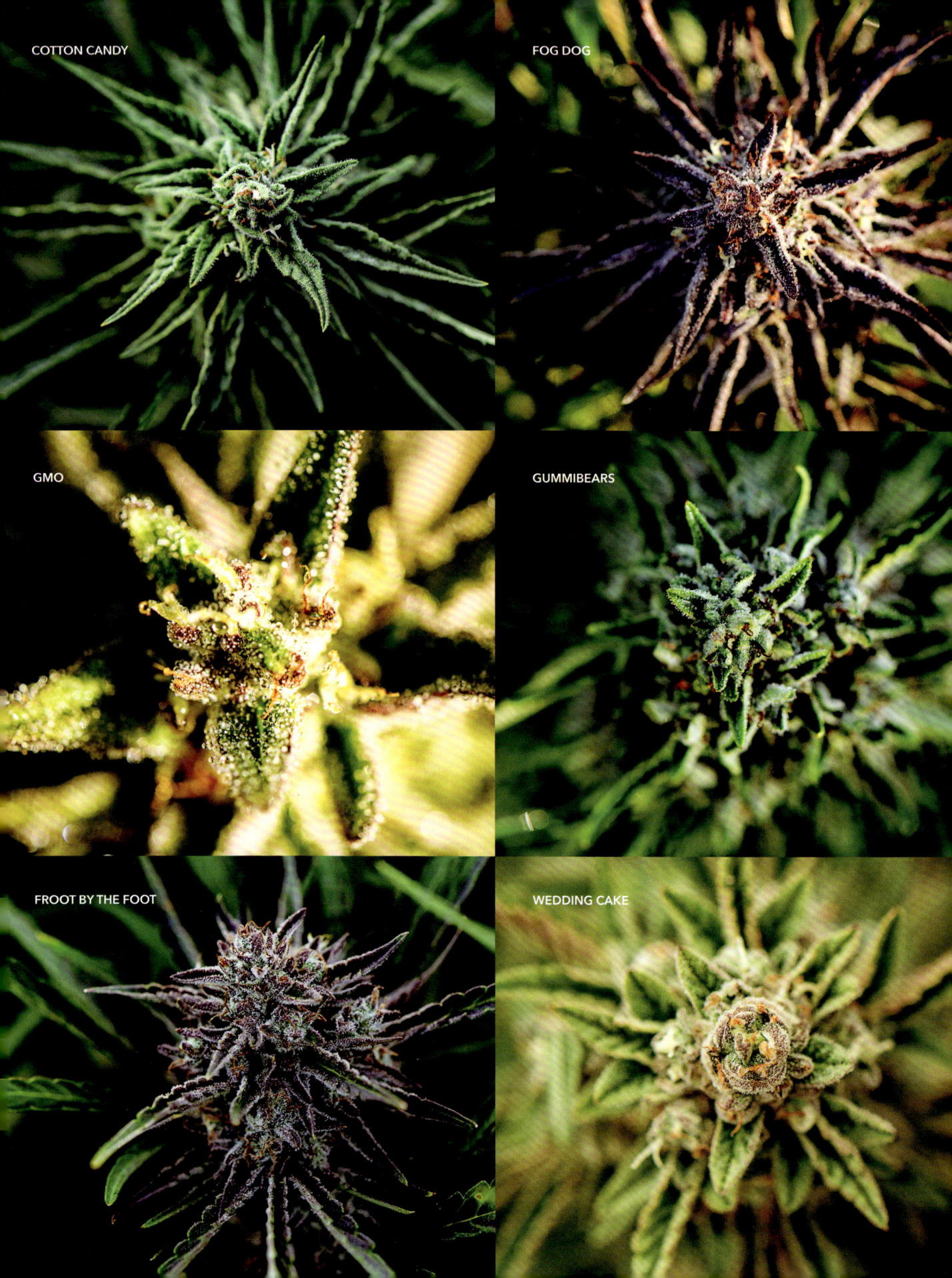

COTTON CANDY

FOG DOG

GMO

GUMMIBEARS

FROOT BY THE FOOT

WEDDING CAKE

Cannabis Aroma Families

Understanding and Categorizing Cannabis Varieties by Aromas, Terpenes, Smell Compounds, and Genetic Lineages

Cannabis aroma families are an Atlas Seed framework that we've created both to understand our own growing and breeding work better and to convey to customers the information they need to decide what cannabis varieties they want to grow.

We've modeled our framework after the work of collaboration between SC Labs and the Emerald Cup to define terpene classes, as well as research from Abstrax Tech on flavorants, which are essentially non-terpene smell compounds, in addition to numerous other articles and conversations. These companies' work, like ours, is built on an understanding of existing cannabis lineages from the past 50 years of contemporary cultivar development, specifically in the Type I, THC-dominant, recreational, and medicinal varieties.

Cannabis plants produce a wide array of smells, and the most straightforward way to describe those is in terms of other familiar aromas: apples and chamomile; sandalwood and blueberries; pineapple and lighter fluid; etc. The system we've created is simple: If a variety smells like a thing, then it gets categorized accordingly!

Gassy, skunky, funky, chemical, and various types of wacky weed smells go in the OG/Chem/Kush category. Mango, papaya, pineapple, and guava weed smells go in the Tropical category. Cakes are included in the Cream/Cake/Cookies/Candy category. And if it's jack, with its characteristic piney scent, it belongs with the Jacks/Hazes. We've earmarked strains that have dominant rare terpenes as Exotics.

The brilliance of the SC Labs terpene class system, which categorizes varieties strictly based on terpene content, is that it begins to make sense of what terpenes offer in modern cannabis cultivars. But as much as it highlights truly unique terpene

Opposite: A selection of the natural variation present in the cannabis genome

201

contributions (i.e., any strains that don't contain the more prevalent myrcene, beta-caryophyllene, and limonene terpenes), the existence of varieties with aromas that don't match their terpene classes indicates that other compounds we don't currently know about or test for in commercial lab settings are also contributing to the overall aroma of a plant.

For example, the Purple Punch variety has a very tropical smell, but if you were to categorize by terpene class, it would belong with the desserts because it is generally beta-caryophyllene and limonene dominant. It likely smells tropical due to some presence of tropicannasulfurs, which are sulfur-based compounds that have a fruity smell, or to some other trace compounds that we don't or can't currently test for. In the Atlas Seed framework, we chose to classify it based on its olfactory presentation rather than put it in a category based solely on the terpenes we were seeing in lab results.

We also thought the SC Labs' Sweets and Dreams category was confusing, and since their Tropical/Floral and their Sweets and Dreams terpene classes were both generally myrcene dominant, we combined the two categories into what we simply call Tropical/Floral. We also renamed their Dessert as Cream/Cake/Cookies/Candy, and their OG/Gas category we're calling OG/Chem/Kush. The SC Labs' Jacks and Haze and their Exotics remain the same in our framework.

What follows is our take on what we're calling aroma families.

The Aroma Families

OG/Chem/Kush

Aromas
Diesel, fuel, gas, sweet, citrus, skunky, earthy, musky

Effects
Uplifting, stimulating, relaxing, analgesic (pain relieving), sedative

Terpenes and smell compounds
Codominance of myrcene, beta-caryophyllene, limonene, volatile sulfur compounds, indoles/skatoles (feces compounds), various flavorants—aldehydes, esters, alcohols

Genotype
Hybrid

Common Varieties
Chemdog, Fatso, GG4, GMO, Gorilla Glue, Grease Monkey, Headband, Jet Fuel, Motorbreath, OG Kush, Original Glue, Sour Diesel

Description

This aroma family is based on crosses between chem and kush lines that established the iconic smell realm that we now think of most commonly as "gas." It is classically a myrcene, limonene, and beta-caryophyllene codominant aroma family, though we believe that some of the more pronounced smells of this category come from volatile sulfur compounds and other mysterious factors that are as yet untested for.

Volatile sulfur compounds are not currently being tested for in market-ready cannabis labs, but they have been identified as active contributors to particularly pungent smells in cannabis aromatics as well as in a number of other aromatically pronounced foods such as garlic, durian, and hops.

Limonene can be the least identifiable and reliable terpene in determining the end-result smell of a variety, but it is limonene that gives this aroma family an extra-energizing boost and provides the consistent notes of citrus common in gas lines.

Myrcene can possibly cross the blood-brain barrier, which is what can cause these varieties to have major sedative effects and psychoactive properties. Myrcene also acts as a potent analgesic, and its pain-relieving properties may be due to its interactions with the opiate system.

Beta-caryophyllene is normally noted for its spice notes, and it can enhance pain-relieving and anti-inflammatory effects.

Though this aroma family doesn't tend to test quite as high as the Cream/Cake/Cookies/Candy aroma family in terms of overall THC potency, it seems on average to have some of the best lines for hash production, and for solventless extraction (i.e., washing strains), OG/Chem/Kush is the way. The most likely reason for this is due to the strong Afghani influence in this aroma family exemplified in the kush lines. After all, it is Afghanistan's cannabis landrace and hash-producing culture that has led the way in hashish output for as far back as anyone can seem to remember. Producing cannabis for smokable flower and artisanal extracts is a very recent and truly American phenomenon!

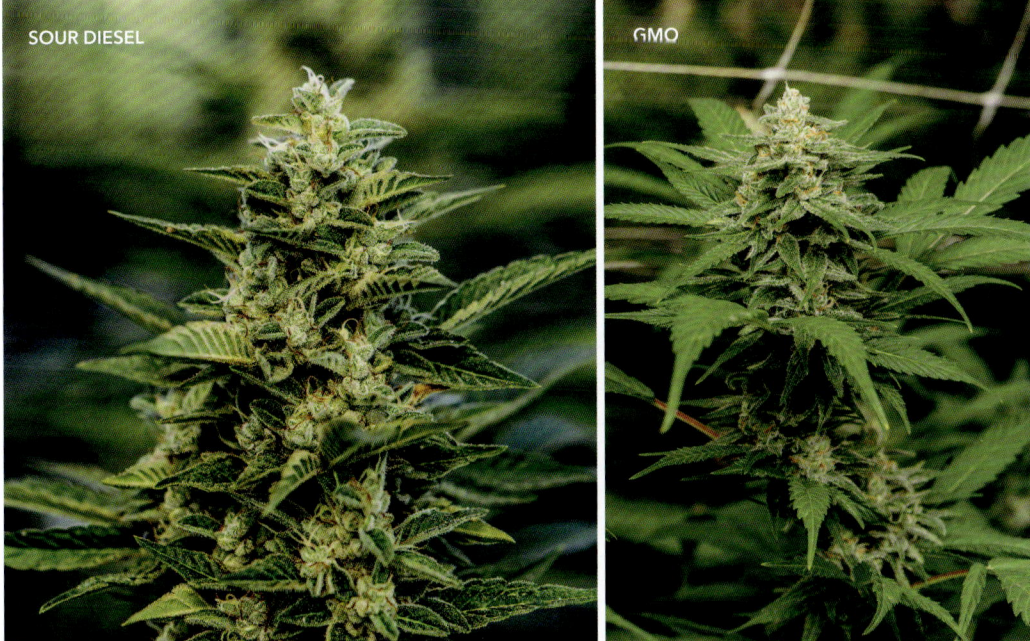

SOUR DIESEL

GMO

Cream/Cake/Cookies/Candy

Aromas
Dessert, candy, fruit, sweet, dough, crust, cream, citrus, spice, ice cream

Effects
Stimulating, uplifting, comforting

Terpenes and smell compounds
Codominance of limonene and beta-caryophyllene, various flavorants—aldehydes, esters, alcohols

Genotype
Hybrid

Common Varieties
Banana OG, Berry White, Bubba Kush, Cakes, Cherry Pie, Cookies, Do-Si-Dos, Gelatos, Girl Scout Cookies, Ice Cream Cake, MAC, Runtz, Strawberry Banana, Sundae Driver, Wedding Cake, Wedding Crasher, Zkittlez

Description

This is one of the more popular aroma families these days—there's something comforting about growing cannabis varieties that smell like our favorite desserts. Most of the varieties in the Cream/Cake/Cookies/Candy aroma family are defined by a codominance of limonene and caryophyllene. Varieties like Ice Cream Cake, Wedding Cake, and Gelato all have more or less equal amounts of limonene and caryophyllene. GSC and Cherry Pie are caryophyllene dominant, and Berry White, Banana OG, and Strawberry Banana are limonene dominant.

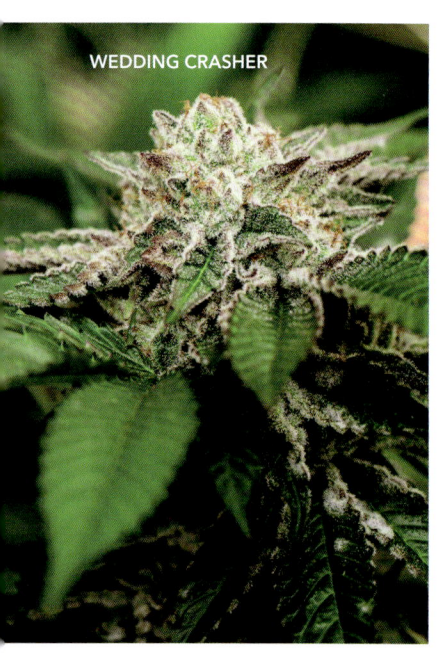

WEDDING CRASHER

This aroma family leads the way in overall highest potency, and for this reason it has become the most dominant aroma family in the cannabis industry. Many boutique growers cultivate only dessert terpene strains, no doubt in an attempt to stretch the boundaries of what's possible as far as high-THC varieties. We like a Girl Scout Cookies or Runtz as much as the next grower but tend to think the overemphasis on high THC in the industry is misguided, annoying, and potentially even harmful, certainly to creative and medicinal breeding programs, and possibly also to consumers' health. Breeding strictly for potency tends to restrict or even eliminate other valuable compounds in the plant over time, since to fill more of the plant with THC you must make room by eliminating other compounds. THC is not the most important component of the plant—it relies on the other cannabinoids/terpenes to guide the psychoactive effect and/or medicinal properties. We would argue that breeding exclusively for THC potency has been one of the most destructive trends in the recent history of the plant. Whatever your taste, tread lightly in this category if you can't hold your smoke, so to speak.

Jack/Haze

Aromas
Fruity, pine, Pine-Sol, woody, haze, jack, Juicy Fruit chewing gum

Effects
Energizing, cerebral, inspiring

Terpenes and smell compounds
Terpinolene dominant, beta-caryophyllene, myrcene, various flavorants—aldehydes, esters, alcohols

Genotype
Sativa

Common Varieties
Black Jack, Clementine, Critical Jack, Durban Poison, Ghost Train Haze, Jack Herer, Platinum Jack, Super Lemon Haze, Trainwreck, White Durban

Description
Perhaps it is due to the ubiquitousness and obvious loudness of jack terps that this aroma family seems to fall in and out of favor among longtime California growers, or perhaps there's something to the terpinolene scent that triggers the same aversion certain people have to cilantro. At Atlas Seed, we are huge fans of the jack smell, and though we don't have a dominant jack catalog, we love encountering it in field walks as either a dominant note or back-end base note that seems to amplify the other smell compounds.

Terpinolene is the most identifiable and determinant terpene of all, meaning that if it's present on an olfactory level, you better believe the lab testing will back that up, and vice versa. Terpinolene is also found in apples, lilacs, and nutmeg. Of note, Jack Herer was made by crossing Northern Lights #5 with Haze. And the Cookies lines were originally created by crossing Durban Poison with OG Kush and Cherry Kush. Also of note: Aroma families will always have imperfections, since certain varieties seem to straddle categories. Would we put Blue Dream in the Jack/Haze category or Tropical/Floral? Since we think it hits hard with berry mango, we put it squarely in the tropical arena. But it has foundational haze lineage and is an instrumental variety in the sensual experience of the haze aroma. Sometimes you just have to make a tough choice and stick with it.

Tropical/Floral

Aroma
Sweet, herbaceous, fruity, woody, hoppy, tropical, tropical fruit

Effects
Soothing, calming, sedative, analgesic (pain relieving), relaxing

Terpenes and smell compounds
Myrcene dominant, sometimes ocimene dominant, pinene, beta-caryophyllene, tropical VSCs (a.k.a. tropicannasulfurs), various flavorants—aldehydes, esters, alcohols

Genotype
Indica

Common Varieties
Agent Orange, Blue Dream, Cherry AK, Dream Queen, Forbidden Fruit, Grape Ape, Green Crack, Hawaiian, Mango Puff, Panama Red, Papaya, Passion Orange Guava, Pink Lemonade, Super Skunk, Sweet Tooth, Tangie; purps: Granddaddy Purps, Purple Punch, Purple Urkle, Tropical Sleigh Ride

Description
This class has two subgroups: the more common myrcene-dominant varieties, and the ocimene-dominant varieties. Tropical Sleigh Ride and Passion Orange Guava are ocimene dominant. Super Skunk, Pineapple, Green Crack, and Dream Queen are high in myrcene with just a little bit of ocimene. But when ocimene is present, even in small amounts—even if it's a secondary or tertiary terpene—the smell is so strong that it naturally groups together with ocimene-dominant strains.

Varieties high in myrcene and paired with small amounts of anything else but ocimene include Tangie, Forbidden Fruit, Cali O, and Agent Orange. High myrcene with a little bit of caryophyllene includes all the purples—Granddaddy Purps, Grape Ape. High myrcene with a little bit of pinene includes Blue Dream.

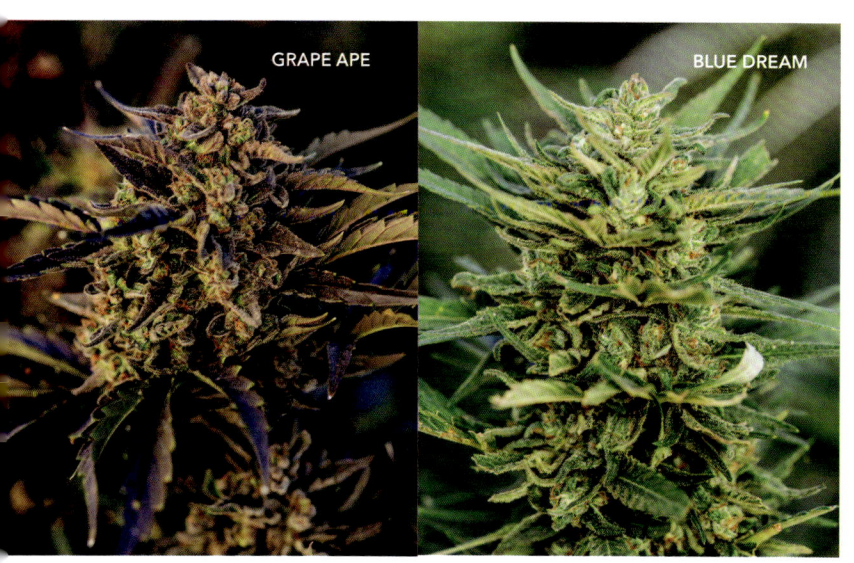

GRAPE APE

BLUE DREAM

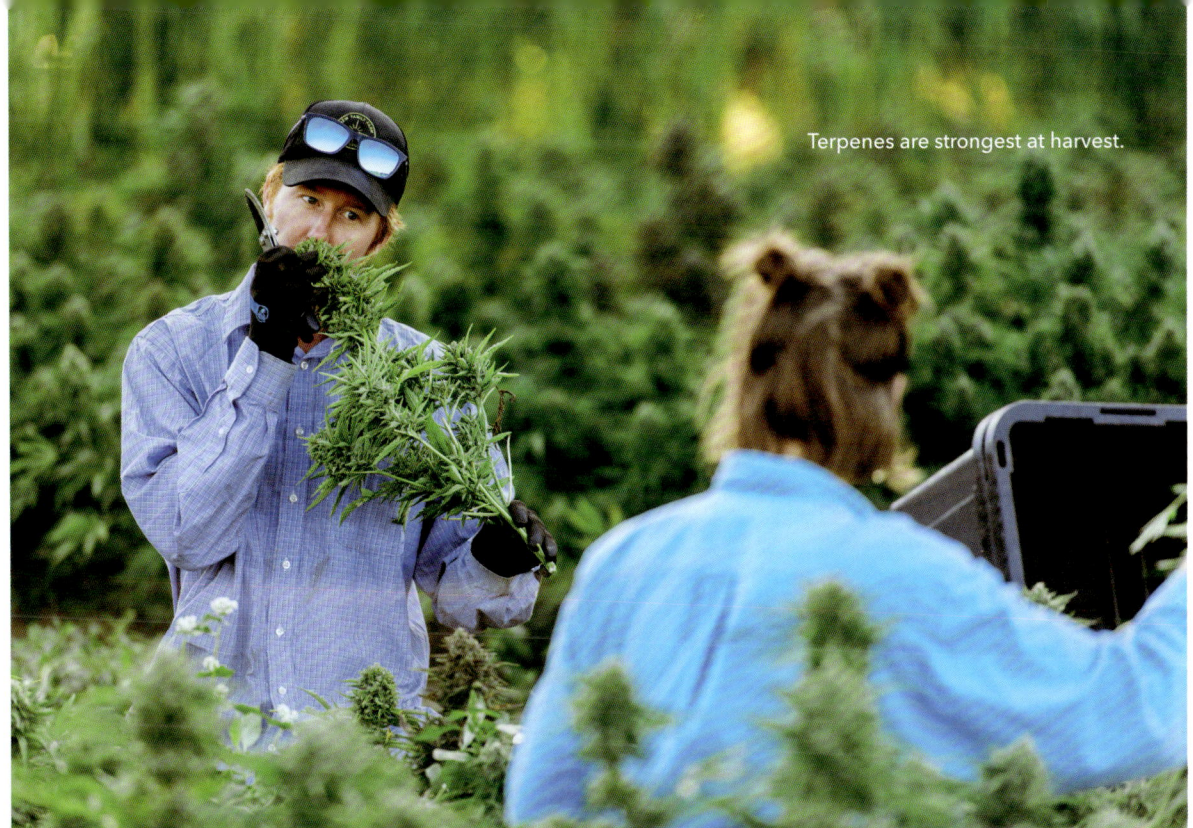

Terpenes are strongest at harvest.

Exotics

Aroma
Eclectic!

Effects
Vary

Terpenes and smell compounds
Rarest terps, not part of myrcene/limonene/beta-caryophyllene family

Genotype
Varies

Common Varieties
Strawberry Cough, Sour Carmelo, Juicy Gushy, and Laffy Taffy

Description
This class encompasses the rarest profiles and all the diverse outliers that don't fall into one of the other major categories. This includes strains dominant in linalool, alpha-pinene, and beta-pinene or ocimene without myrcene present. Better-known Exotics cultivars include Strawberry Cough, Sour Carmelo, Juicy Gushy, and Laffy Taffy.

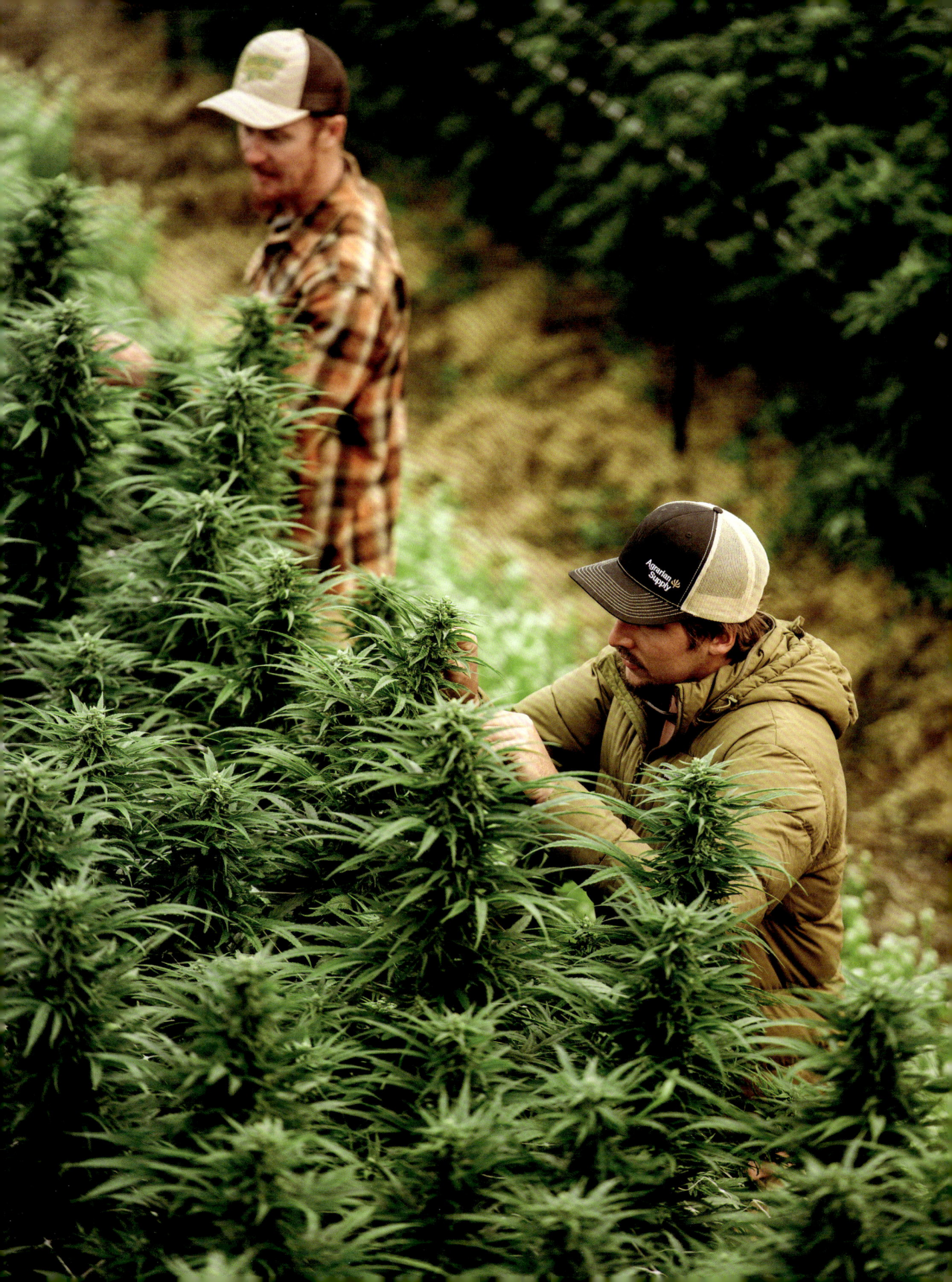

Acknowledgments

It was not easy launching scaled cannabis projects at the rollout of legalization. We had a lot of help along the way, without which we would have failed. Thank you to Al Schmidt for starting this whole thing with us. Big thanks to Mike McCarthy for the support, advice, and camaraderie. Thanks to Darren Story for the consistent successful attitude. Elan Goldbart, a true farmer at heart, has been instrumental in our success and the success of the entire industry, really. Gratitude to Nick Stromberg, who helped us harness the power of seed. Thanks to Vinh and Melissa Huynh for being such strong allies in the beginning. Thanks and love to Gabe Nelson for showing us how to truly grow beautiful plants. We all miss you. We thank Max LaMonte, who worked and lived with us for the entirety of this project and whose help was paramount. Thanks to Robert and Marcel, Stuart Schroeder, Eddie and Wendy Gelsman, Jeffrey Westman, Jim and Linda Morton, and Tim Page. The whole farm wouldn't have been possible without you. To our core crew, thanks: Rogelio Castro, Alex Kuhn, Ezra Acker for fixing everything, Elliot Marshall for keeping it all wet, Drew Garner, Jose Ines and Rocibel. Thanks to Dawne Gilmore for handling all the details. Gratitude to Patrick Numair for facilitating a good arrangement, and to Christopher Holcomb. Thanks to Andrew Smith for assisting, supporting, and helping us get started in an unfriendly regulatory environment. Joe Ullman got us through the first foray with confidence and kindness, for which we are grateful. Jake and Andy of Ladybug Farms—thanks, mates. A huge and special thanks to Liam Hancock, who was a master catalyzer for the entire project. Without his initial encouragement and consistent contribution, this book would never have happened! Liam provided real-time editing, reflection, and structure to this book, and we are grateful for his marked contributions. And huge gratitude to Charlie Dubbe for taking this farm to the next level with us and leaving it turnkey.

There is a long list of folks who wouldn't want their names in a publication but whose help got us to where we are: You all know who you are, and we thank you.

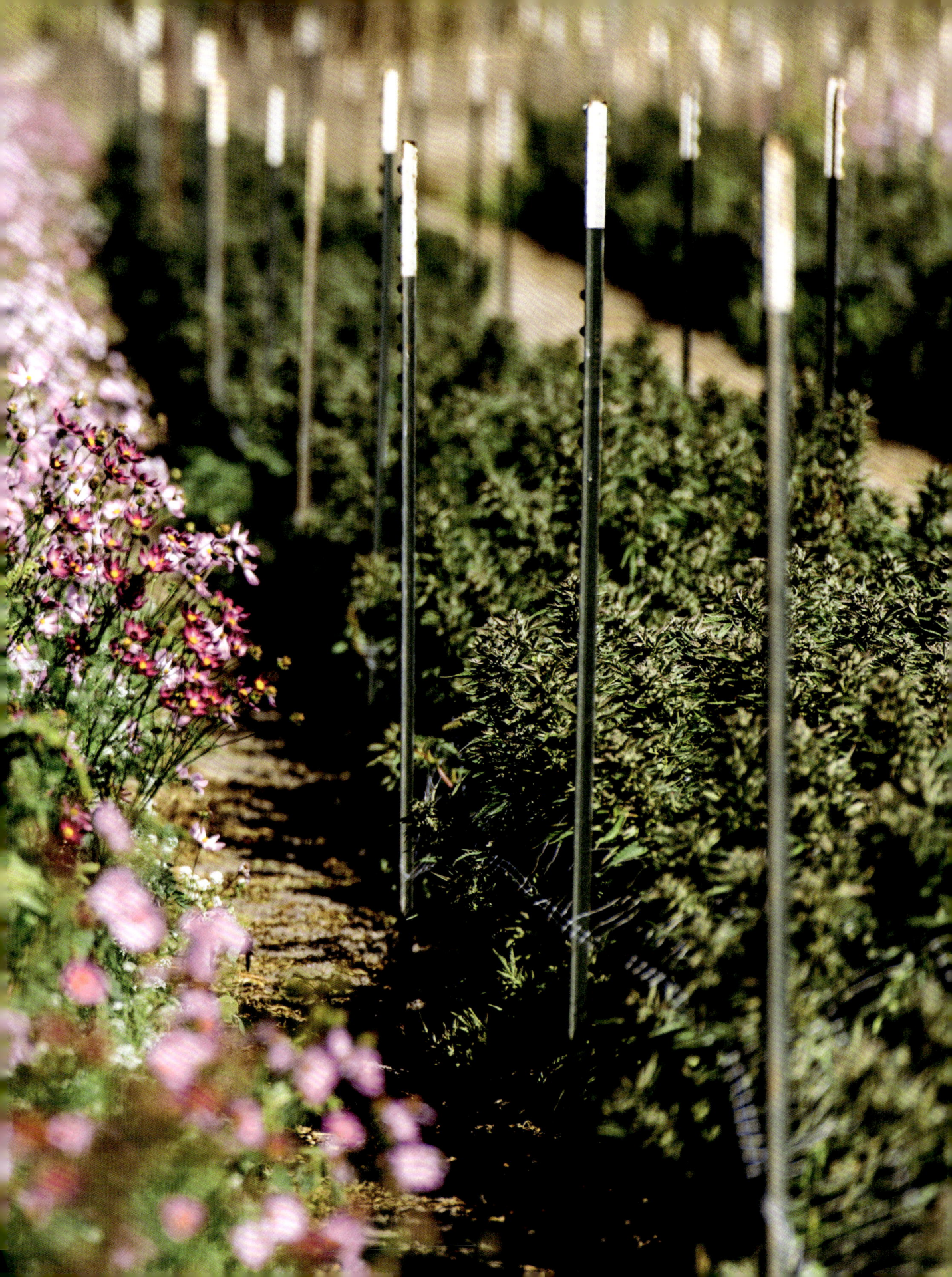

Glossary

agronomic. Qualities related to the holistic study of crop production, including plant genetics, plant physiology, meteorology, and soil science.

apical dominance. The propensity of a plant to energetically prioritize the tallest shoot, which in turn limits branching and the quality and size of flowers on lower branches.

autoflowering. Refers to *Cannabis ruderalis* or day-neutral cannabis genetics. Autoflowering cannabis initiates its flowering cycle automatically, regardless of changes in day length.

big-leaf. The act of removing the biggest fan leaves from cannabis to encourage more airflow, reduce the chance of mold growth, and make harvest easier. Big-leafing occurs during the plant's final phases of flowering and leading up to its harvest.

bioaccumulator. A plant or other living organism that efficiently absorbs substances from the soil, including chemicals, pesticides, heavy metals, and minerals.

biomass. Harvested, unmanicured cannabis flowers.

bioremediator. An organism that captures or breaks down organic contaminants.

botrytis. A fungus in the genus *Botrytis* that infects cannabis flowers in humid conditions. Also referred to as mold, gray mold, or bud rot.

bucking. The process of removing dry plant material (the flowers) from the cannabis plant stem, using scissors for hand-trimmed flowers. See also *wet bucking*.

cannabinoid. A diverse group of chemical compounds found in the cannabis plant, often associated with a medicinal action.

CBD. Cannabidiol, a naturally occurring cannabinoid found in cannabis plants. Unlike its counterpart THC (delta-9-tetrahydrocannabinol), CBD is generally thought to be nonintoxicating and does not produce a psychoactive "high" effect.

clone. In cannabis production, a replica made from sexually mature plants.

cola. A single flowering stalk of cannabis.

cotyledon. The first leaf of a germinating plant. It is a part of the plant embryo and has a nutrient storage role during germination. Also referred to as the seed leaf.

crop production system. A highly organized view of crop production from planning to planting to growing to harvest and post-harvest.

damping-off. A fungal disease that affects newly germinated plants or young seedlings, causing them to rapidly wilt or rot.

day-neutral cannabis. See *autoflowering*.

days to maturity. The number of days from when a seed is planted or a clone is taken to the day of harvest.

de-leaf. See *big-leaf*.

dioecious. Refers to plants that are either male or female. Male plants produce pollen that fertilizes flowers on female plants, resulting in a seeded crop.

dry/cure. The phase in cannabis post-harvest where cannabis sweats its free or nonchemically bound water and enzymatically metabolizes its chlorophyll.

dudding. Stunted and irregular flower growth.

emergence. The point when a plant's first leaves break through the soil into the light.

entourage effect. The synergistic interaction of various compounds found in cannabis plants, particularly cannabinoids, terpenes, and other plant chemicals. It suggests that the combined effect of these compounds working together is greater than the effect of each compound in isolation, and it implies a preference for whole-plant, full-spectrum products.

extraction. The conversion of target molecules in cannabis raw material into a usable form. The process removes the oil found in the trichomes of the cannabis plant and targets and collects the most potent compounds from the plant, including THC, CBD, and terpenes, among others.

fertigation. The delivery of fertilizer or nutrients in liquid form through irrigation processes.

finish time. The calendar date of plant maturity.

floating medium. A substance that physically holds the potting soil within the cell tray, allowing growers to pull plugs out without damaging plant roots.

flowering time. The length of time from when a plant begins to form flowers to when it has mature flowers ready to harvest.

F₁ hybrid. The first-generation cross of two genetically dissimilar, inbred (homozygous) parent lines. When done properly, the cross produces a stable, vigorous, and uniform plant expression.

germination. Refers to the moment when the first root, called a radicle, emerges underground from the seed itself.

hardening off. The process of moving seedlings from the protected conditions of the greenhouse and into conditions closer to those they will be exposed to in the field.

herming. Colloquial shorthand for the expression by plants of intersex or hermaphrodite traits; in the case of cannabis, when male parts present on a female plant.

hop latent viroid (HLVd). An organism known to cause dudding disease in hemp and cannabis. It is a noncapsulated strand of RNA and an obligate parasite that requires the presence of a compatible host for its survival.

initiation. The point at which plants begin to form flowers.

internodal spacing. The space between the plants' growth nodes.

leaf mass. The leaf/bud ratio; that is, the volume of leaves relative to flowers on a plant.

mids. Referring to cannabis flowers of a size between smalls and tops. Also called mid-grade.

nonfeminized seed. Cannabis seed that has not been treated to give rise to only female plants, and thus produces a 50/50 ratio of male and female plants when grown. Often referred to as regs.

percent capacity. The percentage of field capacity, which is the amount of soil moisture or water content held in the soil after excess water has drained away and the rate of downward movement has materially decreased.

photoperiod. An environmental response tendency of plants to initiate their flowering period when the duration of daily light decreases below a critical threshold. Photoperiod cannabis is the most commonly grown.

polyhybrid. A cross between two highly heterozygous cannabis plants, resulting in a highly unstable and varied plant expression.

polyploidy. The condition in which a normally diploid (having two sets of chromosomes) cell or organism has acquired one or more additional sets of chromosomes.

potency. In the context of cannabis market dynamics, the percentage of THC and CBD in flowers.

propagation. The process of germinating seeds and preparing them for transplant.

quicks (quiks). The first-generation cross between autoflowering and photoperiod cannabis parents, which produces vigorous plants that flower two to three weeks earlier than their photoperiod counterparts. Also known as semi-full-term, fast-flowering, and fast-finishing cannabis.

roguing. Removing male flowers.

row cropping. Field-scale agriculture in which crops are planted in straight rows for ease of access and efficiency.

short-day cannabis. Plants that initiate reproductive cycles as days get shorter.

sinsemilla. From the Spanish for "without seeds," sinsemilla is a contemporary cultural trend applied to cannabis production whereby flower pollination is avoided to produce more chemically potent cannabis.

smalls. Referring to cannabis flowers smaller than a dime.

terpene class. Refers to the unique smell and taste of cannabis flowers.

terpenes. A diverse group of organic compounds found in various plants, including cannabis, conifers, and citrus fruits; responsible for the distinct aromas and flavors as well as medicinal benefits.

THC. Stands for delta-9-tetrahydrocannabinol, the primary psychoactive compound found in cannabis. It is responsible for the "high," or intoxicating effects associated with cannabis use, among other medicinal effects and benefits.

tissue culture. The growth of tissues or cells in an artificial medium separate from the parent plant. Also known as micropropagation.

tops. The upper parts of the cannabis plant, which receive the most sunlight and thus exhibit the most growth; in particular, the uppermost flowers.

trichomes. The crystalline, sticky, smelly substance on mature flowers.

water activity. The amount of chemically bound water held in an organic substance, expressed as a percentage or decimal from 0.01 to 1. Ideal cannabis water activity is right around 0.6.

wet bucking. The process of removing fresh flowers from the cannabis stems. See also *bucking*.

Bibliography

Cho, Youngsang. *JADAM Organic Farming*, 2nd edition. JADAM, 2016.

Cohen, Sidney, and Richard Stillman, eds. *Therapeutic Potential of Marihuana*. Plenum Press, 1976.

Coleman, Eliot. *The New Organic Grower: A Master's Manual of Tools and Techniques for the Home and Market Gardener*, 3rd edition. Chelsea Green Publishing, 2018.

Gershuny, Grace. *Start with the Soil: The Organic Gardener's Guide to Improving Soil for Higher Yields, More Beautiful Flowers, and a Healthy, Easy-Care Garden*. Rodale, 1993.

Herer, Jack. *The Emperor Wears No Clothes: A History of Cannabis/Hemp/Marijuana* (Leslie Cabarga, ed.). Ah Ha Publishing, 1998.

Herndon, G. Melvin. "Hemp in Colonial Virginia." *Agricultural History* 37, no. 2 (1963): 86–93. www.jstor.org/stable/3740780.

Magdoff, Fred, and Harold van Es. *Building Soils for Better Crops: Ecological Management for Healthy Soils*. Sustainable Agriculture Research and Education (SARE), 2009.

Mikuriya, Tod, ed. *Marijuana: Medical Papers, 1839–1972*. Medi-Comp Press, 1973.

White, T. C. R. "The Abundance of Invertebrate Herbivores in Relation to the Availability of Nitrogen in Stressed Food Plants." *Oecologia* 63, no. 1 (July 1984): 90–105. Doi: 10.1007/BF00379790.

Wiswall, Richard. *The Organic Farmer's Business Handbook: A Complete Guide to Managing Finances, Crops, and Staff—and Making a Profit*. Chelsea Green Publishing, 2009.

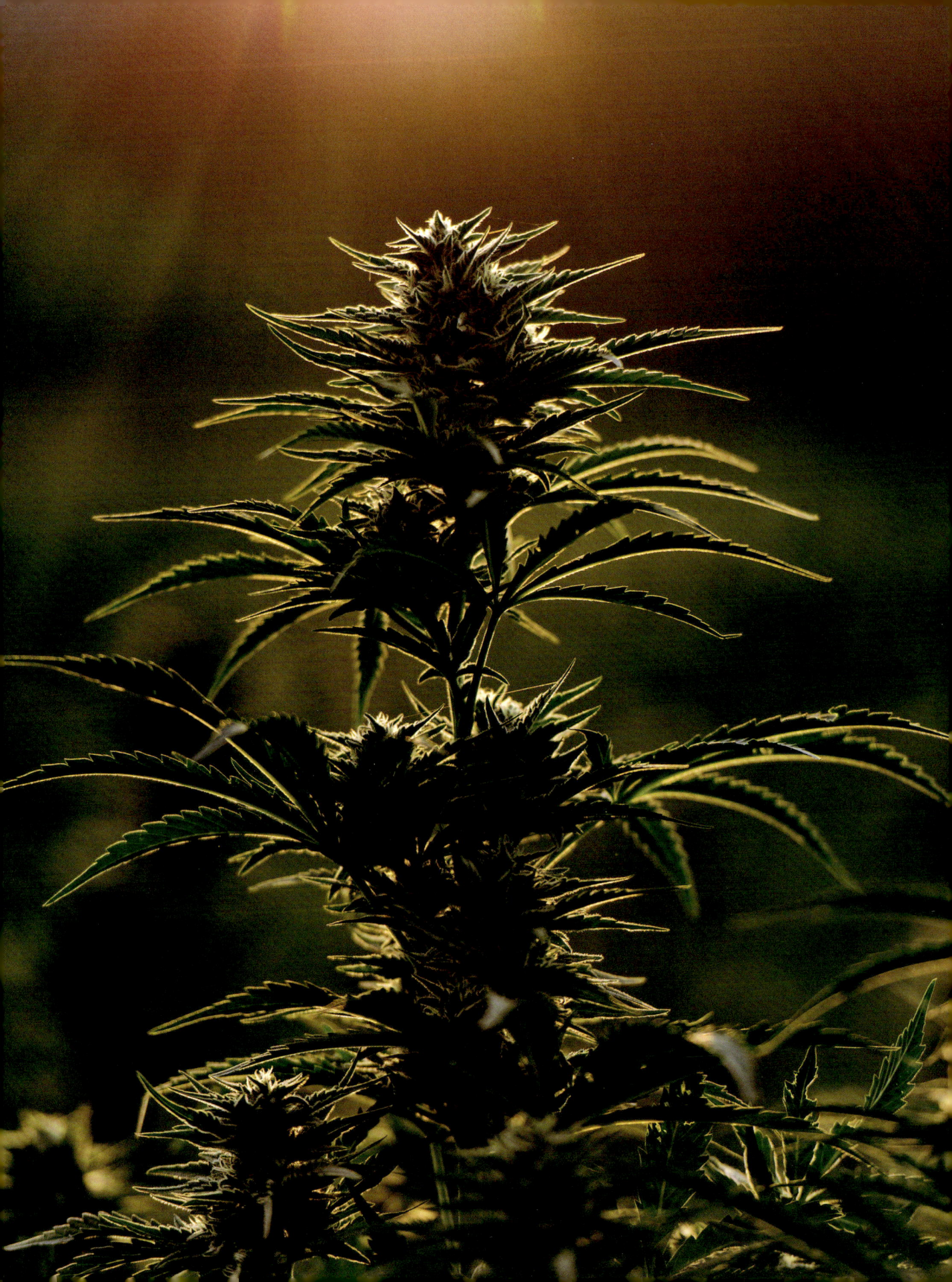

Index

Page numbers in *italics* indicate photos; numbers in **bold** indicate charts.

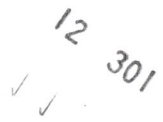